# Essentials of Acupuncture

*By*

Prof. Dr. Debasish Kundu

M.D.H., F.F.Hom, F.I.H.M.S., Ph.D.(U.S.A.), D.Sc.(Colombo)

Dr. Choo Led Sin

Ph.D. of Chinese Medicine (China)

**Originals**

**Delhi-110052**

First Published 2026



ISBN 13: 978-81-8454-160-1
ISBN 10: 81-8454-160-0

**Published By**
**Originals**
A-6, Second Floor, Nimri Commercial Centre,
Ashok Vihar Phase-4, Delhi - 110 052 (India)
Tel. + Fax: 011 4706 1936
website: www.Lppindia.com
e-mail: info@Lppindia.com



**Printed At**
D K Fine Art Press P Ltd.
Delhi-110052

**PRINTED IN INDIA**

**Prof. Dr. Debasish Kundu**

M.D.H., F.F.Hom, F.I.H.M.S., Ph.D.(U.S.A.), D.Sc.(Colombo)

Fellow of International Holistic Medical Society, CA, U.S.A.

Fellow of Foundation of Homeopathy, NY, U.S.A.,

Fellow of World E.Homeopathy System of Medical Council, Hong Kong,

Faculty, International Holistic Medical Society, CA, U.S.A.,

Vice-President, American Nutritional Medical Association, CA, U.S.A.

Foreign Bureau Chief (India), Holistic Medical Hylite International, CA, U.S.A.,

Visiting Professor, Khulna Homeopathic Medical College & Hospital, Khulna, Bangladesh.

Author, Principles & Art of Cure in E.Homeopathy, Materia Medica & Drug Pathogenesy in E.Homeopathy, Materia Medica Pharmacy & Practice of Medicine in E.Homeopathy, Diseases of Women, Natural Medicines, A Clinical Treatise on Cancer, Aids & Homeopathy, Pharmacodynamics in E.Homeopathy, A Treatise on E.Homeopathic Pharmacy, Aids & Your Sex Life, Materia Medica for the New Age Man, Aids & Homeopathy, etc.

Recipient, Royal Assyrian Order of Merit

Laureate, Dag Hammarskjold Award for Medicine

**Prof. Dr. Choo Led Sin**

Ph.D. of Chinese Medicine (China)

Vice Chairman of the World Manipulative Medical Association

Vice Chairman of TCM Diagnosis Specialty Committee of World Federation of Chinese Medicine Societies

President of World Spinal Health Association of Singapore

Vice Chairman of International Fu Yang Health Association

Visiting Professor of World Spinal Health Science Research Institute

Chairman of Singapore Association of Manipulative Medicine

President of Fu Yang Health Association (Singapore)

Assistant Secretary of Singapore Acupuncture Association

Education Director of Health Management Academy Singapore

Member of American Nutritional Medical Association, CA, USA

Life Honorary President of Professional Manipulative Therapist Association (Singapore)

Manipulative Medicine Consultant of Professional Manipulative Therapist Association (Singapore)

Vice Chairman of National Spinal Manipulative Therapist Academic Committee of China

Senior Researcher of Malaysia Chinese Medical Sciences Research Centre

Academic Consultant of Malaysia Acupuncture Academy

Academic Consultant of TCM Training Centre of Penang Malaysia

Academic Consultant of Indonesia Chinese Medicine Society Jakarta TCM College

Life Honorary Consultant of Japan Holistic Manipulative Therapy Association

# Dedication

This work is Dedicated to all seekers of truth of every class, age and race

Authors

# *Contents*


Preface 9

Chapter

1 Introduction 19

2 History of Acupuncture 31

3 Philosophy of Acupuncture 65

4 Five Elements Theory 117

5 Diagnosis in Traditional Chinese Medicine 129

6 Evaluation and Diagnosis 169

7 The Concept of Qi 215

8 Management & Research on Some Disorders 243

9 How Acupuncture Works 261

10 Acupuncture Anesthesia 273

11 Laser Acupuncture 303

12 Auriculotherapy 313

13 Atlas of Acupuncture Points 324

14 Therapeutics of Common Ailments 371

15 Therapeutics of Common Ailments 373

16 Infertility, Impotence and Acupuncture 379

17 Acupuncture in Hairfall 395

18 Does Acupuncture Hurts 397

19 Related Therapies 405

20 Explanation of Some Terms 413

21 Marmapuncture 435

# *Preface*

After ten years of the study of (medical) books<br>
(one believes) that there is no incurable disease.<br>
After ten more years of study of (medical) books<br>
(one is certain) that there is no curable disease.

- Huai Yuan

The Chinese healing art of acupuncture is one that can be dated back at least two thousand years. Some authorities maintain that acupuncture has been practiced in China for even four thousand years. Though its exact age is vague, what is certain is that up until the recent twentieth century, much of the population of the world was uninformed about acupuncture, its origins, and its capacity to promote and maintain good health. Even today in relatively "advanced" nations such as the United States there are many who hold acupuncture under the stereotype of a new or radical medicine, one which would almost always be a second choice after more familiar Western approaches to handling illness. Following a brief synopsis of the theory of acupuncture, the following text will, to a limited extent, elucidate the vast history of this ancient medicine and assert that it is neither new nor radical.

According to Chinese Embryology when two people come together for sex, there is an exchange and blending of sexual energies. When a man and a woman have sex and conception results, the sexual energy blends to form "Pre-Heaven Jing" in the newly conceived individual. Both the father and the mother supply Jing.

The developing embryo and fetus has no independent Jing of its own. It's totally dependent on the Pre-Heaven Jing supplied by the mother and father and on nourishment from the mother's Kidneys. One of the functions of Jing is it acts like a blueprint and master control. It turns things on an off during development.

**1st month** – The newly conceived being is like a drop of essence (jing), like a pearl of dew on a leaf. The mother experiences morning sickness, dizziness, and a lack of appetite. Her pulse is floating and tight. She should eat nourishing and easily digestible cooked foods. She is allowed to eat some sour foods if cravings arise. Barley, which makes the fetus grow normally, is beneficial at this time. Avoid acupuncture on the Liver meridian during this time as the fetus is nourished through this meridian. Blood circulation of the mother is impaired so she should be careful not to over exert herself physically. She should avoid becoming anxious and fearful. The fetus feels pain when the mother is exposed to cold and fear when the mother is exposed to heat.

**2nd month** – The fetus is now like a peach flower and is situated at Zhong ji – Ren 3 (just above the pubic hairline). The placenta is being formed at this time and the mother may experience dizziness, blurred vision, nausea, vomiting, lack of appetite and slight fatigue. The mother should not eat pungent/spicy foods and should avoid excessive sexual activity and physical work. Joint pain is quite common at this time. The fetus is now nourished through the Gallbladder channel and therefore should not be needled. This is also the time that the Original Qi of the fetus comes into being so the mother should stay relaxed, breath properly and meditate. Exposure to excessive cold may bring about miscarriage and exposure to excessive heat may make the fetus weak.

**3rd month** – The fetus is now like a cocoon. It begins to look like a silkworm, large at one end and small at the other. The mother experiences nausea and vomiting and should avoid extreme cold or heat. Included now with any treatment of the mothers disease should be that of 'calming the fetus'. The fetus's body shape and sex are still changing and are under the influence of external stimuli of the mother. If she wants a son she should practice shooting arrows, if she wants a daughter she should spend time with jewellery and pretty things. For a nice looking child she should spend time feasting her eyes on jade and for a good hearted child she should spend as much time as possible sitting quietly. During this month the fetus is nourished through the Heart channel and therefore should not be needled.

**4th month** – The fetus and the placenta this month collect the Field of Elixir (Dan Tian). The mother should not eat Rabbit and should not be exposed to cold. During this time the fetus begins to absorb essence from the mother's Kidneys to form blood vessels. The mother should now eat rice, fish or wild goose, this makes the fetus's Qi and blood strong, its ears and eyes sensitive and bright, and its channels free from obstructions. In this month the fetus is nourished from the San Jiao meridian and should not be needled. The Yang organs are formed this month. The mother should keep herself calm and free from any emotional disturbance, and be moderate in her eating.

**5th month** – It is in this month that the gender differentiation occurs. A strange test; if one stands behind the pregnant woman and calls her, if she turns to the left it is male; if she turns to the right it is a female. Also if she is carrying a boy she will prefer sour foods. At this time the fetus is firmly embedded in the uterus and is steady. It is the 5th month that the fetus begins to receive Essential Qi of the Heart from the mother. This is to establish temperament. It is therefore advisable to sleep long hours, bathe and change clothes often, stay away from strangers, wear enough clothes and get exposure to sunshine. The mother should eat wheat, beef and lamb. She should also balance sweet with sour foods and bitter with salty. The fetus is nourished this month through the Spleen meridian and should not be needled there. The limbs are formed. The mother should not eat too much or go hungry. She should not eat drying foods or have Moxibustion or hot compresses or water bottles applied.

**6th month** – In this month the muscles and hair grow. If it is a boy his movements will be felt more on the left and if it is a girl the feeling will be more on the right. The fetus is now described as being like a fish in the mother's abdomen. During this month the fetus receives the mother's Lung Qi, which forms sinews and gives the child its Corporeal (physical) soul, great care should be taken with this in mind. The mother should take light exercise and not stay indoors all the time. She should go to the countryside to look at horses or dogs running around and should eat meat of wild animals. Doing this will make the fetus grow strong sinews, muscles, skin, and spine. The fetus is nourished through the Stomach meridian and should not be needled there. The mouth and eyes are formed and the mother should eat sweet foods but not in excess. The fetus will now move more which may lead to restlessness.

**7th month** – In the seventh month the fetus grows big, the eyes are bright, the nose has Qi, the ears are open and the mouth can taste. At this time the mother is usually very healthy, but if there is any problem one should implement 'calming the fetus'. The fetus begins to receive Essential Qi from the mother's Liver to form bones. The mother should take enough exercise to promote the circulation of Qi and blood by flexing and extending her joints. Her bedroom should be dry. She should avoid cold foods and eat rice, which will nourish the fetus's bones and teeth. The Lung meridian nourishes the fetus this month and therefore should not be needled. The skin and hair develop, the mother should not shout or speak in loud tones or wear too thin clothes. She should also bathe less often.

**8th month** – This month the Qi of the fetus becomes active and this may cause some irritability with a feeling of oppression in the chest, lack of appetite and all food may taste sweet or stale. Problems at this time should be checked by regulating the Stomach and 'calming the fetus'. The Essential Qi from the mother's Spleen now promotes the growth of the skin. At this time the mother should avoid emotional upsets and practice quiet breathing to maintain her Qi, which will promote a moist lustrous skin on the fetus. The Large Intestine meridian nourishes the fetus this month and therefore should not be needled. The mother should avoid over eating and getting angry.

**9th month** – Now the fetus is very large, reaching into the hypochonrial regions. The mother still may feel oppression in the chest and a lack of appetite. This is the time when the fetus receives Essence from the mother. All the organs are formed. The mother should eat sweet foods, wear loose clothes and not live in dampness. The fetus is now nourished through the Kidney meridian and therefore should not be needled.

**10th month** – The fetus is now ready to emerge. The limbs stretch as it naturally turns and starts its downward descent. All Yin organs are developed and the Yang organs are free from obstructions. The mother should concentrate her Qi on the lower Dan Tian below the umbilicus to promote the growth of the fetus's joints and mental faculties. The fetus is now nourished through the Bladder meridian and therefore should not be needled. 'When the melon is ripe it falls off the plant'. The mother goes into labor.

Basic to traditional Chinese medicine is the dualistic cosmic theory of the yin and the yang. The yang, the male principle, is active and light and is represented by the heavens; the yin, the female principle, is passive and dark and is represented by the earth. The human body, like matter in general, is madeup of five elements: wood, fire, earth, metal, and water. With these are associated other groups of five, such as the five planets, the five conditions of the atmosphere, the five colours, and the five tones. Health, character, and the success of all political and private ventures are determined by the preponderance, at the time, of the yin or the yang; and the great aim of ancient Chinese medicine is to control their proportions in the body.

One of the most important concepts of Chinese medicine is that of natural balance. From this idea of balance arises the fundamental theory of yin and yang. According to this theory, life takes place in the alternating rhythm of yin and yang.

Day gives way to night, night to day; a time of light and activity (Yang) is followed by darkness and rest (Yin). Flowers open and close, the moon waxes and wanes, the tides come in and go out; we wake and sleep, breathe in, breathe out. Yin/Yang is a constant, continual flow through which everything is expressed on the one hand and recharged on the other. They are an inseparable couple. Their proper relationship is health; a disturbance in this relationship is disease.

The paradoxical nature of yin and yang is further illustrated in an excerpt from the Huang Di Nei Jing, or "The Yellow Emperor's

Canon of Internal Medicine," which is considered to be the best known and earliest of Chinese medical texts:

Yang has it's root in Yin
Yin has it's root in Yang
without Yin, Yang cannot arise
Without Yang, Yin cannot be born
Yin alone cannot arise; Yang alone cannot grow
Yin and Yang are divisible but inseparable.

The well-known symbol of the yin-yang further demonstrates that nothing is pure Yin or pure Yang; black and white embrace and intertwine in perfect symmetry, each side containing a small seed of its opposite. The conclusion drawn from this theory is that good health entails the balance and harmony of all that is yin and all that is yang within the body.

When such a proper balance of forces exists, the body has achieved a healthy circulation of the life force qi (roughly pronounced "chee"). In Chinese medicine it is theorized that the human body, as well as every other living thing, has a natural flow of qi throughout it. Qi is said to travel the body along channels called "meridians," of which there are mainly fourteen. Qi flows constantly up and down these pathways, and when the flow of qi is insufficient, unbalanced, or interrupted, yin and yang become unbalanced, and illness may occur. An understanding of the relationship between the body, yin and yang, and qi is necessary to understand the utility of acupuncture.

Acupuncture can be described as the insertion of very fine needles (sometimes in combination with electrical stimulus or with heat produced by burning specific herbs, called Moxibustion) into the skin at specific acupuncture points in order to influence the functioning of the body. Traditionally, there are 365 acupoints on the body, most of which have a specific energetic function. Some are the meeting of meridian pathways while others are junctions with an internal pathway of the meridian. Some points tend to move qi towards the interior of the body while others bring energy to the surface. The choice of acupuncture points varies from patient to patient and from treatment to treatment and relies on very careful diagnoses of different kinds. Diagnosis entails the observation of the body through looking, touching, smelling and listening. In diagnosis, detailed questions are asked about the history ofthe illness and about such things as the patient's taste, smell, and dreams. Conclusions are drawn from the quality of the voice, and note is made of the colour of the face and of the tongue. The most important part of the investigation, however, is the examination of the pulse. Wang Shu-ho, who wrote the "Pulse Classic," lived in the 3rd century BC, and innumerable commentaries were written on his work. The pulse is examined in several places, at different times, and with varying degrees of pressure. The operation may take as long as three hours. It is often the only examination made, and it is used both for diagnosis and for prognosis. Not only are the diseased organs ascertained but the time of death or recovery may be foretold.

One of the primary and fundamen tal diagnostic methods of traditional Chinese medicine is pulse taking, which is far more intricate than pulse taking in the West.

It has been said to take upwards of fifteen years to master this diagnostic art.

Today Acupuncture enjoys what may be its greatest popularity to date. It is important to note that this popularity, however, is a fairly recent achievement of the medicine. In the early 20th century, China, as the rest of Asia, experienced a flood of Europeans and American influence. As early as the late 1890's the European germ theories of Koch, List, and Pasteur were starting to arrive in China, marking the beginning of Western medicine in the Far East. By 1912, acupuncture was in precipitous decline, barely able to counter this growth of biomedicine. At the same time, traditional Chinese medicine had gained a small hold in Europe and North America but was far from accepted, and by the beginning of the First World War, the art of acupuncture was close to cultural extinction in China.

Only a handful of background information is required to understand this sharp decline of acupuncture. What Europeans first introduced to China was not medicine or culture; it was a narcotic drug called opium. Designed to profit the Westerners who organized it, the opium trade grew exponentially throughout the 19th century, having appalling effects on Chinese society. It was a social horror, and it very aptly illustrated the subhuman status in which many Westerners held the Chinese as well as the creations of Chinese culture, including acupuncture. To add to the trauma, a famine in 1878-1879 left 9 million people in unimaginably horrifying conditions. There was no public sanitation, and open sewers and garbage-laden streets were the standard urban scene. It was in this atmosphere of decline, loss of self-determination, and inconceivable human suffering that the Republic of China was formed in 1911. China quickly developed a desire to modernize, and its people began to turn to Western medicine. Given this background information, it is not difficult to understand why the beginning of the 20th century was a devastating time for acupuncture, theoretically as well as practically. In the fall of 1915, an order was issued demanding that medical, pharmacy, and veterinary students meet the qualifications established by Western nations. By 1929, registration of traditional doctors was ceased, and an announcement was made by the Ministry of Health proposing the abolishment of traditional medicine altogether.

Though in rapid decline, not everyone stood for the disappearance of traditional Chinese medicine. In the 1920's a group of traditional practitioners formed the zhong yi ("Chinese medicine") movement seeking to salvage their medicine. Through this movement, the group attempted to create a force that could resist the enroachment of xi yi, "Western medicine." Though unsuccessful at the time, this movement laid the foundation for the reappearance and modernization of traditional medicine following the Second World War.

The resurgence of acupuncture in China after the Second World War had a relatively simply understood cause, namely "the greatest and most intractable public health problem of any nation in the world," as stated by the United Nations Relief Organization. Among the first tasks of the People's Republic was coming up with a way to provide health care for a huge society. China found itself with less than 40,000 Western physicians and approximately 500,000 disorganized and crudely trained traditional practitioners attempting to serve a population of a half billion people. Thus, the clear and pragmatic reason for the post-war promotion of traditional medicine: there was no other choice.

A compromise had to be reached. Conservative politicians saw traditional medicine as an aspect of Chinese culture to preserve against the onslaught of Western enroachment. Meanwhile, political modernists saw it as, at best, "a collection of empirical tricks, some of which might be useful". With the help of a general feeling of preserving the essence of Chinese culture, traditional medicine was saved from abandonment or possible prohibition, but not without being scientifically modernized. And so, starting in the 1950's, traditional medical schools with standardized curricula were established to teach basic biomedical sciences, traditional pharmacotherapy, and acupuncture. It was then, too, that the zhong yi movement triumphantly re-emerged. For the first time in the 20th century, Chinese medicine had "a firm cultural position, a clear economic role, and a powerful political patron"

Efforts to integrate Western and Chinese medicines continued through the 1950's with limited success. Having neither money nor prestige, traditional practitioners, who were not themselves united, feared eventual elimination. Furthermore, "popularization and expansion had further diluted what had never been a homogenous system". Despite these drawbacks, the late 1950's did experience one of the most important developments of acupuncture, at least from the viewpoint of Western physicians. It is during this time that aggressive acupuncture techniques were developed and that acupuncture was first utilized as an anesthetic and analgesic during surgery.

When Westerners started flooding China after Nixon's visit, it was these techniques they were shown. They brought these back to the West, where they were popularized and became a primary focus for research. Another factor that greatly contributed to the westward migration of acupuncture appeared in the 1970's in the form of acupuncture programs sponsored by the World Health Organization. Physicians from many countries came to China to take advantage of these programs, and since the early 1980's many similar programs have been established for non-physician acupuncturists as well. Today, affiliations exist between many Western acupuncture schools and traditional medical schools in China, allowing students to travel abroad to partake in pre- and post-graduation programs. In the 1980's by the so-called "three roads" policy allowed for the individual development of traditional medicine, biomedicine, and their combination, integrated medicine. Since then, more than 2000 Chinese physicians have graduated with a thorough training in both traditional and Western medicine.

It is evident that this medicinal art is indeed one of the oldest and most complex that exists, based on ideas and theories formulated over hundreds of years. Acupuncture has come a long way since its origins and has won an uphill battle against time, misunderstanding, and criticism to gain the great popularity that it enjoys today. Despite its successes, however, there are still many legislative and public opinion battles to be fought in terms of its acceptance and utilization as a modern medicine. It is hoped that within the next several years, acupuncture will break through the remaining political barriers and that the world will see practitioners of traditional Chinese medicine as primary care providers with licensing in all states, much the way chiropractors are today. Much of the friction arises from the western need to see hard scientific evidence of how acupuncture works. Advocates of the practice are optimistic that western science will eventually catch up to the complexities of acupuncture and provide a logical explanation for its consistent success. Traditional Chinese medicine offers a comprehensive, integrated and well-tested theory for its application in acupuncture, which is inexpensive, non-invasive, safe and effective, is surely a key form of treatment for the future.

We are indebted to Dr. Choo Led Sin, eminent Acupuncturist. for his untiring effort of editing and revising the entire text, to Dr Fabio R Ambrosi(Italy) for his suggestions for compilation of this work.

**July 30, 2013**

**Dr. Debasish Kundu**

**Dr. Choo Led Sin**

# *Chapter One*

# Introduction

Acupuncture: Latin word 'Acus' means needle and 'Punctura' means insertion. Acupuncture is an ancient chinese science and art of therapeutics in which needles are inserted into specific points or nerve endings or nerve junctions of the body to create a stimulation or 'deqi' to optimize energy levels, which reduces pain and improves the functions and vitality of the internal organs concerned.

Acupuncture needles dating from 4,000 years ago have been found in China. The first needles were stone; later, bronze, gold, or silver were used, and today needles are usually made of steel. Initially, needles were used only to prick boils and ulcers

Acupuncture grew out of ancient Chinese philosophy's dualistic cosmic theory of the yin and the yang. The yin, the female principle, is passive and dark and is represented by the earth; the yang, the male principle, is active and light and is represented by the heavens. The forces of yin and yang act in the human body as they do throughout the natural universe as a whole. Disease or physical disharmony is caused by an imbalance or undue preponderance of these two forces in the body. An imbalance of yin and yang results in an obstruction of the vital life force, or ch'i, in the body. The fundamental energy of the ch'i flows through 12 meridians, or pathways, in the body, each in turn associated with a major visceral organ (liver, kidney, etc.) and with a functional body system. Acupuncture is designed to affect the distribution of yin and yang in these channels so that the ch'i will be enabled to flow freely and harmoniously.

Acupuncture was developed in response to the theory that there are special meridian points on the body connected to the internal organs and that vital energy flows along the meridian lines. According to this theory, diseases are caused by interrupted energy flow, and inserting and twirling needles restores normal flow.

According to classical chinese doctrine, the acupuncture points follow a series of 'life force' lines called 'Meridians' which circles the body longitudinally (14 Meridians).

In western countries there is a misleading conception that it could only be effective in certain conditions, such as, pain or weightloss, whereas, it is found effective in a wide range of disease conditions through it's power to stimulate the body's own healing powers.

Acupuncture is one aspect of Traditional Chinese Medicine that has flourished in China for over 2,500 years. Presently, it is practiced widely throughout Asia and Europe. The United States has followed suit, and Acupuncture is now accepted as one of the newest forms of health care in this country. Some insurance plans pay for acupuncture treatments. The Texas State Board of Medical Examiners regulates the practice of Acupuncture in this state.

Acupuncture treats diseases and its syndromes, strengthens the immune systems and the physical body, prevents diseases and achieves longevity. A lot of research has confirmed that acupuncture can regulate and balance the endocrine system and hormone levels. So, it is useful to treat reproductive disorders. Acupuncture is not however a cure all and does not take the place of surgery.

Acupuncture is based on the knowledge of vital energy flow to the whole body. This energy travels through pathways called meridian, etc. Once this energy is deficient or blocked, then the body stops functioning normally and will eventually become sick. An Acupuncturist is trained to find these deficiencies or blocks. Through complex diagnostic techniques, he or she determines if the energy supply is ample, if it is flowing the correct direction and speed. Then, with the application of needles and needling techniques, he or she is able to restore the flow of energy back to normal. The body returns to its normal function, pain is relieved, other symptoms disappear, vital energy and health is restored.

As a side effect of the restoration of ample and correct energy flow in the body, studies have shown that Acupuncture could influence the central and peripheral nervous systems. Evidence indicates that it releases endorphins from the brain making it particularly effective in pain control. Among a host of factors, acupuncture also affects the metabolism and production of sugar levels in the blood, as well as affects the endocrine system, and digestive system.

In the Chinese medical paradigm, all the major organs in the human body have corresponding energetic pathways along the surface of the body which are called channels or meridians, and these meridians have points which have certain energetic functions. In Chinese medicine this disease is considered to be a disturbance of prenatal qi (energy), what we in the West would call our genetic makeup. Prenatal qi governs a person's organization, creation, and continuing re-creation. This qi originates in the kidneys, therefore the kidney channel or meridian must be considered in treatment. There is also the factor of stagnation of dampness and coldness in the body, which Chinese medicine considers to be an excessive yin or deficient yang condition. Put in simpler terms, the qi is too cold and not moving well, therefore the qi must be warmed to help it move. A technique called moxibustion is used to alleviate the dampness and cold, and bring warmth (yang energy) into the body. Moxibustion is the burning of a wool-like herb called mugwort near the skin's surface on preselected points along meridians.

Acupuncture is the practice of puncturing the skin with needles at certain anatomical points in the body to relieve specific symptoms associated with many diseases. The anatomical points (acupuncture points) are thought to have certain electrical properties, which affect chemical neurotransmitters in the body.

Acupuncture is one of the oldest, most commonly used medical practices in the world. Originated in China more than 2,500 years ago, acupuncture gained attention in this country in the 1970s, when China and the US opened relations. The practice has been growing in popularity since.

The first record of Acupuncture is found in the 4,700 year old Huang Di Nei Jing (Yellow Emperor's Classic of Internal Medicine). This is said to be the oldest medical textbook in the world. It is said to have been written down from even earlier theories by Shen Nung, the father of Chinese Medicine. Shen Nung documented theories about circulation, pulse, and the heart over 4,000 years before European medicine had any concept about them.

As the basis of Acupuncture, Shen Nung theorized that the body had an energy force running throughout it. This energy force is known as ***Qi*** (roughly pronounced Chee). The Qi consists of all essential life activities which include the spiritual, emotional, mental and the physical aspects of life. A person's health is influenced by the flow of Qi in the body, in combination with the universal forces of Yin and Yang. (I will discuss Yin and Yang a little later). If the flow of Qi is insufficient, unbalanced or interrupted, Yin and Yang become unbalanced, and illness may occur. Qi travels throughout the body along "Meridians" or special pathways. The Meridians, (or Channels), are the same on both sides of the body (paired). There are fourteen main meridians running vertically up and down the surface of the body. Out of these, there are twelve organ Meridians in each half of the body (remember they are in pairs). There are also two unpaired midline Meridians. The acupuncture points are specific locations where the Meridians come to the surface of the skin, and are easily accessible by "needling," Moxibustion, and Acupressure. The connections between them ensure that there is an even circulation of Qi, a balance between Yin and Yang.

Energy constantly flows up and down these pathways. When pathways become obstructed, deficient, excessive, or just unbalanced, Yin and Yang are said to be thrown out of balance. This causes illness. Acupuncture is said to restore the balance.

Yin and Yang is an important theory in the discussion of Acupuncture treatment, in relation to the Chinese theory of body systems. As stated earlier Qi is an energy force that runs throughout the body. In addition, Qi is also prevalent throughout nature as well. Qi is comprised of two parts, Yin and Yang. Yin and Yang are opposite forces, that when balanced, work together. Any upset in the balance will result in natural calamities, in nature; and disease in humans. Yin is signified by female attributes, passive, dark, cold, moist, that which moves medially, and deficient of Yang. Yang is signified by male attributes, light, active, warm, dry, that which moves laterally, and deficient of Yin. Nothing is completely Yin or Yang. The most striking example of this is man himself. A man is the combination of his mother (Yin) and and his father (Yang). He contains qualities of both: This is the universal symbol describing the constant flow of yin and yang forces. You'll notice that within yin, there is Yang, and within Yang, there is the genesis of Yin. Whether or not you believe in Taoist philosophy, (which all this is based on), one thing is indisputable: Acupuncture works.

Acupuncturists can use as many as nine types of Acupuncture needles, though only six are commonly used today. These needles vary in length, width of shaft, and shape of head. Today, most needles are disposible. They are used once and disgarded in accordance with medical biohazard regulations and guidlines. There are a few different precise methods by which Acupuncturists insert needles. Points can be needled anywhere in the range of 15 degrees to 90 degrees relative to the skin surface, depending on the treatment called for. In most cases, a sensation, felt by the patient, is desired. This sensation, which is not pain, is called deqi (pronounced dah-chee). The following techniques are some which may be used by an Acupuncturist immediately following insertion: Raising and Thrusting, Twirling or Rotation, Combination of Raising/Thrusting and Rotation, Plucking, Scraping (vibrations sent through the needle), and Trembling (another vibration technique). Once again, techniques are carefully chosen based on the ailment.

There are a few related procedures that fall into the range of Acupuncture treatments. The first is Electro-Acupuncture. This is the using of very small electrical impulses through the Acupuncture needles. This method is generally used for analgesia (pain relief or prevention). The amount of power used is only a few micro amperes, but the frequency of the current can vary from

5 to 2,000 Hz. The higher frequencies are generally used for surgery (usually abdominal), and the lower frequencies for general pain relief. The first reported successful use of Electro-Acupuncture was in 1958 in China for a tonsillectomy. Today, it is a common method of surgical analgesia used in China. Other methods for stimulating Acupuncture points have used Lasers and sound waves (Sonopuncture). A very commonly used treatment in the United States is Auriculotherapy or Ear Acupuncture. The theory is that since the ear has a rich nerve and blood supply, it would have connections all over the body. For this reason, the ear has many Acupuncture points which correspond to many parts and organs of the body. Auricular Acupuncture has been successful in treating problems ranging from obesity to alcoholism, to drug addiction. There are numerous studies either completed, or currently going on which affirms Auricular Acupuncture's effectiveness. (These will be mentioned in detail later on in the concerned chapter.)

Another popular treatment method is Moxibustion, which is the treatment of diseases by applying heat to Acupuncture points. Acupuncture and Moxibustion are considered complimentary forms of treatment, and are commonly used together. Moxibustion is used for ailments such as bronchial asthma, bronchitis, certain types of paralysis, and arthritic disorders.

Cupping is another type of treatment. This is a method of stimulating Acupuncture points by applying suction through a metal, wood or glass jar, in which a partial vacuum has been created. This technique produces blood congestion at the site, and therefore stimulates it. Cupping is used for low backache, sprains, soft tissue injuries, and helping relieve fluid from the lungs in chronic bronchitis.

One of the most popular alternatives to Acupuncture is Acupressure. This is simply Acupuncture without needles. Stimulation of the Acupuncture points is performed with the fingers or an instrument with a hard ball shaped head. Another variation of Acupressure is Reflexology (also called Zone Therapy). This is where the soles of the feet and the posterio-inferior regions of the ankle joints are stimulated. Many diseases of the internal organs can be treated in this manner.

There are many diseases that can be treated successfully by Acupuncture or its related treatments. The most common ailments currently being treated are: lower backache, Cervical Spondylosis, Condylitis, Arthritic Conditions, Headaches of all kinds (including migraine), Allergic Reactions, general and specific use for Analgesia (including surgery) and relief of muscles spasms. There have also been clinical trials in the use of Acupuncture in treating anxiety disorders and depression. Likewise, very high success rates have been found in treating addictions to alcohol, tobacco (nicotine) and "hard' drugs. Acupuncture can rid the body of the physical dependency, but can not rid the mind of the habit (psychological dependency). For this reason, Acupuncture treatment of addictions has not been fully successful.

A report issued through the National Institutes of Health concluded that acupuncture is a safe, effective, and painless treatment for a number of medical conditions. The report encouraged patients and physicians to consider acupuncture as an alternative or complementary treatment for some common health problems, including nausea associated with pregnancy and chemotherapy and pain after dental surgery, but said that larger and better studies were needed to fully establish its benefits and limitations.

According to theories of traditional Chinese medicine, the human body has more than 2,000 acupuncture points connected via pathways, or meridians. These pathways create an energy flow (Qi, pronounced "chee") through the body that is responsible for overall health. Disruption of the energy flow can cause disease. Acupuncture may correct these imbalances when applied at acupuncture points and improve the flow of Qi.

Acupuncture theories today are based on extensive laboratory research, and have become widely known and accepted. In addition, controlled studies have shown evidence of the effectiveness of acupuncture for certain conditions. Acupuncture is not for everyone. If you choose to see an acupuncturist, find a practitioner who is licensed with appropriate training and credentials.

Several studies have documented acupuncture's effects on the body, but none has fully explained how acupuncture works within the framework of Western medicine. Researchers have proposed several processes to explain acupuncture's effects, primarily on pain.

In general, acupuncture points are believed to stimulate the central nervous system, which, in turn, releases chemicals into the muscles, spinal cord, and brain. These chemicals either alter the experience of pain or release other chemicals that influence the body's self-regulating systems. These biochemical changes may stimulate the body's natural healing abilities and promote physical and emotional well-being.

Attention has been focused on the following theories to further explain how acupuncture affects the body:

Evidence suggests that acupuncture points are strategic conductors of electromagnetic signals. Stimulating these points enables electromagnetic signals to be relayed at greater-than-normal rates. These signals may start the flow of pain-killing biochemicals, such as endorphins, or release immune system cells to specific body sites.

Considerable research supports the claim that acupuncture releases opiods, synthetic or naturally-occurring chemicals in the brain that may reduce pain or induce sleep. These chemicals may explain acupuncture's pain-relieving effects.

Joined at the base of the brain, the hypothalamus and pituitary glands are responsible for many body functions. The hypothalamus activates and controls part of the nervous system, the endocrine processes, and many bodily functions, such as sleep, regulation of temperature, and appetite. The pituitary gland supplies some of the body's needed hormones. Stimulation of these glands can result in a broad spectrum of effects on various body systems.

Studies suggest that acupuncture may alter brain chemistry in a positive way. This is accomplished by changing the release of neurotransmitters (biochemical substances that stimulate or inhibit nerve impulses) and neurohormones (naturally-occurring chemical substances that can change the structure or function, or impact the activity of, a body organ).

People seek acupuncture treatment for relief of chronic pain, such as arthritis or low back pain. Acupuncture, however, has expanded uses in many parts of the world. The exact data for in which disease conditions that may benefit from acupuncture is however not available.

The ever-increasing concern of drug side effects reminds us why some people have come in for acupuncture, and it makes me think about who else gets acupuncture.

Acupuncture isn't only for the people who are worried about drug side effects (short term-long term/life threatening-annoying). Who else gets acupuncture? People who actually experienced undesirable side effects to their medications. People who are sensitive to drugs or herbs. People who don't want to take drugs. People who cannot take drugs (pregnant woman who need help with other symptoms). People who became addicted to their medications. There are those who found their medications stopped working, while some found their drugs never worked. Some people no longer want to take drugs to counter side effects of another drug. There are those who refused to have an invasive procedure, where they'd be placed on medications the rest of their lives, knowing that these drugs would cause other problems.

Some people get acupuncture as their primary health maintenance, using western medicine if drastic intervention is needed. Who else? People who want to prepare for surgery or want to recover from surgery more quickly. People with wild and weird problems. People who are old. People who are very young. People who want overall health improvement instead of masking a symptom. People who think that exploratory surgery is not their next option. People come to acupuncture when they don't want two years of biweekly allergy shots.

Why else? People come because nothing else has worked. People come because they want to try acupuncture before trying anything else. People come because their symptoms cannot be explained in western terms. People come because the battery of tests show that nothing is wrong, but they just don't feel right. Some come because they just feel off balance.

People come because their doctor prescribed acupuncture. Doctors come. Nurses come. Physical therapists, nutritionists, psychotherapists, massage therapists, and dentists come. A few patients have reported that their doctor said he wouldn't do anything else for them until they finally followed his prescription for acupuncture. They were so reluctant yet so surprised and pleased after finally complying that they asked for their acupuncture prescriptions to be refilled. There are also people who have come in for acupuncture because their insurance paid for it.

Today our bodies have to deal with unnatural levels of pollutants, toxins, heavy metals, antibiotics, hormones, over-the-counter medications and self-prescribed supplements. The acupuncture approach is to tune up the organs instead of adding more for the organs to process. It may take time to clear out toxins and re-energize the organs, but it is a logical approach.

Most of us do not know how to listen to our bodies. Many have gotten used to routinely taking sleeping pills, caffeine, laxatives, pain killers, aspirin, and antacids. This leads to a constant drugging to deal with living life out-of-balance, shutting down the body, interfering with natural healing processes and other basic functions.

There was a recent study of over 80,000 women without high blood pressure. The women and their use of pain-relief medication, such as ibuprofen (found in Advil), acetaminophen (found in Tylenol) or naproxen (found in Alieve), were tracked over a two-year period. The researchers found that women who took these medications more than 22 times a month were almost twice as likely to have high blood pressure. Other studies have shown how these drugs also contribute to heart and kidney failure. How many of us take medication with no idea that it could eventually cause another problem?

I often see patients who complain of fatigue, headache, and malaise. It turns out that they are taking in too much (vitamins, medications, etc.) overtaxing their liver and kidneys. In these cases, it is not sensible to add more demands on overtaxed organs in an attempt to purge or balance the person.

Instead of looking for ways to get the toxins out, why not reduce what goes in. Try a nap to see if it helps your headache; hydrate regularly; chew your food adequately to see if it aids digestion; do a TV news fast; create a white space in your schedule; say "NO" to reading newspaper headline stories; go for a walk without driving to a place to walk. Especially during the holidays, we should all check to see if we have "hurry" sickness, and eliminate optional stressors.

The technologies of our time have created additional stresses not present for our ancestors. This makes it harder for us to follow our bodies' rhythms and cycles. Instead, we artificially cause sleep, waking, digestion, and relaxation.

Acupuncture helps the body to return to natural wellness. Needling, moxa, rest, carefully balanced diet, and specific exercises are used to address the root cause of problems, while calming down the overall system. This brings about normal function without overpowering, costly intervention.

The World Health Organization (WHO) lists dozens of conditions that acupuncture treats, and medical journals discuss conditions not mentioned by the WHO. So, acupuncture isn't just for pain relief. It is a whole-person medical system that has been used for thousands of years. It directs the patient's body to heal and naturally move toward health. The physical or psychological conditions that bring people to acupuncture are as varied as their general reasons for coming.

# *Chapter Two*

# History of Acupuncture

Acupuncture is believed to be one of the oldest medical science in the world. It is originated in China and in later years spread all over the world. Researchers have now established that there was existence of Acupuncture like treatment in the stone age, in which sharp or pointed stones are used in place of needles, which are known as 'Bian', 'Chan' or 'Zhen', thereafter needles made of bones or bamboos are being used, during the 'Shang' dynasty (1600 to 1046 B.C.) bronze needles are brought to use, and the concept of 'Channel' or 'Meridian' is developed. During the regime of 'Han Emperors' (2697 to 2596 B.C.) the "Yellow Emperor's Classic of Internal Medicine" or 'Huang Di Nei Jing' was written. It is believed to be the first book written on Classical Chinese Medicine. It is presented in the form of a questionnaire between the Yellow Emperor Huang Di and his Prime Minister and Royal Physician Chi Po. It is in two parts, part one 'Su Wen' means simple questions on principles of traditional Chinese medicine and part two 'Ling Shu' means magic gate which deals with therapeutics.

## Foundations

Examination of Chinese history will begin in a period known as the Early Zhou. This period, taking place from -1027 to -772, was a period of classic feudalism in China. The Zhou dynasty was established through military conquest, whose success was a result not only of inadequate opposing defense, but also of the Zhou's superior agricultural productivity. An increased production of crops due to communally managed irrigation systems allowed for more of the population to be fed by fewer laborers, which in turn allowed for the conscription of larger armies from the peasantry and a victory over the Shang.

The Early Zhou has little connection to acupuncture. In fact, the predominant feature of the period was the rise of the idea that demons were a harmful influence on humankind. Human health was left to supernatural powers and demonology. Popular belief maintained that a group of shaman leaders were possessed of magical powers and were responsible for "provision of rain, quieting violent storms, and purging poisonous creatures and evil influences". This is not to say that the Early Zhou was unimportant in the genesis of acupuncture or Chinese medicine in general. The era is accredited with setting the stage for the next period in Chinese history, in which medicine began to establish itself as a valuable independent entity.

In 771 the feudal arrangement of the Early Zhou was disrupted when a foreign alliance backfired, forcing the Zhou capital further east and thus giving rise to a new period known as the Middle Zhou (772 to-480). While it is safe to conclude that Chinese arts did not flourish in the midst of the ruthlessness of this new "farm and fight" state, this period did see a significant advancement in medicine. It is during the Middle Zhou that medicine, although still dominated by magical correspondences and demonology, began to develop as a separate activity and take a place distinct from religion in the social order. Evidence of this progression in medicine can be found in the descriptions of four different kinds of doctors in Zhou archives, including physicians, surgeons, dieticians, and veterinary surgeons. Another notable achievement of this period was the appearance of evidence of what would become the theory of the six environmental evils. This evidence appeared in a story of a physician's attendance on the prince of Jin, wherein yin and yang were represented as hot and cold. Together with wind, rain, darkness and brightness, the six comprised the influences that can cause disease. This concept of evil influences is referenced today when acupuncturists speak of "cold damp wind" et cetera during diagnosis.

By far the most important outcome of the Middle Zhou was the establishment of Confucianism as the first of the Three Pillars of Chinese thought (Confucianism, Daoism [Taoism], and Buddhism). Among the significant contributions to Chinese culture by Confucianism was the establishment of a solid connection between "responsible human behavior and desirable outcomes". This social connection found parallel expression in the progression of medicine by developing a link between human well-being and human action, a link which was important for the origin of the qi paradigm because it shifted thinking away from demonic causation of illness. Though Confucianism is not solely responsible for the rise of the medicine of qi, qi could not have existed without this link.

While the Middle Zhou is noted for the birth of Confucianism, the Late Zhou (480 to 221) is accredited with the rise of Daoism. At this time in China there were two movements in medicine. Aspects of the older magico-demonic tradition were being survived as magical correspondence while new ideas of prior periods were the groundwork of the new systematic correspondence. The interesting point to note regarding the simultaneous existence of two systems of medicine is that neither system required the elimination of the other. Unlike Western intellectual history where success of a new model involves the replacement of a previously dominant model, Chinese thinkers tended to accumulate their models, retaining previous ideas. Such behavior permitted the application of whatever model worked best in a particular situation. This also permitted the unbiased acceptance of new ideas. Thus, the emergence of the five-phase doctrine, which is a crucial concept in acupuncture, and of Daoism during this period in Chinese history eliminated neither Confucianism nor any earlier religious traditions. It is in this period, with the power of Confucianism and Daoism, that medicine began its development as an institution.

The subsequent period in Chinese history is the Qin dynasty (221 to 206), also known as the period of book burning. This period was marked by unceasing unrest and witnessed little progress in the field of medicine. Though wealth- and power-driven, China's new Legalist government did have its triumphs, without which future advancement in medicine might not have been possible. Emperor Shi Huang-di ended China's long tradition of small, self-reliant towns and unified an empire of interdependent, currency-driven population centers. His government standardized weights, measures, and writing, set the value of coinage, and imposed the construction of a transportation system throughout this kingdom. Through his ruthless drive to wealth and power, Shi Huang-di inadvertently laid the foundations for the prosperity and creativity of the Han.

The Han dynasty (206 to 220), the period of systemization, was certainly a very climactic and exciting period in the history of acupuncture. Socially, too, and especially after the harshness of the Qin, the Han was a period of a thriving Chinese culture. Taxes were lowered, government control was loosened, power was decentralized, policies were humanized, and the social and political elite was broadened to include more of the population. Cultural barriers were eliminated, and all classes of society benefited from an increasing wealth from trade and ordered economic interdependence.

In the midst of this flourishing society, medicine, too, advanced in leaps and strides. The Ma Wang-dui scripts, the Nan Jing (The Classic of Difficult Issues), and the Huang Di Nei Jing were all products of this period. These three documents collectively trace over four hundred years the development of the major conceptual features and theories of the medicine of systematic correspondence including anatomy, physiology, and pathology.

Traditionally dated from 2698 to 2598, but now agreed to have been completed in the 2nd to the 1st century, the Nei Jing is truly a cornerstone of acupuncture. It is comprised of 162 articles divided into two sections, each composed of multiple books. In the first book, Su Wen, or "Fundamental Questions," the conversation clarifies points of medical theory. The second book is named Ling Shu, or "Spiritual Axis/Pivot" and is essentially an acupuncture manual. These two texts together not only explain the assimilation and extension of the yin-yang theory and the incorporation of the five-phase doctrine, they also provide a focus on individual symptoms as somatic rather than supernatural events. By the time of the Nei Jing, all of the currently defined 12 regular channels as well as 135 bilateral acupoints were identified. Together, about 295 of the 670 presently accepted acupoints were known.

Furthermore, the channels were illustrated as carrying qi, described partly as a product of the body and partly as a product of the environment. Either the disruption of "healthy" bodily qi or the "evil" external qi were said to induce illness.

Assigned to a date between the 1st and 2nd centuries, the Nan Jing is a composition of 81 articles and is considered "the mature development of the medicine of systematic correspondence, because it integrates for the first time all aspects of health care into the yin-yang and five-phase doctrines" . By the time of this text, two front and back midline channels expanded the 12 regular channels to 14, the channel system itself was further elaborated, and the idea of circulation of qi took a dominant role in the medicine. Moreover, the art of pulse diagnosis finds its origin in the Nan Jing. The author of the text structured the idea that the "hand great yin channel," the channel associated with the lung, was the key junction of all the channels of the body. Careful assessment of the many qualitatively distinct patterns at the radial arteries near both wrists consequentially provided diagnosis of the entire body. Although today a more generalized pulse diagnosis is taught where classroom teaching is dominant, classical Nan Jing pulse diagnosis survives today, especially in Japan where acupuncture training retains more of the apprentice tradition.

It is during the Han that the human body came to be seen as relationships between functional units (organs). "The organs were divided into zang ("depots" in the language of the time) and fu ("palaces"), reflecting their role in a complex system of functional interactions". The idea was developed and accepted that qi is the ground substance of the human organism and of all that is, and that human well-being relied on the balanced flow of qi in channels throughout the body. It is clear that by the end of the Han, the essentials of disease and treatment had reached maturity, and the medicine of systematic correspondence had come of age.

Since then, with its basic practical and philosophical tenets in place, acupuncture could only further develop and expand. Though it would go through oscillating periods of expansion and decline, acupuncture would ultimately become a staple of Chinese medical and social tradition. The following is a brief summation of acupuncture's innovations and developments and their socio-political context from the end of the Han dynasty through modern times.

Between 220 and 589, China underwent another period of political turmoil and instability. Buddhism was introduced to China, though it had relatively little influence over traditional Chinese medicines. It did, however, provide new theories for maintaining the body's health through physical exercise and psychological healing methods.

Acupuncture continued to develop throughout the period. In 282, Huang-fu Mi completed the Zhen Jiu Jia Yi Jing (The Systematic Classic of Acupuncture and Moxibustion) text, "the oldest extant technical book devoted to acupuncture and moxibustion". This text was responsible for reporting 649 of the 670 presently known acupoints. It was also the first text to emphasize acupuncture as a means of disease prevention. It provided the framework for the fundamental idea that with the proper knowledge, disease can be treated before it arises. The text gave detailed descriptions of "the channels, naming the points on each, and listing their locations and how deeply each should be needled. It also records the length of time for which needles should be retained, the number of moxa cones to be applied to each point, and what each point is known to treat". The Jia Yi Jing clearly marked the early progression of the healing art of acupuncture.

The ideas brought forth during this period would largely remain in place through modern times. The understanding of qi circulation was further developed and refined; "the principles of correspondence, yin-yang, and the five phases were totally incorporated into the fabric of the art". This formation and unification of ideas also proved useful in the precise application of diagnoses and choice of acupoints. Concurrently, the three major schools of religious thought, Confucianism, Daoism, and Buddhism, were contributing to the already established institution of Chinese medicine as well.

By around 562, this knowledge was beginning to spread to the neighboring lands of Korea, Vietnam and Japan. Particularly in Japan, the fundamental texts of acupuncture were imported, absorbed and studied with great care.

The short but notable Sui dynasty ran from 590 to 617. During this period, China was re-centralized, and again its medicines continued to develop. The medicine man Sun Si-miao contributed greatly to the history of acupuncture, combining Daoism and Buddhist theory with that of systematic correspondence. His published works touched on a broad variety of different medicines. Most importantly, "Sun Si-miao is regarded as having systematized the measurement system that is still used to describe the positions of acupoints". In addition, he reported several different types of points not located on channels, which are still described among acupuncturists today. Although there were not any profound innovations during the Sui dynasty, it set the stage for the following Tang era, where the principles of systematic correspondence would receive more widespread acceptance.

The Thang dynasty (618 to 907) is often referred to as the second golden age of China. "The empire was united; the three philosophical pillars and contact with neighboring cultures created an atmosphere of intellectual richness". Moreover, the economic resources of the Chinese nation were abundant, creating an ideal setting for population and culture to flourish. Despite these conditions, acupuncture and the general knowledge base of traditional Chinese medicines developed minimally. The one major contribution to acupuncture during this time was through an updated edition of the Huang Di Nei text; the practice of acupuncture was, for the first time, related to seasonal and other such cycles of the Chinese calendar. The greatest concern of the emperors, however, was not advancing medicine, but rather a pseudo-scientific search for an elixir to produce immortality. Nevertheless, acupuncture remained stable as a practiced medicinal art.

In Korea and Japan, meanwhile, knowledge of acupuncture was largely increasing. In 702, the first Imperial medical college was founded in Nara, Japan. Its studies comprised mainly the traditional texts, Nei Jing, Nan Jing, and Jia Yi Jing. Schools were eventually established in both countries, which would become accepted and remain in place through modern times.

After a period of decline, the Tang dynasty collapsed in 906. For the next fifty years, China underwent yet another period of social and political disorder during which acupuncture neither advanced nor declined significantly. The country's financial resources were depleted, and it was forced to respond to external threats and aggressions from its surrounding neighbors.

Early Shang thought was based upon a cyclic notion of time, corresponding to the seasons. This notion, which remained relevant throughout Chinese history, represents a fundamental distinction from western philosophy, in which the dominant view of time is a linear progression. During the Shang, fate could be manipulated by the great deity Shang Di (ch. 上帝 ; py shàngdì), most frequently translated as "Lord on High". Ancestor worship was also present, as was human and animal sacrifice.

When the Shang were overthrown by the Zhou, a new political, religious and philosophical concept was introduced called the "Mandate of Heaven". This mandate was said to be taken when rulers became unworthy of their position, and provided a shrewd justification for Zhou rule. During this period, archaeological evidence points to an increase in literacy and a partial shift away from the faith placed in Shang Di, with ancestor worship becoming commonplace and a more worldly orientation coming to the fore.

In around 500 BC, after the Zhou state weakened and China moved in to the Spring and Autumn Period, the classic period of Chinese philosophy began (it is an interesting fact that this date nearly coincides with the emergence of the first Greek philosophers). This is known as the Hundred Schools of Thought (bǐijiâ). Of the many schools founded at this time and during the subsequent Warring States Period, the four most influential ones were Confucianism, Daoism (often spelled "Taoism"), Mohism and Legalism. The short founder Qin Dynasty, where Legalism was the official philosophy, quashed Mohist and Confucianist schools. Legalism remained influential until the emperors of the Han Dynasty adopted Daoism and later Confucianism as official doctrine. These latter two became the determining forces of Chinese thought until the 20th century, with the introduction Buddhist philosophy (mostly during Tang Dynasty) negotiated largely through perceived similarities with Daoism.

The respective influences of Daoism and Confucianism are often described this way: "Chinese are Confucianist during the day, while they are Daoists at night". Moreover, many Chinese mandarins were government officials in the daily life and poets (or painters) in their spare time.

During the Shang dynasty, 960 to 1264, China went through a stage named the period of Neo-Confucianism. The qi paradigm was again popularized, proposing that "that qi had always existed and that all things came in and out of existence as gatherings or dissolutions of qi". Finally, these basic principles viz. yin-yang, the five phases, the celestial stems, and the six climactic influences introduced 1000 years before in the Nan Jing, found universal acceptance in all fields of Chinese medicine. (The Nan Jing was studied enthusiastically in Japan and Korea during this time as well.)

Other important contributions to acupuncture took place during this period. One of these was the publication of Dou Han-jing's Zhen Jing Zhi Nan. "This text described zi-wu, or noon and midnight cycles, and monthly, seasonal and annual cycles of qi according to which acupuncture could be performed". Additional texts with similar concepts, including "nai jia fa, a 10-day biorhythmic cycle used in acupuncture treatment", arose at the same time. The development of these time- and cycle-oriented ideas introduced during the Tang dynasty added considerably to the foundation of acupuncture theory.

The Yuan dynasty (1264 to 1368) was a period when China became a subject of Genghis Khan's vast Mongolian empire. The Khan were fairly lenient rulers of the Chinese, allowing the free exchange of knowledge and the continued spread of Neo-Confucianism. Medicine became increasingly specialized and the understanding of acupuncture was further detailed. The most notable new text of the time was Hua Shuo's Shi Si Jing Fa Hui (An Elucidation of the Fourteen Channels), published in 1341. This text described "303 points on the 12 regular channels, and 51 on the two medial channels - a total of 657 of the now-accepted 670 acupoints." There were other important aspects of the text as well.

Hua Shuo realized that the governing vessel and conception vessel were the only extra channels to have their own points, and created many of the modern waterway analogies used to describe the circulation of qi. ä His edition of the Nan Jing is considered by some to be the best of those that survived.

In 1368, the Chinese regained control of their land. The Ming dynasty lasted from 1368 until 1643. Confucian education became available to members of the many lower classes who would have formerly been excluded. Opportunity and prosperity increased in abundance for the masses. There were more books and a more widespread sharing of information. These factors combined encouraged the Chinese intellectual community to expand far beyond its previous limits: "orthodoxy lost its power and diversity took its place". Medicine, too, was thoroughly diversified. Many new schools were formed based on this resultant broad variety of ideologies.

Though primarily stable, acupuncture experienced a slight decline in popularity during this period, mainly due to criticism toward the formerly dominant yun-qi stem-branch biorhythmic system. Nonetheless, new innovations in the field continued to arise. One example is Xu Feng's Zhen Jiu Da Quan, "the first text to systematically describe the eight extraordinary vessels and the daily, 10-day and 60-day biorhythm treatment methods". Another is Gao Wu's Zhen Jiu Ju Ying, which introduced the use of supplementing and draining acupoints.

The most famous work of the era, however, is Yang Ji-zhou's Zhen Jiu Da Cheng, published in 1601. This text reported 667 of the known 670 acupoints. The Zhen Jiu Da Cheng and Li Shi-zhen's Ben Cao Gang Mu together comprise the most comprehensive volumes of Chinese medical knowledge before modern times. Particularly significant about these works is that they were not merely individual or personal theories, but a reflection of the consensus of the medical community. Thus they remain "the strongest representative[s] of classical clinical acupuncture".

The final dynasty, the Qing, lasted from 1644 to 1911. For almost three centuries, China was subject to the rule of Manchurians. The Manchu, too, had adopted the "Confucian social model," so China's "cultural continuity" was preserved. They ruled relatively peacefully, though the empire was destined to collapse due to a number of circumstances. By the 19th century, the population explosion caused a shortage of food supplies; a number of wars and rebellions finally led to the dismantling of the empire and the chaotic birth of the new Chinese Republic.

Meanwhile the increasing infiltration of Western thought brought about a severe decline in all traditional Chinese medicines. In the entire Qing dynasty, there were few new books or innovations in the field of acupuncture. By 1912, the vast majority of China had given up altogether on the traditional medicinal methods of the past. The once dominant qi paradigm was reduced to "a tangled web of details and complexities.

The few who still believed in traditional medicine turned to what is considered the Han-Xue movement. Proponents of this movement looked toward the early Han dynasty for the pure and untainted knowledge of the earlier wise men. Xu Da-chun, the most avid and articulate supporter of this movement, criticized the modern acupuncturists "for incorrect channel and point location, over-reliance on formula acupuncture, ignorance of the generic five-phase points, loss of supplementation and draining theory and technique, and ignorance of seasonal correspondences and the methods of internal medicine" .

Despite the efforts of this fleeting movement, by the 1930's acupuncturists in China were a dying breed: "there was only one acupuncturist in all of Canton".

In contrast, during the regime of 'Han' Emperors the famous acupuncturist Hua Thuo developed much this science of therapeutics. The unit for measuring bodily distance in acupuncture treatment 'cun' is also believed has been introduced during this period.

The 'Tang' dynasty (618 to 907) witnessed the establishment of the first acupuncture teaching institution of the world. In this institution there were ten demonstrator-teachers, one chief professor, one assistant professor and twenty needle makers.

In the era of 'Ming' Emperors (1368 to 1644) several literatures were written on acupuncture and hollow human bodies of bronze with pores in the specific acupuncture points for demonstration and teaching were made.

In sixth century it spread to Japan followed by Middle East and Europe.

Beginning in AD 608, when young Japanese physicians were sent to China for a long period of study, Chinese influence on Japanese medicine was paramount. In 982, Tamba Yasuyori completed the 30-volume Ishinhô, the oldest Japanese medical work still extant. This work discusses diseases and their treatment, classified mainly according to the affected organs or parts. It is based entirely on older Chinese medical works, with the yin and yang concept underlying the theory of disease causation.

In 1570 a 15-volume medical work was published by Menase Dôsan, who also wrote at least five other works. In the most significant of these, the Keitekishû (a manual of the practice of medicine, 1574), diseases—or sometimes merely symptoms—are classified and described in 51 groups; the work is unusual in that it includes a section on the diseases of old age. Another distinguished physician and teacher of the period, Nagata Tokuhun, whose important books were the I-no-ben (1585) and the Baika mujinzo (1611), held that the chief aim of the medical art was to support the natural force, and consequently that it was useless to persist with stereotyped methods of treatment unless the physician had the cooperation of the patient.

During the regime of 'Manchu' Emperors (1644 to 1911) it's practice has been banned, after the opium war (1840-1842) it declined due to official patronage to western allopathic medicine and legal ban on the practice of traditional chinese medicine, however, the ban was lifted after the salvation war in 1949 and hailed as a heritage or ancient culture in free china. When the Communist Party took over power, previous schools of thought, excepting notably Legalism, were denounced as backward, but their influence on Chinese thought remains.

**Great Philosophical Figures of China:**

*Confucius*, seen as the Great Master but sometimes ridiculed by Taoists.

*Mencius*, Confucius' follower having idealist inspiration.

*Xun Zi*, another Confucius' follower, closer to realism.

*Zhu Xi*, founder of Neo-Confucianism

*Wang Yangming*, most influential proponent of xinxue or "school of mind."

*Lao Zi*, the chief of Taoist school.

*Zhuang Zi*, said to be the author of the Zhuangzi.

*Lie Zi*, said to be the author of the True Classic of Perfect Emptiness.

*Mozi*, the founder of Mohist school.

*Han Feizi*, one of the theoricians of Legalism

*Lin-chi*, a great Buddhist Ch'an thinker and teacher, essentially shaped what would become one of the largest schools of Buddhism (Rinzai school of Zen)

**Concepts within Chinese Philosophy:**

Although the individual philosophical schools differ considerably, they nevertheless share a common vocabulary and set of concerns.

*Among the Terms Commonly Found in Chinese Philosophy are:*

*Tao* (the Way, or one's doctrine)

*De* (virtue, power)

*Li* (principle)

*Qi* (vital energy or material force)

The Tai Ji (Great Heavenly Axis) forms a unity, from which two antagonistic concepts, Yin and Yang originate. The word Yin originally referred to a hillside facing away from the sun. Philosophically, it stands the gloomy, passive, female concept, whereas Yang (the hillside facing the sun) stands for the bright, active, male concept. Both concepts, though antagonistic, are also complementary and the present domination of one implies the future rise of the other, as moon's phases (this is one of the meanings of the well-known Yin-Yang figures).

**Among the Great Controversies of Chinese Philosophies are:**

The relation between matter and principle

The method of discovering truth

The nature of human being (good or bad?)

**Among the Commonalties of Chinese Philosophies are:**

Epistemological optimism. The belief that the big questions can be answered even if the answers are not currently known.

The tendency not to view man as separate from nature.

The tendency not to invoke a unified and personified supernatural power. Questions about the nature and existence of God which have profoundly influenced Western philosophy have not been important in Chinese philosophies.

The belief that the purpose of philosophy is primarily to serve as an ethical and practical guide.

The political focus: most scholars of the Hundred Schools were trying to convince the ruler to behave in the way they defended.

Archeologists have unearthed acupuncture needles that are 3,000 B.C. and earlier.

Written records tell us that acupuncture was being practiced in China at least as early as the Culture Heroes Period that ended with Emperor Huang Di (around 2,700 B.C.). Sometime since its development, acupuncture spread beyond the boundaries of China. Lineages of multiple styles developed in China, Korea, Japan, Vietnam, other Asian countries, and the West.

The Japanese, having a talent for innovation and refinement, developed a unique acupuncture style called meridian therapy. Meridian therapy is taught in hundreds of different schools with many variations in this style. The Japanese use thinner needles, fewer needles, and insert to a shallower depth.

The Japanese also have discovered that the blind are well suited to be acupuncturists.

They use their heightened sense of touch for diagnosis and treatment. They learn to feel many subtleties: circulation,

circulation blocks, skin temperature, skin texture, pulse qualities, and how to actually feel chi.

With their palpation skills, the blind acupuncturists developed an elegant technique of touch needling: non-insertion of a silver needle that directs chi in specific ways. This technique is taught in the Toyohari schools. (Toyo=Asia, hari=acupuncture or acupuncture needle.)

In toyohari touch needling technique, first, the practitioner forms a diagnosis based on signs, symptoms and acupuncture theory, next, she palpates meridians to check the potential effect of treating a particular meridian, then, "alive" acupuncture points are located and lightly needled (typically without puncturing the skin) and finally, she checks for desirable changes in pulses and other physical signs. As with all meridian therapies, this "root" treatment is supplemented with other techniques aimed at improving symptoms, providing an overall treatment for wellness while addressing specific complaints. The supplemental technique may be moxibustion, bodywork, exercise, or other needling techniques.

The Japanese generally follow the notion that "less is more." Instead of overwhelming the nervous system with deep insertion of thicker needles, these techniques give the patient's body a gentle nudge in the right direction. The patient's natural healing ability responds to the subtler hint. Having overloaded nervous systems, our society is better suited to these gentler styles of acupuncture. With acupuncture, we do not treat or cure diseases, we treat the whole person, promoting self-healing. The Toyohari style offers an effective, less invasive approach to this end.

In 1976 scientists of Germany and Hungary introduced needleless acupuncture technique by invention of Acu-Laser Apparatus, other electronic devices which use ultrasonic ray, magnetic impulses, etc. inplace of needles are developed.

## The History of Medical Acupuncture

According to Chinese medical theory medical acupuncture is understood to work via the modern understanding of anatomy, physiology and biochemistry.

The principal differences between the traditional and medical acupuncture schools can be summarized as follows:

| Traditional | Medical |
|---|---|
| Follows procedures based on past experience | Largely ignores the traditional theories and technique |
| Based on pre-scientific observations and theory | Based on modern anatomy andphysiology |
| Described with Taoist metaphor | No element of mysticism |

These differences are theoretical, but there may are also practical differences. Whereas traditional acupuncture practitioners, at least today in the West, tend to insert large numbers of needles and leave them in place for at least 20 minutes, sometimes longer, some Western acupuncturists use many fewer needles (sometimes only one) and practise brief insertion (from two or three minutes right down to one second). This modern technique is also used by those traditionally trained, though it may be less common.

Medical acupuncture lends itself to use in a busy practice where there is little time to spend on each patient. It also has the advantage that it can be learned much more easily than traditional acupuncture by modern health practitioners such as doctors, physiotherapists, osteopaths, chiropractors, and podiatrists. Such people do not have to learn another system of thought or technique; rather, they see acupuncture as an extension of what they are already doing.

For traditionalists, medical acupuncture appears to be a watered-down version of "real" acupuncture, having at best a limited degree of effectiveness in certain situations. However, there is little good research evidence to support the use of any form of acupuncture, traditional or modern, and even less to show that one kind is better than the other. To some extent, therefore, choosing which version to use, whether as patient or practitioner, comes down to subjective choice.

If acupuncture is not to be based on the traditional ideas, how can we choose where to insert the needles? There are several possibilities. One popular idea is to use the concept of trigger points. These are tender areas, mostly in muscles, from which pain and other sensations may radiate to distant areas. Some studies have shown a considerable degree of correspondence between the locations of trigger points in the Western literature and classic acupuncture points.

Another idea is to base the needling on body segments. The spinal cord is arranged segmentally, with pairs of nerve roots emerging from it along its length. These nerve root pairs supply the skin in a series of stripes, so that it is possible to say which spinal segments supply sensation to different parts of the body. A similar arrangement exists at deeper levels, so that we may speak of myotomes (related to the muscles) and sclerotomes (related to the bones and joints). In some versions of medical acupuncture the needles are inserted in segments that are related to the internal organs that one wishes to treat.

Other ways of choosing where to needle also exist. However, some medical acupuncturists think that it often makes relatively little difference where the needles are inserted, at least in quite broad terms. Certainly there seem to be some patients who react very strongly to needling and in whom the actual site of treatment is not very important. A traditionally-trained acupuncturist, however, might consider this belief heresy, and consider this random approach dangerous.

Considering that acupuncture has more than a placebo effect, how can we explain its action? Two main kinds of scientific medical explanation have been suggested:

The gate theory of pain, first put forward some thirty years ago by Patrick Wall and Robert Melzack, postulates the existence of gates or filters in the spinal cord that can modulate (increase or decrease) transmission of pain information within the nervous system.

The second explanation is based on the existence of natural opiates (pain-relieving substances such as endorphins and enkephalins) in the central nervous system and elsewhere in the body.

Although both these mechanisms may well be involved, they are probably not the whole story. Science has yet to be able to fully understand acupuncture. There is increasing evidence today to suggest that various areas of the brain, such as parts of the limbic system (especially the anterior cingulate cortex) are important. Another idea which is currently attracting attention is the role of oxytocin, a pain-relieving hormone that also causes feelings of relaxation and tranquillity.

In contrast, while it is possible to put forward a reasonably plausible explanation for how acupuncture may work, we have to acknowledge that much of this theorizing may be wrong or based on inadequate information. One difficulty to date is that much of the experimental work has been done on short-term pain relief in animals, whereas what happens when acupuncture is used clinically in humans is different in a number of ways. For example, in clinical acupuncture the pain relief may take several hours or even days to develop, but may then continue for long periods or even permanently. There is also a build-up effect with repeated treatments. And whereas the animal experiments have mostly used strong electrical stimulation of the needles, much clinical acupuncture is brief and gentle, using minimal manual stimulation. For all these reasons it is doubtful how far the available research into acupuncture mechanisms is really applicable to clinical acupuncture in humans.

### The Relationship Between TCM and Western Medicine

The Chinese materia medica has always been extensive and consists of vegetable, animal (including human), and mineral remedies. There were famous herbals from ancient times; but all these, to the number of about 1,000, were embodied by LiShih-chen in the compilation of Pen-ts'ao kang-mu (the "Great Pharmacopoeia") in the 16th century AD. This work, in 52 volumes, has been frequently revised and reprinted and is still authoritative. The use of drugs is mainly to restore the harmony of the yin and the yang and is also related to such matters as the five organs, the five planets, and the five colours. The art of prescribing is therefore complex.

Among the drugs taken over by Western medicine from the Chinese are rhubarb, iron (for anemia), castor oil, kaolin, aconite, camphor, and Cannabis sativa (Indian hemp). Chaulmoogra oil was used by the Chinese for leprosy from at least the 14th century, and about a century ago it began to be used for this purpose by Western physicians. The herb mahuang (Ephedra vulgaris) has been used in China for at least 4,000 years, and the isolation of the alkaloid ephedrine from it has greatly improved the Western treatment of asthma and similar conditions.

The most famous and expensive of Chinese remedies is ginseng. Western analysis has shown that it has diuretic and other properties but is of doubtful value. In recent years reserpine, the active principle of the Chinese plant Rauwolfia , has been isolated; it is now effectively used in the treatment of high blood pressure and some emotional and Within China, there has been a great deal of cooperation between TCM practitioners and Western medicine, especially in the field of ethnomedicine. Chinese herbal medicine includes many compounds which are unused by Western medicine, and there is great interest in those compounds as well as the theories which TCM practitioners use to determine which compound to prescribe. For their part, advanced TCM practitioners in China are interested in statistical and experimental techniques which can better distinguish medicines that work from those that do not. One result of this collaboration has been the creation of peer reviewed scientific journals and medical databases on traditional Chinese medicine.

The relationship between TCM and Western medicine in the West is more contentious. While more and more medical schools are including classes on alternative medicine in their curricula, older Western doctors and scientists are far more likely than their Chinese counterparts to skeptically view TCM as archaic pseudoscience and superstition. This skepticism can come from a number of sources. For one, TCM in the West tends to be advocated either by Chinese immigrants or by those that have lost faith in conventional medicine. Many people in the West have a stereotype of the East as mystical and unscientific, which attracts those in the West who have lost hope in science and repels those who believe in scientific explanations. There have also been experiences in the West with unscrupulous or well-meaning but improperly-trained "TCM practitioners" who have done people more harm than good in many instances.

As an example of the different roles of TCM in China and the West, a person with a broken bone in the West (i.e. a routine, "straightforward" condition) would almost never see a Chinese medicine practitioner or visit a martial arts school to get the bone set, whereas this is routine in China. As another example, most TCM hospitals in China have electron microscopes and many TCM practitioners know how to use one.

This is not to say that TCM techniques are considered worthless in the West. In fact, Western pharmaceutical companies have recognized the value of traditional medicines and are employing teams of scientists in many parts of the world to gather knowledge from traditional healers and medical practitioners. After all, the active ingredients of most modern medicines were discovered in plants or animals. The particular contribution of Western medicine is that it strictly applies the scientific method to promising traditional treatments, separating those that work from those that do not. As another example, most Western hospitals and increasing numbers of other clinics now offer T'ai Chi Ch'uan or qigong classes as part of their inpatient and community health programs.

Most Chinese in China do not see traditional Chinese medicine and Western medicine as being in conflict. In cases of emergency and crisis situations, there is generally no reluctance in using conventional Western medicine. At the same time, belief in Chinese medicine remains strong in the area of maintaining health. To put it simply, you see a Western doctor if you have acute appendicitis, but you do exercises or take Chinese herbs to keep your body healthy enough to prevent appendicitis, or to recover more quickly from the surgery. Very few practitioners of Western medicine in China reject traditional Chinese medicine, and most doctors in China will use some elements of Chinese medicine in their own practice.

A degree of integration between Chinese and Western medicine also exists in China. For instance, at the Shanghai cancer hospital, a patient may be seen by a mutlidisciplinary team and be treated concurrently with radiation surgery, Western drugs and a traditional It is worth noting that the practice of Western medicine in China is somewhat different from that in the West. In contrast to the West, there are relatively few allied health professionals to perform routine medical procedures or to undertake procedures such as massage or physical therapy.

In addition, Chinese practitioners of Western medicine have been less impacted by trends in the West that encourage patient empowerment, to see the patient as an individual rather than a collection of parts, and to do nothing when medically appropriate. Chinese practitioners of Western medicine have been widely criticized for overprescribing drugs such as corticosteroids or antibiotics for common viral infections. It is likely that these medicines, which are generally known to be useless against viral infections, would provide less relief to the patient than traditional Chinese herbal remedies.

It is almost certain that acupuncture has been known and used in the West since the seventeenth century, but the first recorded use of acupuncture was by Dr. Berlioz at the Paris medical School in 1810. He treated a young woman suffering from abdominal pain. The Paris Medical Society described this as a somewhat reckless form of treatment, but Dr. Berlioz continued to use acupuncture, and claimed a great deal of success with it.

Acupuncture is not new to England, the first known British acupuncturist being John Churchill who, in 1821, published a series of results on the treatment of tympany and rheumatism with acupuncture. John Elliotson, a physician at St Thomas' Hospital, also use acupuncture widely in the early part of the nineteenth century. In 1823 acupuncture was mentioned in the first edition of the Lancet and in 1824 Dr. Elliotson began to use this method of treatment. In 1827 he published a series of results on the treatment of forty-two cases of rheumatism by acupuncture, and came to the conclusion that this was an acceptable and effective method of treatment for these complaints.

In the context of Western medicine, the development of acupuncture points on the body demonstrates an interesting story of re-discovery. Over the last fifty years many Western physicians have discovered independently that pressing, stimulating or injecting various superficial body points can help to relieve pain. This is particularly true of muscular or rheumatic-like pains. These points are not necessarily at the site of pain, but often over distant areas. For instance, neck pain is frequently referred to the shoulder or arm and can present to the doctor as shoulder or arm pain. On close examination of the patient it is quite easy to define the origin of the pain, and to show that the neck is the cause of the problem. Injection, or stimulation of the painful points around the shoulder or arm, will often relieve the pain and free the movement of the neck.

These points have a variety of names, such as trigger points (for pain), or motor points. In 1977 Dr. Melzack, who has been awarded the Nobel prize for his work in the field of pain, correlated these trigger points with acupuncture points, and found that most of the trigger points were already well known as acupuncture points. There are a number of explanations for the existence of trigger points but, as yet, there is no clear answer to this phenomenon. It is interesting to note that the Chinese realized this fact at least some three thousand years ago, and the Ling Shu summarises this approach when it says 'In pain, puncture the tender points".

Acupuncture is now quite widely used in Europe and North America, both as a method of therapy and, in a few centers, as a method of anesthesia. Operations with acupuncture as the main anesthetic have been carried out in France and Austria, and the results have been comparable with those of the Chinese. Since its intimate contact with the Chinese in the 1950's, the USSR has also been using and researching into acupuncture, although the relationship between Russia and China could not be described as good. In 1972 a Russian researcher published work suggesting that acupuncture points were points of low electrical resistance on the body. He also found a network of low resistance points in both animals and plants. The use of acupuncture in the USSR steadily increased during the 1970's and in 1972 acupuncture clinics were planned for all the major medical centers in the Soviet Union. The Russians claim they are using acupuncture for a wide variety of conditions such as asthma, stomach ulcers, raised blood pressure and angina, as well as for pain. In the West, acupuncture has been used mainly for pain relief. This is primarily because acupuncture for pain is easy to learn, and does not require a knowledge of traditional Chinese concepts in order to obtain results. The concepts of traditional Chinese medicine can seem alien and unacceptable to Western doctors and they are therefore rejected in favor of a simpler and probably less efficient method of treatment, in spite of the value of many of the traditional concepts. Some doctors practicing acupuncture in the West are simply puncturing tender points as this seems a rational and logical approach.

Acupuncture has become very popular in North America since President Nixon reopened relationships with the Chinese. There are many research clinics evaluating the effectiveness of acupuncture, and also investigating the basic physiological mechanisms involved. The research output from North America is prolific and some excellent work has been done much of which re-emphasizes that acupuncture is an effective form of therapy for many conditions, especially pain, although it is not a guaranteed cure. Over the last twenty years the West has developed a great deal of technological hardware which is now being applied in the field of acupuncture. The chapter on modern acupuncture techniques describes briefly the use of a variety of electrical machines and sources of stimulation, such as lasers and electroacupuncture. Many of these techniques are still in their infancy and some will be rejected whilst others may prove to be important.

China is a poor nation without enough resources and trained manpower to research and develop acupuncture adequately. Until fairly recently few useful statistics were available from the acupuncture clinics in China, and most of the research into the basic mechanism of acupuncture had come from Western research institutes. Within this context it is probable that many of the major advances in acupuncture will come from the West rather than from the East.

The World Health Organization (WHO) in their 'Inter Regional Seminar on Acupuncture, Moxibustion and Acupressure' held in Peiking in june 1979 published a list of 40 conditions that may benefit from acupuncture. These conditions include the following: Abdominal pain, Constipation, Diarrhoea, Hyperacidity, Indigestion, Cataracts, Gingivitis, Poor vision, Tinnitis, Toothache ,Arthritis, Back pain, Muscle cramping, Muscle pain and weakness, Neck pain, Sciatica ,Asthma, Bronchitis, Common cold, Sinusitis, Smoking cessation, Tonsillitis ,Anxiety, Depression, Insomnia, Nervousness, Neurosis, Infertility,Menopausal symptoms, Premenstrual symptoms ,Headaches, Migraines, Neurogenic bladder dysfunction, Parkinson's disease, Postoperative pain, Stroke , Addiction control, Athletic performance, Blood pressure regulation.

It is almost certain that acupuncture has been known and used in the West since the seventeenth century, but the first recorded use of acupuncture was by Dr. Berlioz at the Paris medical School in 1810. He treated a young woman suffering from abdominal pain. The Paris Medical Society described this as a somewhat reckless form of treatment, but Dr. Berlioz continued to use acupuncture, and claimed a great deal of success with it.

Acupuncture is not new to England, the first known British acupuncturist being John Churchill who, in 1821, published a series of results on the treatment of tympany and rheumatism with acupuncture. John Elliotson, a physician at St Thomas' Hospital, also use acupuncture widely in the early part of the nineteenth century. In 1823 acupuncture was mentioned in the first edition of the Lancet and in 1824 Dr. Elliotson began to use this method of treatment. In 1827 he published a series of results on the treatment of forty-two cases of rheumatism by acupuncture, and came to the conclusion that this was an acceptable and effective method of treatment for these complaints.

In the West, Traditional Chinese Medicine (TCM) is often considered alternative medicine, however in mainland China and Taiwan, TCM is widely considered to be an integral part of the health care system. The term TCM is sometimes used specifically within the field of Chinese medicine to refer to the standardized set of theories and practices introduced in the mid-20th century under the government of Mao, as distinguished from related traditional theories and practices preserved by people in Taiwan, Hong Kong and by the overseas Chinese. The more general sense is meant in this article.

TCM developed as a form of noninvasive therapeutic intervention (also described as folk medicine) or traditional medicine, rooted in ancient belief systems, including traditional religious concepts. Chinese medical practitioners before the 19th century relied essentially on observation, trial and error. Like their counterparts in the West, they had a very different understanding of infection which predated the discovery of bacteria, viruses (germ theory of disease) or cellular structures and little knowledge of organic chemistry, relying mainly on distinctly personal medical theory describing the nature of infections and remedies. Traditions associated with three millennia of practical experience guided their courses of treatment and instruction in diagnostic principles.

Unlike other forms of traditional medicine which have largely become extinct, traditional Chinese medicine continues as a distinct branch of modern medical practice, and within China, it is an important part of the public health care system. There are thousands of years of empirical knowledge about TCM on its own terms, and in recent decades there has been an effort to place traditional Chinese medicine on a firmer Western scientific empirical and methodological basis as well as efforts to integrate Chinese and Western medical traditions.

That this effort has occurred is surprising to many for a number of reasons. In most of the world, indigenous medical practices have been supplanted by practices brought from the West, while in Chinese societies, this has not occurred and shows no sign of occurring. Furthermore, many have found it peculiar that Chinese medicine remains a distinct branch of medicine separate from Western medicine.

Zang– Fu Theory: As Traditional Chinese Medicine (TCM) is holistic, each organ cannot be explained fully unless the TCM relationship/homeostasis with the other organs is understood. TCM also looks at the functions of the organs rather than fixed areas and, therefore, describes different organs that are not actually physical, like the Triple Burner (San Jiao). This also leads to controversy about the validity of TCM, which comes a lot from the difficulty of translating and lack knowledge about TCM concepts and Chinese culture. So, to avoid conflict and to keep an open mind, please realize that these notions evolved in a different culture and are a different way of viewing the human body.

Zang-Fu theory translates roughly into "theory about solid organ-hollow organ". It is a concept within traditional Chinese medicine and part of the TCM model of the body. There are five zang (pinyin zang1) and six fu (pinyin fu3).

The association between the zangfu and particular souls or spirits is a later accretion and has been largely absent from the discourse of traditional Chinese medicine for at least the past 200 years.

This theory treats each of the Zang organs as organs that nourish the body. The Zang systems include organs, senses, emotions, and the musculoskeletal system—essentially, the entire person divided into five categorical systems. Zang organs are also known as yin organs, and each has a Fu partner, a yang organ (see Yin Yang). Fu organs can be viewed as hollow organs that aid in digestion. In addition to bodily functions, each Zang organ is the home of an aspect of the spirit.

With a thorough understanding of the Zang Fu organs, practitioners can achieve therapeutic results accordingly. The theory is always in service of practical, therapeutic application, with the goal of an "elegant" treatment. An elegant treatment uses the least amount of force for the greatest therapeutic benefit, and requires true mastery of the art of traditional Chinese Medicine.

The five elements are associated energetically with the following Zang-Fu organs:

Wood: Liver, home of the Hun (Ethereal Soul), paired with the Gall Bladder

Fire: Heart, home of the Shen (Aggregate Soul) paired with the Small intestine (and secondarily, the San Jiao or Triple burner and Pericardium)

Earth: Spleen, home of the Yi (Intellect), paired with the Stomach

Water: Kidney, home of the Zhi (Will), paired with the Bladder

Metal: Lung, home of the Po (Corporeal Soul), paired with the Large Intestine

## The Concept of Meridians

The concept of meridians (Chinese: "jing-luo") arises from the techniques and doctrines of traditional Chinese medicine including acupuncture and acupressure. According to these practices, the body's vital energy, "qi", circulates through the body along specific interconnected channels called meridians. Disruptions of the body's energy flow are thought to cause emotional and physical illness. To release those disruptions, specific points on the meridians called tsubo are stimulated via needles, pressure or other means.

The aligned water theory of meridians conjectures that meridians are made up of clusters of "aligned water" in the body that allow ions, light, and sound waves to flow more readily. Aligned water clusters are said to occur where large numbers of water molecules align electrically to form a stable cluster. These have supposedly been photographed outside the body with an electron microscope by Shui-Yin Lo, who calls them IE crystals. These aligned water molecules are said to flow between the cells, forming a chain that completes a circuit around the body. When these water molecules "fall out of alignment" this supposedly has a negative impact on health.

The chinese meridians have their counterpart in the mayan acupuncture techniques practiced in the Yucatan. The analogous concept is that of wind channels. Curiously, most of the key points in Mayan acupuncture correspond exactly with key acupuncture points in the chinese meridian model. Aside from speculation and *ad hoc* hypothesising, there is little objective scientific evidence to suggest that meridians or "aligned water" exist, and indeed their existence is not compatible with a conventional understanding of physics, anatomy and physiology. Some experts consider these conjectures to be pseudoscience.

In 1950 Yoshio Nakatani demonstrated that in specific organ disease a number of acupuncture points along that organ's acupuncture meridian had a markedly decreased electrical resistance compared with the surrounding skin. (e.g. in Kidney disease several of the kidney points had a lowered skin resistance). He found the resistance values for these points varied with the time of the day, ambient temperature Acupuncture, activity and emotional state of the subject.

In the late 1970's Dr. Robert Becker and associates similarly identified lowered resistance values for over 50% of acupoints along the Large Intestine meridian. Becker suggested that the acupoints acted as amplifiers of a semi conducting Direct Current traveling along the perineural cells which wrap around each and every nerve in the body. This D C system became more negative as it traveled to the ends of fingers and toes and more positive as it returned to the trunk and head (i.e. a Yin - Yang flow).

It was known that the skin acted as a battery (outside of skin is negative and inside was positive) and Becker found the acupuncture point was more positive than the surrounding skin. The insertion of a needle would short circuit this battery and generate a current of injury lasting for several days. Further electrical activity occurred because of:

1. Ionic reactivity between the metal needle and body fluids

2. Low frequency pulses of electricity from twirling the needle.

This generated electrical energy would flow along this DC system to the brain and would be analogous to the Qi described by classical acupuncture.

In 1978 Luciani produced Kirlean photographs of the LED (light emission diode) effect of acupoints along the small intestine meridian and the large intestine meridian.

The existence of the meridian system was further established by French researcher Pierre de Vernejoul, who injected radioactive isotopes into the acupoints of humans and tracked their movement with a special gamma imaging camera. The isotopes traveled thirty centimeters along acupuncture meridians within four to six minutes. Vernejoul then challenged his work by injecting isotopes into the blood vessels at random areas of the body rather than into acupoints. The isotopes did not travel in the same manner at all, further indicating that the meridians do indeed comprise a system of separate pathways within the body.

Although reports of acupuncture have been recorded in the west since the 1800's, it wasn't until the 1970's that this method of therapy became well publicized. A reporter for the "New York Times" became ill with appendicitis while traveling in China and had an appendectomy without anesthesia, but with the use of acupuncture. This was widely reported in the western press. Doctors tried to explain the technique by saying it was the "placebo affect". This is the phenomenon in which 30% of people will be shown to be able to self heal in experiments when given a sugar pill instead of the "real medicine". However, this was shown to be a false belief because animals (who couldn't possibly respond to suggestion) also responded to the analgesic properties of acupuncture.

In the 1960s, western scientists developed a special tissue-staining technique that allowed him to identify these meridians in rabbits. Western scientist ignored this research until the 1980s when two French researchers, Drs. Claude Darras and Pierre De Vernejoul repeated Dr. Hans experiment using radioactive tracers on human beings.

They injected and then twirled radioactive technetium into the acupoints of patients and used nuclear scanning equipment to follow the flow of technetium. They also injected non-acupoints. At non-acupoints, the radioactive tracer diffused outward from the injection site into circular patterns. When the true acupoints were injected, the radioactive technetium followed the exact pathways as the acupuncture meridians in the ancient charts of the human body! They also found that when acupuncture needles were inserted into distant acupoints along the same tracer-labeled meridians and the twirled, a change was produced in the rate of flow of the technetium through the meridians. This research supported the ancient Chinese claim that the acupuncture needle stimulation affected the flow of ch'i through the body's meridians.

In 1951 Dr. Yoshio Nakatani presented his theory of Ryodoraku Acupuncture. Dr. Nakatani had found that there were a series of low electrical resistance points (or high electrical conductivity) running longitudinally up and down the body. When linked together these points closely matched the acupuncture meridians. Dr. Nakatani called these lines (or meridians) "Ryodoraku" (ryo = good, 'do is (electro) conductive, 'raku = line).

The points along the Ryodoraku he named Ryodoten.

Dr. Nakatani was the first person to measure the electrical activity of acupuncture points and the first to formulate diagnostic and treatment criteria from these measurements. Nakatani was the first recorded acupuncturist to use electrical stimulation of acupuncture points. Point location and electrical stimulation has become the norm for most acupuncturists world wide but the Ryodoraku detection, analysis and point selection for electrical stimulation is much less popular. This is unfortunate as Nakatani's concepts provide an accurate pulse-organ diagnosis, accurate location of required treatment points and a very time efficient treatment regimen (generally only 7 seconds stimulation of each point is required. A classic acupuncture treatment lasting an average of 30 minutes would only take 2 - 3 minutes using Ryodoraku!).

The indications for Ryodoraku are identical to those for acupuncture, but the results are often faster. In particular acute pain and acute traumatic swelling e.g. sports injury will often respond during the initial treatment.

A Ryodoraku unit called a "Neurometer" uses a constant voltage of 12V (occasionally 21V will be used in ear acupuncture) and a variable current (this current is set to 200uA for treatment) . To provide consistency and avoid artefacts because of dryness/ wetness of skin a moist electrode is used to locate the points of lowered electrical resistance i.e. Ryodoten or Electro permeable Points (EPP).

The moist electrode consists of a small cup containing a plug of cotton wool soaked in saline (sometimes alcohol is used). This is run lightly over the skin until a high reading is seen on the meter i.e. this area of low resistance, high conductivity allows current to flow. An increase of 20-50 uA is expected. As in other forms of electro acupuncture practice is required to achieve consistent results. Too much pressure or repeated checking of a point can change the electrical properties of the skin in that area and lead to error. Computerised measuring Ryodoraku units are available in Japan. These give a steady 3g electrode pressure to the skin.

This EPP can then be located exactly by using the fine probe in the two or three headed point locater on the Ryodoraku unit.

Nakatani discovered that the number of electro permeable points not only varied with any disease process but also with the voltage of the detector probe. Most of the traditional acupoints could be located if a 21 volt circuit was used. However if a 12 volt circuit was used, there were other electrically conductive points over the body, not associated with any specific acupuncture points. He called these Responsive Ryodo-points or Reactive Electropermeable points (REPPs). These points often correspond with trigger points or Ah Shi (tender to touch) points. Nakatani theorised that they occurred along tracts of the Autonomic Nervous system and were representative of internal disorder/ dysfunction and/or disease.

Nakatani showed that needling these REPP, and stimulating them for 7-10 sec with a 200uA charge would render them electrically inert and produce symptom relief. Headaches, neck aches, back aches and acute pains would often be relieved - sometimes in minutes, sometimes over several days. This is a very effective form of local or regional acupuncture but Nakatani developed it further.

Using his knowledge of the Ryodoraku pathways Nakatani formalised Ryodoraku acupuncture. He used the same concepts of the twelve paired acupuncture meridians or organ systems (Heart, lungs, triple warmer,pericardium, large intestine, small intestine on the upper limbs and gall bladder, stomach, liver,kidney, bladder and spleen on the lower limb ) and the two single midline meridians (anteriorly, Conception Vessel and posteriorly, Governing Vessel). However he did not use the classical names. He assigned the letters "H" to each of the six Ryodoraku on the upper limbs numbering them from one to six.

Similarly he assigned the letter "F" to each of the six Ryodoraku on the lower limbs, numbering them from one to six. Thus H3 represented the Heart meridian on the upper limb; F6 represented the stomach meridian on the lower limb.

To further confuse the issue (at least as far as traditional acupuncturists were concerned) Nakatani did not use either the Chinese name nor the more commonly accepted, international numbering of acupuncture points. [He numbered his Ryodo points starting at the end of each limb]. Acupuncture uses the Yin-Yang energy flow concepts to number its acupuncture points. Thus energy flows outwards towards the end of a limb along one meridian and back to the trunk along another meridian i.e. the meridians are paired off. In the paired meridians Lung and Large Intestine energy starts on the trunk in the Lung meridian so L1 (the first Lung meridian acupuncture point) is on the anterior chest. The first point for the Large Intestine meridian (LI. 1) is on the index finger. In Nakatani's Ryodoraku system both H11 (the first Ryodo point on the large intestine Ryodoraku) and H51 (the first Ryodo point on the lung Ryodoraku) are on the finger tips.

Nakatani believed this was a much simpler way of representing and teaching acupuncture. No knowledge of the complex acupuncture nomenclature, philosophy and mnemonics was required. In fact a therapist theoretically did not even have to memorise the exact position of the acupuncture points. He/She could use the Ryodoraku Neurometer to locate the points.

In a further departure from traditional acupuncture Nakatani compared readings from Ryodoraku on the right side of the body with those of the same Ryodoraku on the left side of the body. If one side showed higher (or lower) reactivity than the other, he would use a specific needling procedure to bring the EPP readings to the same level. When the right and left paired Ryodoraku [eg. right and left H1 (Lung) Ryodoraku] had the same electrical reactivity, the body was balanced for that organ system.

Initially, Nakatani measured the electrical resistance of each and every EPP along a meridian, added them together and divided by the total number of EPP. This gave him an average energy value for that meridian. This was obviously very time consuming and, eventually, Nakatani discovered that there was a point on each meridian that was representative of the energy in that meridian. He named this point a Representative Measuring Point (RMP). Thus there are 24 RMP - six on each wrist and six on each foot.

These twenty four points were measured and charted on a special chart, the left side being compared with the right side for the paired meridians.

The Traditional Chinese Medicine (TCM) analysis for the the meridian system is based on pulse diagnosis. This involves taking pulse readings, twice on each wrist; the first three lightly, and the next three deeply (for a total of 12 readings). Each pulse reading must be analyzed for 28 separate pulse characteristics! The Asian masters of acupuncture and pulse diagnosis, who palpate the 12 pulse positions, take as long as 15-20 minutes per wrist. Thus, they can only treat 6 to 8 patients a day by the "traditional method".

All this changed in the early 1950s, with the development of Ryodoraku by Dr. Yoshio Nakatani of Japan. Nakatani developed his procedure of electronic evaluation by measuring skin conductance at the yuan (source) points of the wrist and ankle. He created one of the most significant acupuncture diagnostic methods yet created in either contemporary or traditional acupuncture. When one compares the findings of Asian masters of pulse diagnosis with the findings of ryodoraku, they are most often identical or extremely close.

With ryodoraku, you take 12 measurements on each side of the body. Then, one plots the "readings" on a graph, as below:

To make a graph, one would take and plot all 24 measurements, which will range from zero to 200. Then, you divide that sum by 24, to get the "average", or "median" reading. The accepted "standard deviation" is 15. In this graph, the average is 75, with a range from 60-90. Notice how many of the meridians are out of balance in this individual! Readings outside the "range" are out of balance. If a meridian is too full of energy, it needs to be sedated. If it is deficient in energy, it needs to be tonified.

The greatest achievement of ryodoraku over pulse diagnosis was realizing that there could be a third balance issue. Traditionally, meridians are evaluated by comparing them with each other. The diagnosis was that a particular meridian had "too much" or "not enough" Qi energy, as compared to the other meridians. BUT, there are 12 meridian pathways on each side of the body! With ryodoraku, it became apparent that a particular meridian could be out of balance with itself, that is, from one side of the body to the other! The early rydoraku procedure was time consuming, but very accurate.

In 1976 scientists from Germany and Hungary introduced needleless acupuncture technique by invention of acu-laser apparatus, other electronic devices which use ultrasonic rays, magnetic impulses, etc. are also developed.

## *Chapter Three*

# Philosophy of Acupuncture

According to classical chinese acupuncture, a force or energy is active in the universe, our bodies are smaller versions of the universe and during lifetime a similar force or energy acts in our bodies, which is often called the vital energy or life energy, in chinese it is called 'qi', Theories of traditional Chinese medicine assert that the body has natural patterns of qi associated with it that circulate in channels called meridians in English. Symptoms of various illnesses are often seen as the product of disrupted or unbalanced qi movement through such channels (including blockages), or imbalances of qi in the various Zang Fu organs. Traditional Chinese Medicine seeks to relieve these imbalances by adjusting the flow of qi in the body using a variety of therapeutic techniques. Some of these techniques include herbal medicines, special diets, physical training regimens (qigong), massages to clear blockages, and acupuncture, which uses fine metal needles inserted into the skin to reroute or balance qi. Traditional Asian martial arts also discuss qi. For instance, internal systems attempt to cultivate and direct qi during combat as well as to ensure proper health. Many other martial arts include some concept of qi in their philosophies.

The nature of qi is highly controversial, and the old controversy among Chinese philosophy as to the nature of qi still exists. Among some TCM practitioners, qi is merely a metaphor for biological processes similar to the Western concept of the soul, and there is no need to invoke new biology, much less new physics, to account for its effects. Others argue that qi involves some new physics or biology. Attempts to directly connect qi with some scientific phenonomena have been attempted since the mid-nineteenth century. The philosopher Kang Youwei believed that qi was synonymous with the later abandoned concept of lumeniferous ether. In the early 21st century, attempts have been made to link the concept of qi to biophotons or inner biological energy flow. As of yet, science considers these claims of qi as an independent force to be unconvincing. Claims that control of qi allows one to transcend normal physical and biological processes are widely regarded as pseudoscience by the scientific establishment.

Views of qi as an esoteric force tend to be more prominent in the West, where it has sometimes been associated with New Age spritualism. These views are less prominent in China, where traditional Chinese medicine is often practiced and considered effective, but in which esoteric notions of qi are considered to contradict Marxist notions of dialectic materialism. Many traditional martial arts schools also eschew a supernatural approach to the issue, identifying "external qi" or "internal qi" as representative of the varying leverage principles used to improve the efficacy of a well trained, healthier than normal body with a given work load.

The ancient chinese acupuncturists believed that an ailment is the expression of excessive (shi) or inadequate ( xu) work of the corresponding part or organ of the body. Chronic diseases often referred to have link with xu and acute diseases with shi. In diseases related to shi, Xie (reducing or sedation of energy) and alternately, in diseases related to xu, Bu (reinforcing or tonification of energy) is required.

In ancient times gold and silver needles were used respectively for Bu and Xie.

The classical procedure of needling according to this law in comparison is as under:

| **Bu** | **Xie** |
|---|---|
| Insert during inspiration | Insert during expiration |
| Along the direction of the energy flow | Against the direction of the energy flow |

| | |
|---|---|
| Rotate needle anti-clockwise | Rotate needle clockwise |
| Rotate with little force | Rotate forcefully |
| Retain needle for long period | Retain needle for short period |
| Remove needle slowly | Remove needle rapidly |
| Close the hole (to retain vital energy) | Leave the hole open (to let free vital energy) |
| Massage after needling | No massage |

Most complementary and alternative medicine (CAM) researchers not only assume the existence of vital energy but believe that the purported subtle energy running through and surrounding the body can be manipulated so as to cultivate increased physical, psychological and spiritual health. Acupuncture along with other practices of traditional Chinese medicine (TCM), homeopathy, ayurveda and many other traditional disciplines worldwide provide examples of similar beliefs. Properly funded, conducted and repeated empirical research is necessary to determine if the success rate of these CAM approaches is due to the existence of subtle energy, the placebo effect, or various other factors.

Skeptically minded followers of the scientific method have to assume the possibility that the results claimed by martial arts students and patients of traditional Chinese medicine practitioners can be explained without invoking esoteric or supernatural processes. In answer, most proponents of the effects of the cultivation of qi maintain that since modern scientific technologies have to this point been unable to create life out of organic chemicals in their laboratories, and that as qi is a metaphor for the energy of life itself, it is to be thereby demonstrated that the mechanisms of how the subject of such a metaphor would work so far elude the abilities of the scientific community to describe. Opponents argue that qi is merely a form of vitalism, a theory that was largely abandoned in the early 19th century.

The concept of qi appears often in Chinese fiction, in which a stock character is that of the kung fu master who has gained control of qi, to the point that he can alter the forces of nature.

There are qigong masters who claim to be able to manipulate their students from a distance with qi.

In contrast to the strictly scientific Western approach, individuals harnessing their qi would explain the qi cultivation process as a combination of repetitive movements, concentration and breathing. For example, in swinging an axe muscle control is initially all-important, but once the basic movement is learned the mind will naturally start to concentrate on the back foot, moving swiftly up through the body and down the arm to the axe rather than simply trying to get the body to perform the movement. Qi will go wherever the mind concentrates, and so the axe will start to swing effortlessly.

Qì is the pinyin romanisation of what is sometimes transliterated, using the older Wade-Giles romanisation, as ch'i (and frequently mis-spelled as chi). The Japanese form is ki while the Korean form is gi.

Sometimes qi is compared with electricity, as like electricity it is not visible but the physical presence and activity of 'qi' can be felt easily. In the flow of electrical energy there are two poles negative and positive, similarly, in the flow of vital energy there are two poles 'yin' and 'yang'. Yin is negative and feminine by nature and yang is positive and masculine by nature, for the maintenance and proper functioning of the body, balance between the energy levels of yin and yang is necessary. If due to some reasons any imbalance is caused in the energy levels of yin and yang that is reflected in the body by means of ailments, balance can be restored by insertion of needles to the specific acupuncture points of the internal organs or body parts concerned. By which line the specific points related to an internal organ or body part is linked is called a 'Channel' or 'Meridian' of that internal organ or the body part concerned. The vital energy or 'qi' flows through these channels. There are six regular superficial channels each for yin and yang in the body besides two additional channels and six extra channels. These regular channels together with additional channels form the basic fourteen channels. The vital energy flows from downwards to upwards in the yin channels and vice-versa in the yang channels.

**Yin Channels:**

Lung Channel

Spleen Channel

Heart Channel

Kidney Channel

Pericardium Channel

Liver Channel

There are eleven points in lung channel, twenty one points in spleen channel, nine points in heart channel, twenty seven points in kidney channel, nine points in pericardium channel and fourteen points in liver channel.

**Yang Channels:**

Large Intestine Channel

Stomach Channel

Small Intestine Channel

Urinary Bladder Channel

San Jiao Channel

Gall Bladder Channel

There are twenty points in large Intestine channel, fourty five points in Stomach channel, nineteen points in Small Intestine channel, sixty seven points in Urinary Bladder channel, twenty three points in San Jiao channel ( imaginary channel linked with the cavities in between Pericardium and Umbilical channel) and fourty four points in Gall Bladder channel.

**Additional Channels:**

Du Channel (Governing)

Ren Channel (Conception)

There are twenty eight points in Du channel and twenty four points in Ren channel.

**Extra Channels:**

Chong Channel (Vital Channel)

Dai Channel (Gridle Channel)

Yang Qiao Channel (Motility Channel of Yang)

Yin Qiao Channel (Motility Channel of Yin)

Yang Wei Channel (Regulating Channel of Yang)

Yin Wei Channel (Regulating Channel of Yin)

There are eleven points in Chong channel, three points in Dai channel, twelve points in Yang Qiao channel, three points in Yin Qiao channel, sixteen points in Yang Wei channel and seven points in Yin Wei channel.

**Extra Ordinary Points:**

These are the points introduced in the process of redefining during the centuries, while most fall outside the fourteen channels, some are located on the course of a regular channel, and few coincide with regular channel points.

Commonly used Extra Ordinary Points are:

Head – Ex 1 to 10

Trunk – Ex 17, 20, 21

Upper Limb – Ex 28, 30

Lower Limb – Ex 31, 32, 33, 35, 36

**Ah-Shi points:**

These points are used for treatment of pain in the localised or concerned area of these points. These points are first brought in to practice by Chinese physician Sunjho Miao (618-907) of Tang dynasty. Ah-Shi means 'Oh Yes' in chinese. Ah-Shi is the reaction of the patients when these points are touched and tenderness is felt.

**The Eight Influential Points:**

The Influential Points are eight important points where qi of the respective body tissues is infused into the body surface, namely zang, fu, qi, blood, tendons, vessels, bones and marrow. "Hui" means influential in particular. The earliest record of the Eight Influential Points is found in the book "*Nanjing: Question Forty-five.*"

The Eight Influential Points regulate the function of the zangfu organs, promote the circulation of qi and blood, release tendons and nourish marrow.

Zhangmen (Liv.13), the Influential Point of zang organs;

Zhongwan (Ren 12), the Influential Point of the fu organs;

Shanzhong (Ren 17), the Influential Point of qi;

Geshu (U.B.17), the Influential Point of blood;

Yanglingquan (G.B.34), the Influential Point of tendons;

Taiyuan (Lu.9), the Influential Point of the vessels;

Dashu (U.B.11), the Influential Point of the bones; and

Xuanzhong (G.B.39), the Influential Point of the marrow.

Respective Influential Points can be selected for treating disorders associated with the above eight parts of the body. Explanation of the actions of the Eight Influential Points are as follows:

Zhangmen (Liv.13) is the Influential Point of zang organs and is also the Front-mu point of the spleen. The functional activities of the five zang organs originate from spleen qi. This point can be used in the treatment of disorders of zang organs, such as spleenomegaly, hepatomegaly, hypochondriac pain or jaundice.

Zhongwan (Ren 12) is the Influential Point of the fu organs and is also the Front-mu point of the stomach. The functional activities of the six fu organs originate from stomach qi. This point can be used for treating disorders of the six fu organs such as epigastric distention, abdominal pain, constipation or diarrhea, as well as some other gastrointestinal disorders.

Shanzhong (Ren 17) is the Influential Point of qi, being located in the centre of the chest where Zong qi js formed (Zong qi is the qi of the thorax, formed from respiratory qi and food essence). Internally, this point is in close proximity to the lung, the organ which dominates qi. This point, also called Upper-Qihai, can be used for treating disorders of qi derangement such as chest pain, shortness of breath, asthma and hiccup.

Geshu (U.B.17) is the Influential Point of blood, being located between Xinshu (heart point) and Ganshu (liver point). The liver stores blood while the heart dominates blood. This point is situated between the two organs and has the function to promote the manufacture of blood. It is used for treating disorders of blood such as anemia, stasis of blood, bloody vomiting, bloody stool or cough with bloody sputum.

Yanglingquan (G.B. 34) is the Influential Point of the tendons and is also the He-sea point of the Gall Bladder Meridian of Foot-Shaoyang. The gall bladder and the liver are internally-externally related organs. The liver dominates the tendons. Besides, Yanglingquan (G.B.34) is below the knee joint, the convergent place of the tendons. It is used for treating disorders such as spasm and painful tendons, hemiplegia or numbness.

Taiyuan (Lu.9) is the Influential Point of vessels. Taiyuan (Lu.9), also the Yuan (source) point of the Lung Meridian of Hand-Taiyin, is located at cunkou (at the wrist where the pulse is palpated). The lung is associated with the pulses and cunkou is the major converging place of the qi of the vessels. This point can be used for treating disorder of the vessels, such as vasculitis, acrotism and arteriosclerosis.

Dashu (U.B.11), lateral to the spinal column, is the Influential Point of bones. Bone arises from marrow while marrow flows down to Dashu (U.B.11) from the brain, and further to the bones and joints. This point, the convergent place of qi of the bones, is located superior to all of the Back-shu points. It can be used for treating disorders of the bones such as pain in the shoulder, scapula or back.

Xuanzhong (G.B.39) is the Influential Point of marrow. It was considered in ancient times that marrow was a part of the bones. Marrow is thought of as helping the growth of bones. Thus, it is an essential factor in the ability to walk normally. It is used in the treatment of disorders of the marrow, such as myo-asthenia and anemia.

Clinically, the Influential Points can be used as main points, secondary poinrs being prescribed according to the varying symptoms and signs. For example, Taiyuan (Lu.9), as the main point, could be used in combination with Neiguan (P.6) and Shanzhong (Ren 17) for treating acrotism. Geshu (U.B.17), as the main point, could be used in combina tion with Xuehai (Sp.10) and Qihai (Ren 6) for treating chronic hemorrhage. Palpation of the Influential Points can also be a useful aid to diagnosis, tenderness at a given point indicating a disorder of the related tissue.

## The Twelve Primary Channels:

In this chapter we will briefly review the twelve primary Qi channels along with the eight extraordinary meridians. You should also know the organ's Yin and Yang. In our body, there are six Yang organs and six Yin organs. Each Yang organ is associated with a Yin organ by a special Yin/Yang relationship.

Paired Yin and Yang organs belong to the same phase in the Five Phases. Their channels are sequential to each other in the circulation of Qi, their functions are closely related, and disease in one usually affects the other. In Chinese medicine, the channel corresponding to the Yang organ is often used to treat disorders of its related Yin organ.

In the limbs, the Yang channels are on the external side of the limbs while the Yin channels are on the internal side. Generally speaking, the outsides of the limbs are more Yang and are more resistant and prepared for an attack, while the internal sides are more Yin and weaker.

The organs are further subdivided in order to distinguish the different levels of the Yin/Yang characteristics. The Yang organs are divided into Greater Yang (Taiyang), Lesser Yang (Shaoyang), and Yang Brightness (Yangming). The Yin organs are divided into Greater Yin (Taiyin), Lesser Yin (Shaoyin), and Absolute Yin (Jueyin). In the following discussion, all of the classifications will be shown in the title, for example: the Lung Channel of Hand Greater Yin.

## The Lung Channel of Hand — Greater Yin

The lungs (Yin) and the large intestine (Yang) are considered paired organs. They belong to Metal in the Five Phases, the westerly direction, the season of autumn, the dry climatic condition, the color white, the pungent taste, the rank odor, the emotion of sadness, and the sound of weeping. Their opening is the nose, and they govern skin and hair.

In Qigong practice, since the lungs belong to Metal, they are able to regulate heartburn. The heart belongs to Fire. Whenever the heart has excess Qi, deep breathing is able to lead the heart's fire to the lungs, and therefore cool the heartburn. When the weather is changing from damp, hot summer into dry and cool autumn, lungs are the first organ to sense the change. If your lungs are not able to readjust themselves to fit the new situation smoothly, you will catch a cold. The lungs access the outside world through your nose. The lungs are responsible for taking Qi from the air, and for the energy (Qi) state of the body.

Breathing is considered a strategy for leading Qi to the extremities such as skin and hair. When your breathing is regulated properly, you are able to strengthen your body's Guardian Qi and generate an expansive Qi shield to protect your body. You are also able to raise or lower your Qi state through your breathing. For example, when you are angry, deep breathing is able to calm your excited Qi state.

The lungs are sensitive to emotional changes, especially when you are sad or angry. They also control that part of the liquid metabolism which distributes liquid to the skin.

Because the lungs are usually the first to be attacked by exogenous diseases, they are called the Delicate Organ. These diseases can also cause what is called the Non-Spreading of the Lung Qi. The main symptom of a problem with the lungs is coughing, which is a form of Rebellious Qi (since the lung Qi normally flows downward). If coughing is also accompanied by lassitude, shortness of breath, light foamy phlegm, and weakness in the voice, it is called Deficient Lung Qi. However, if the cough is a dry one, with little phlegm, a parched throat and mouth, and Deficient Yin symptoms (such as night sweating, low grade fever, red cheeks, etc.), the condition is referred as Deficient Lung Yin.

## The Large Intestine Channel of Hand - Yang Brightness

The lungs (Yin) and the large intestine (Yang) are considered paired organs. From Table 2-1 you can see that they belong to Metal in the Five Phases, the westerly direction, the season of autumn, the dry climatic condition, the color white, the pungent taste, the rank odor, the emotion of sadness, and the sound of weeping. Their opening is the nose, and they govern skin and hair. The main function of the large intestine is the metabolism of water and the passing of water. It extracts water from the waste material received from the small intestine, sends it on to the urinary bladder, and excretes the solid material as stool. Many disorders affecting this organ are categorized as spleen and stomach patterns. Certain abdominal pains are considered manifestations of a blockage of Qi or blood in the large intestine.

In Qigong, the Dan Tian in the lower abdomen is considered the residence of Original Qi. In order to keep this Qi at its residence, this area must be strong and healthy. The Qi circulating around the intestines must not be stagnant. When you practice Qigong you must learn how to regulate your breathing to smooth the Qi flow in the large intestine and the lungs. This will allow you to relax the front of your body and regulate the Qi flow in the other organs.

## The Stomach Channel of Foot - Yang Brightness

The spleen (Yin) and the stomach (Yang) are paired organs. They belong to Earth in the Five Phases, the center, the season of long summer (the end of summer), the climatic condition of damp ness, the color yellow, the emotion of ppnsiveness, the taste of sweet ness, fragrant odor, and the sound of singing. Their opening is the mouth and they control the flesh and the limbs.

The Yin/Yang relationship between the spleen and the stomach is a particularly strong example of the relationship between organs. The stomach receives food while the spleen transports nutrients. The stomach moves things downward while the spleen moves things upward. The stomach likes dampness while the spleen likes dryness.

Though there are some patterns relating to deficiency of the stomach (many of these originate in the spleen), most stomach disorders are caused from excess. Stomach Fire gives a painful, burning sensation in the stomach, unusual hunger, bleeding of the gums, constipation, and halitosis.

Once saliva has begun the process of digestion, food passes to the stomach, located in the middle Sanjiao (middle triple burner) area. The stomach breaks down the food, and then passes it on to the intestines, where the essence is absorbed and converted into Qi, and circulated through the entire body.

The stomach is related to the emotion of pensiveness. When you are upset, the stomach will not function normally. In Qigong, regulating the mind is the first step to maintaining the stomach in a healthy condition. The type of food you eat is the second consideration. The proper amount and quality of food will help you to obtain high quality Qi to circulate in your body.

**The Spleen Channel of Foot - Greater Yin**

The spleen (Yin) and the stomach (Yang) are paired organs. They belong to Earth in the Five Phases, the central direction, the season of long summer (the end of summer), the climatic condition of dampness, the color yellow, the emotion of pensiveness, the taste of sweetness, fragrant odor, and the sound of singing. Their opening is the mouth and they control the flesh and the limbs.

The spleen is the main organ of digestion. Its function is to transport nutrients and regulate the blood (regulate means to keep it within the channels). It is responsible for the transformation of food into nourishment.

When the spleen is weak, the body will not be able to use the nourishment available in food. This will cause general lassitude, fatigue, and a pasty complexion. The upper abdomen is considered the province of the spleen. Deficient spleen Qi is shown by a sense of malaise or fullness in that area. Because it is required that the transportive function of the spleen distribute its Qi upward, weak ness in the spleen will usually cause diarrhea. Spleen Qi is also regarded as the Middle Qi, and it is responsible for holding the viscera in place. Insufficiency of the Middle Qi will presage prolapsed stomach, kidneys, etc. In more serious cases, the spleen Yang Qi will be deficient, which is manifested in diarrhea, cold limbs, and abdominal pain that can be soothed by the warmth of frequent hot drinks.

If any of the above symptoms are accompanied by bleeding, especially from the digestive tract or uterus, it is called Spleen Not Controlling the Blood.

Cold and Dampness Harassing the Spleen is a manifestation characterized by a pent-up feeling in the chest and a bloated sensation in the abdomen, lassitude, lack of appetite and taste, a feeling of cold in the limbs, a dark yellowish hue to the skin, some edema and diarrhea or watery stool. The cold and dampness prevent the spleen from performing its transforming and transporting functions. This leads to a great disturbance in water metabolism and is one of the origins of Phlegm.

In Qigong training, one of the final goals is to regulate the Qi flow to its original (normal) levei in the five Yin organs. Among them, the spleen is the last and the hardest organ to regulate. It is believed that if you are able to regulate the Qi in your spleen to a normal and healthy level, you will have grasped the key to health and longevity.

### The Heart Channel of Hand - Lesser Yin

The heart and the small intestine are paired organs. The heart is considered Yin, and the small intestine is considered Yang, balancing this paired channel. These two organs correspond to Fire in the Five Phases, the southerly direction, the summer season, the climatic condition of heat, the color red, the emotion of happiness, the sound of laughter, the taste of bitterness, and the odor of burning. Their point of entry is the tongue, they control the blood vessels and are reflected in the face.

Almost all of the problems and disorders of the heart are associated with weakness. The four major types of heart weakness are Deficient Heart Qi, Deficient Heart Yang, Deficient Heart Blood, and Deficient Heart Yin.

The main functions of the heart are associated with the spirit and the blood vessels. The heart governs the blood vessels and is responsible for moving blood through them. It also stores the spirit, and is the organ usually associated with mental processes.

Therefore, some forms of emotional distress, dizziness, palpitations, shortness of breath, and lack of vitality are common symptoms of heart ailments. Deficient Heart Qi is symbolized by general lassitude, panting and shallow breathing, and frequent sweating. If the face is swollen and ashen gray or bluish-green, and the limbs are cold, it is called Deficient Heart Yang. The symptoms of restless ness, irritability, dizziness, absentmindedness, and insomnia are typical signs of Deficient Heart Blood. In Deficient Heart Yin cases, developments with a flushed feeling in the palms and face, low grade fever, and night sweating will occur.

The symptom of Heart Excess arises from an excess of Heart Fire. This is manifested by fever, occasionally accompanied by delirium, a racking pulse, intense restlessness, insomnia or frequent nightmares, a bright red face, a red or blistered and painful tongue, and often a burning sensation during urination. The latter symptom is the result of Heat being transferred from the heart to the small intestine, which interferes with the small intestine's role in metabolism and the body's management of water.

In Qigong society, it is believed that the mind is associated with the heart, and that it is also directly related to the spirit. The term heart (Xin) is usually used to represent the emotional mind or ideas. The Middle Dan Tian at the solar plexus is considered the residence of the Fire Qi. This Fire is used to nourish the brain and the spirit (Shen) at its residence, the Upper Dan Tian or third eye. In Chinese medicine it is said that the heart is the temple of the spirit because it supplies Fire Qi and can nourish the spirit without limit.

Generally speaking, the heart is very sensitive during the summertime: The heart is a Yin channel, and when the summer Yang comes it can increase the heart's Qi level and cause problems. Emotional disturbances, such as excitement from happiness, are considered harmful to the heart as well, especially during the summer time. Qigong emphasizes regulating the heart in the summer.

### The Small Intestine Channel of Hand - Greater Yang

The heart and the small intestine are paired organs. The heart is considered Yin, and the small intestine is considered Yang, balancing this paired channel. These two organs correspond to Fire in the Five Phases, the southerly direction, the summer season, the climatic condition of heat, the color red, the emotion of happiness, the sound of laughter, the taste of bitterness, and the odor of burning. Their point of entry is the tongue. They control the blood vessels and are reflected in the face.

The major function of the small intestine is to separate waste material from the nutritious elements in food. The nutritious elements are then distributed throughout the body and the waste is sent on to the large intestine.

The small and large intestines are located in the Lower Dan Tian. In order to store the Original Qi converted from Original Essence, the abdomen must be healthy and the Qi circulation in the area of the intestines must be smooth and natural. The best way to reach this goal is through abdominal breathing exercises. One such exercise is to lead the Original Qi upward following the heart and small intestine Qi channels to cool down the heart Fire.

### The Urinary Bladder Channel of Foot - Greater Yang

The kidneys (Yin) and the urinary bladder (Yang) are paired organs. They correspond to Water in the Five Phases, the winter season, the cold climatic condition, the southerly dicection, the color black, the emotion of fear, the taste of salt, the smell of decay, and the sound of groaning. Their sensory organ is the ear. Their opening is the urethra. They control the bones, marrow, and brain, and their health is reflected in the hair of the head.

The main function of the urinary bladder is to transform fluids into urine and excrete it from the body.

In Qigong, the urinary bladder has never enjoyed serious attention. However, its pairing partner the kidney is cne of the most important organs - one with which all Qigong practitioners are concerned and train most often. The reason for this is simply that the kidneys are the residence of the Original Essence.

### The Kidney Channel of Foot - Lesser Yin

The kidneys (Yin) and the urinary bladder (Yang) are paired organs. They correspond to Water in the Five Phases, the winter season, the cold climatic condition, the southerly direction, the color black, the emotion of fear, the taste of salt, a rotten smell, and the sound of groaning. Their sensory organ is the ear. Their opening is the urethra. They control the bones, marrow, and brain, and their health is reflected in the hair of the head.

The kidneys store Original Essence (Yuan Jing) and are therefore responsible for growth, development, and reproductive functions. They play the primary role in water metabolism and control the body's liquids, and also hold the body's most fundamental Yin and Yang.

Because the kidneys are the repositories of the basal Yin and Yang of the body, any disorder, if sufficiently chronic, will involve the kidneys. More significantly, a disease of the kidneys will usually lead to problems in other organs. Methods of strengthening the kidneys are therefore used by both medical and Qigong societies to increase or maintain vitality and health. The symptoms of Deficient Kidney Yang or Yin are typical symptoms of the disorder, and will appear to a certain extent as Deficient Yang or Yin patterns in any organ.

It is easy to undeistand and memorize the symptoms of Deficient Kidney Yin if one learns the correspondences of the kidneys and remembers that Yin represents the constructive, nourishing, and fluid aspects of the body. Usually, the lower back is weak and sore, there is ringing in the ears and loss of hearing acuity, the face is ashen or dark, especially under the eyes. It is common to feel dizziness and thirst, and to experience night sweats and low grade fevers. In addition, men have little semen and tend toward premature ejaculation, while women have little or no menstruation.

Deficient Kidney Yang symptoms are significantly associated with loss of energy or warmth. Similar to Deficient Kidney Yin, there is commonly ringing in the ears, dizziness, and soreness in the lower back. However, the soreness is characterized by a feeling of coldness, lassitude, and fatigue. Weakness in the legs can be noticed. In men, there is a tendency toward impotence, and in both sexes, clear and voluminous urine or incontinence.

Usually, Deficient Kidney Yin generates similar disorders in the heart and liver, while Deficient Kidney Yang disturbs the functions of the spleen and lungs. The progression could be in the opposite direction. When this pattern is associated with the lungs, it is called "Kidney Not Receiving Qi," a type of wheezing characterized by difficult breathing, mainly during inhalation. In addition to the Deficient Kidney Yang symptoms, this condition is also manifested by a faint voice, coughing, puffiness in the face, and spontaneous sweating.

The kidneys perform an important role in the metabolism of water. If these functions are disrupted, the condition of Deficient Kidneys will lead to Spreading Water.

In Qigong practice, essence (Jing) is considered the most original source of human vitality. Qi is converted from essence, and this Qi supplies the entire body and nourishes the brain and spirit. It is believed by both Chinese medical and Qigong societies that the kidneys are the residence of Original Essence. In order to protect your inherent essence, you must strengthen your kidneys. Only when your kidneys are strong will you be able to keep your essence at its residence. Therefore, keeping the kidneys healthy has become one of the most important subjects in Qigong.

Maintaining the kidneys in a healthy state includes protecting the physical kidneys from degeneration, and maintaining a smooth and correct level of Qi flow. In order to reach this goal, the diet must be considered. For example, too much salt is harmful to the kidneys, and eating too much eggplant will weaken the kidneys. In addition, the condition of the body is also important. Such things as over working without proper rest will increase tension on the kidneys and make the Qi flow stagnant. In winter, the kidneys will have more tension than in summer. Due to this, the Qi flow is more stagnant in the wintertime than in the summertime. Consequently, back pain problems increase in the winter.

In order to protect the kidneys, Qigong practitioners have studied the relationship of the kidneys to nature, food, and even to emotional states. They have developed massage techniques and specific exercises to increase Qi circulation in the kidneys during the winter. Since the health of the kidneys is related to the emotions as well, learning how to regulate the mind in order to regulate the Qi has become one of the major training goals in Qigong.

### The Pericardium Channel of Hand - Absolute Yin

The pericardium (Yin) and the triple burner (Yang) are paired organs. They are said to correspond to the "Ministerial Fire," as opposed to the "Sovereign Fire" of the heart and small intestine. Though the pericardium has no separate physiological functions, it is generally mentioned with regard to the delirium induced by high fevers.

The regulation of Qi in the pericardium is considered a very important subject in Qigong. It is believed that the heart, the most vital organ in your body, must have a proper level of Qi circulation in order to function normally. The Qi level of the heart can be raised easily to an abnormal state by illness, emotional disturbance, exercise, or injury. The function of the pericardium is to dissipate the excess Qi from the heart and direct it to the Laogong cavity (P-8), located in the center of the palm. From Laogong, the excess Qi will be released naturally and hence, regulate the heart's Qi level. The Laogong cavity is used in Qigong massage to reduce the body's temperature during a fever. You can see that the purpose of the pericardium is to regulate the Qi in the heart through the Laogong cavity.

You should understand that in Qigong it is believed that there are five centers (called gates) where the Qi of the body is able to com municate with the surrounding environment, and, consequently, regulate the Qi level in your body. Two of these five centers are the Laogong cavities, and two others are the Yongquan cavities (K-1), used to regulate the Qi in the kidneys. The fifth one is your face. The face is connected and related to many of your organs. Whenever any of your organ Qi is not normal, it shows on your face.

### The Triple Burner Channel of Hand - Lesser Yang

At least as far back as the 3rd century A.D., in the "Classic of Difficulties" (Nan Jing) the triple burner was regarded as "having a name but no form." In the "Inner Classic" (Nei Jing), the triple burner was considered an organ that coordinated all the functions of water metabolism. In other traditional documents, the burners were considered three regions of the body that were used to group the organs. The upper burner includes the chest, neck, and head as well as the functions of the heart and lungs. The middle burner is the region between the chest and the navel, and includes the functions of the stomach, liver, and spleen. The lower burner spans the lower abdomen, and the functions of the kidneys and urinary bladder. Therefore, the upper burner has been compared to a mist which spreads the blood and Qi, the middle burner is like a foam which churns up food in the process of digestion, and the lower burner resembles a swamp where all the impure substances are excreted.

Regulating the Qi to a normally "smooth-flow" state is one of the main Qigong training methods for maintaining health. It is normally done through Wai Dan exercises, and it is believed that the Qi must flow around internal organs smoothly in order for them to maintain their normal functions. This means that in order to keep Qi flow smooth and the organs healthy, you must first learn how to regulate and relax muscles that are holding and related to a given organ. External movements also exercise internal muscles. One of the most common external exercises is regulating the triple burner by lifting your hands up above your head and then moving them down slowly. These up and down arm movements extend and relax the internal muscles and thereby increase Qi flow.

### The Gall Bladder Channel of Foot - Lesser Yang

The liver (Yin) and the gall bladder (Yang) are paired organs. They correspond to Wood in the Five Phases, the direction east, the spring season, the climatic wind, the color green, the emotion of anger, the taste of sourness, the goatish odor, and the sound of shouting. Their point of entry is the eyes. They control the sinews (muscles and joints), and their health is reflected in the finger and toe nails.

The main function of the gall bladder is storing and excreting the bile produced by the liver. Together with the heart, the gall bladder is responsible for decision-making.

The main disease related to the gall bladder is a disorder affect ing the flow of bile, usually caused by Dampness and Heat. This is commonly manifested by pain in the region of the liver, an oppressive sensation of fullness in the abdomen, and yellowish eyes, skin, urine, and tongue.

The gall bladder has never enjoyed serious attention during Qigong training. Its paired partner the liver however, has received much more attention.

**The Liver Channel of Foot - Absolute Yin**

The liver (Yin) and the gall bladder (Yang) are considered paired organs. They correspond to Wood in the Five Phases, the direction east, the spring season, the climatic condition of wind, the color green, the emotion of anger, the taste of sourness, the goatish odor, and the sound of shouting. Their point of entry is the eyes. They control the sinews (muscles and joints), and their health is reflected in the finger and toe nails.

The main task of the liver is spreading and regulating Qi throughout the entire body. Its unique character is flowing and free. Therefore, depression or frustration can disturb the functioning of the liver. In addition, the liver is also responsible for storing blood when the body is at rest. This characteristic, together with its control over the lower abdomen, makes it the most critical organ in regards to women's menstrual cycle and sexuality.

Depression or long-term frustration can stagnate the liver's spreading function and result in continuing depression, a bad temper, and a painful, swollen feeling in the chest and sides. If this condition worsens, it may cause disharmony between the liver and the stomach and/or spleen. This disorder is symbolized by the "rebellion" of Qi in the latter organs, whereby Qi moves in the opposite direction than is normal. For example, the stomach Qi normally descends, so rebellious Qi means hiccoughing, vomiting, etc. In the case of the spleen, the Qi ordinarily moves upward, so rebellious Qi in this organ means diarrhea.

Depression of the liver Qi is the main cause of many women's disorders, including menstrual irregularities, swollen and painful breasts, etc.

One of the most important responsibilities of the liver is the storage of blood with intended emphasis upon nourishing and moistening. Whenever the liver blood is deficient, the liver will not be able to handle the function of moistening. This is generally shown as dry and painful eyes with blurred or weak vision, lack of supple ness or pain in moving the joints, dry skin, dizziness, and infrequent or spotty menstruation. If the Deficient Liver Yin has become serious, the conditions Rising Liver Fire or Hyper Liver Yang Ascending occur. These occurrences are evidenced in ill-temper, restlessness, headache, vertigo, red face and eyes, and a parched mouth. If the liver Yin is so deficient that it is incapable of securing the liver Yang, many of the symptoms appear as disorders of the head. Weakness in the lower joints may also be manifested.

The liver is one of the five Yin organs whose Qi level the Qigong practitioner wants to regulate. Since the liver and the gall bladder are directly connected, when the liver's Qi is regulated, the Qi circulating in the gall bladder will also be regulated. Many methods have been developed for regulating the liver Qi. Wai Dan Qigong works through the limbs. For example, when the arms are moved up and down, the internal muscles surrounding the liver will be moved and the Qi around the liver will be circulated smoothly. In Nei Dan Qigong, it is believed that the liver is closely related to your mind. It is also believed that when your mind is regulated, the Qi circulation in the liver will be normal and therefore the liver will function properly.

The spleen, liver, and heart are the organs with the most direct relationship with the blood. The spleen filters the blood (modifying the blood's structure), the liver stores the blood, and the heart moves it. Any problem associated with the blood will involve at least one of these organs.

The liver and the kidney are closely related. Their channels cross in many places. The liver stores blood; the kidney stores essence. These substances, both of which are Yin, have a consider able influence on the reproductive functions.

The heart (upper burner, Fire) and the kidney (lower burner, Water) keep each other in check and are dependent upon one another. The spirit of the heart and the essence of the kidneys cooperate in establishing and maintaining human consciousness.

The spleen's digestive function is associated with the distributive functions of the liver. Disharmony between these two results in various digestive troubles. The transportive and digestive functions of the splcen (also called the Middle Qi) depend upon the strength of the kidney Yang.

Although the lungs govern Qi, Qi from the lungs must mix with essence from the kidneys before Original Qi can be produced. The lungs govern Qi, the liver spreads Qi, and the kidneys provide its basis.

**The Twelve Yuan Points:**

Each of the 12 regular meridians has a Yuan (Source) point near the wrist or ankle joints of the four extremities through which the vital energy of the zangfu organs passes and to some extent accumulates. "Yuan" means origin, and refers to the source of vital energy through which the pathological changes of zangfu organs are manifested. The chapter on the Nine Needles and the Twelve Sources of the book Lingshu states, "The twelve Yuan (source) points are indicated in disorders of the internal organs." The vital energy of the twelve regular meridians is ciosely associated with the Sanjiao which generalizes the functional activities of the stomach, spleen and kidney and is the manifestation of the function of vital energy. Vital energy, originating from the congen ital qi of the kidneys, is transported all over the body. It goes to the exterior, interior, superior and inferior parts of the body, following the courses of the meridians and maintaining vital functions of the human body. This process is maintained by the Sanjiao.

Clinically, Yuan (source) points are of great significance in treating diseases of the internal organs. Puncturing the Yuan (source) points stimulates the vital energy of the regular meridians, regulates the functional activities of the internal organs, reinforces antipathogenic factors and eliminates pathogenic factors. This method of treating diseases deals principally with the root causes. The Yuan (source) point from the affected meridian is often combined with the Luo (connecting) point of the internally-externally related meridians in use.

This is known as the combination of the main point (Yuan) and the accompanying point (Luo), or simply the combination of the Yuan (source) point and the Luo (connecting) point. Functionally, the Lung Meridian of Hand-Taiyin and the Large Intestine Meridian of Hand-Yangming are internally-externally related. The Yuan (source) point from the primarily affected meridian is combined with the Luo (connecting) point of its externally-internally related meridian. For example, if the Lung Meridian of Hand-Taiyin (interior) becomes diseased, sore throat, cough and asthma will occur. Taiyuan (Lu.9) is chosen as the main point and Pianli (L.I.6) is chosen as the accompanying one in the prescription. If the Large Intestine Meridian of Hand- Yangming (exterior) becomes diseased, e.g. toothache, Hegu (L.I.4), the Yuan (source) point of the Large Intestine Meridian of Hand-Yangming, and Lieque (Lu.7), the Luo (connecting) point of the Lung Meridian of Hand-Taiyin are prescribed.

Clinically, research has shown that pathological changes of the zangfu organs are often manifested at the twelve Yuan (source) points. For example, tenderness at a Yuan (source) point often indicates pathological changes of the associated meridian and the internally related organ.

In researching the meridian over the last few decades, Yuan (source) points were used as the key points to detect changes of cutaneous electrical resistance and to examine the condition of qi and blood of the twelve regular meridians. It was discovered that a significantly accurate estimation of the nature of many zangfu disorders could be made by using these methods.

The 12 Yuan (source) points are within the category of the Five Shu Points. Each Yang meridian has its own Yuan (source) point which is located between the Shu-stream point and the Jing-well point. The 6 Yin meridians do not have separate Yuan (source) points, their Shu-stream points being concurrently the Yuan (source) points, i.e. the Yuan (source) points and Shu-stream points of Yin meridians are actually the same.

## The Twelve Yuan (Source) Meridians Points

| | |
|---|---|
| Taiyuan (Lu.9) | The Lung Meridian of Hand-Taiyin |
| Hegu (L.I.4) | The Large Intestine Meridian of Hand-Yangming |
| Guanchong (St. 42) | The Stomach Meridian of Foot-Yangming |
| Taibai (Sp.3) | The Spleen Meridian of Foot-Taiyin |
| Shenmen (H.7) | The Heart Meridian of Hand-Shaoyin |
| Hand-Wangu (S.I.4) | The Small Intestine Meridian of Hand-Taiyang |
| Jinggu (U.B.64) | The Urinary Bladder Meridian of Foot-Taiyang |
| Taixi (K.3) | The Kidney Meridian of Foot-Shaoyang |
| Daling (P.7) | The Pericardium Meridian of Hand-Jueyin |
| Yangchi (S.J.4) | The Sanjiao Meridian of Hand-Shaoyang |
| QiuXu (G.B.40) | The Gall Bladder Meridian of Foot-Shaoyang |
| Taichong (Liv.3) | The Liver Meridian of Foot-Jueyin |

## The Fifteen Luo Points:

"Luoxue", meaning to connect, is a point where a collateral starts to connect a definite pair of Yin and Yang meridians which are externally-internally related. The 12 regular meridians, externally-internally related in pairs, are linked together by the Luo (connecting) points in order. This establishes a continuous system for the circulation of qi and blood through the 12 regular meridians, as to warm and nourish the entire body. Each of the 12 regular meridians has a Luo (connecting) Point as well as Jiuwei (Ren 15), the Luo (connecting) point of the Ren Meridian (connecting with the abdomen), Changqiang (Du 1), the Luo (connecting) point of the Du Meridian (connecting with the head), and Dabao (Sp.21), the Luo (connecting) point of the major collateral of the spleen (connecting with the hypochondriac region), a total of 15. The Spleen Meridian of Foot-Taiyin has another Luo (connecting) point Dabao (Sp.21) in addition to its original one, Gongsun (Sp.4). This is because the four extremities all acquire vital energy from the stomach. As this can not be obtained directly, the help of the spleen is required. The spleen helps the stomach to transport fluids to the five zang organs and the four extremities through its major collateral which governs both Yin and Yang collaterals of the body. Each of the 15 collaterals has its own course and distribution. Each of them has its own pathological manifestations. Consequently, the Luo (connecting) points are as important as the other specific points.

The Luo (connecting) points are all located below the elbow or knee, where the collaterals of the Yin meridians connect with their respective Yang meridians, and the collaterals of the Yang Meridians connect with their respective Yin meridians. Thus, the respective Yin and Yang meridians are internally-externally related by Luo (connecting) points. The fifteen collaterals are the major ones of the fourteen meridians, with the addition of the small collaterals, superficial ones and the tertiary ones which are divided from, governed by and dominated by the major ones. The Luo (connecting) points are locations at which the qi of the twelve regular meridians converges. Jiuwei (Ren 15), the Luo (connecting) point of the Ren Meridian, dominates the collaterals of the Yin merdians; Changqiang (Du 1), the Luo (connecting) point of Du Meridian, governs the collaterals of Yang Meridians; and Dabao (Sp.21), the Luo (connecting) point of the major collateral of the spleen, governs both the collaterals and blood vessels of the whole body. The concept of the spleen's function in keeping the blood circulation inside the vessels and preventing it from extravasation was based on the above understanding.

All of the fifteen collaterals are the passages through which qi and blood are transported into the zangfu organs and tissues of the body. An injury of the collaterals will inhibit the circulation of qi and blood, giving rise to stagnation of qi and coagulation of blood.

Clinically, Luo (connecting) points are often combined with Yuan (source) points in the treatment of diseases. Observations of the collaterals can sometimes be used as a diagnostic aid. For example, observation of the thenar collateral for diagnostic purposes.

The chapter on meridians in the book Lingshu says,

"The fifteen collaterals are sometimes visable in patients suffering from Shi conditions; but are not apparent in those patients affected by Xu syndromes. Such differences vary from person to person, due to particularity of the collaterals and varying degrees of experience among observers."

"When collaterals are observed, the colour blue suggests cold and pain, while red suggests heat in the body. For example, over-riding blue at the thenar collateral implies cold in the stomach; over-riding red means heat in the stomach; complete blackness implies prolonged stagnation; a mixture of red, blue and green means invasion of pathogenic cold and heat; and light green denotes qi deficiency."

"Pricking at particular collaterals to cause some bleeding once every other day can regulate Xu and Shi conditions in certain diseases."

The application of Luo (connecting) points in general is summarized in the table "Distribution and Indications of the Fifteen Luo (connecting) Points". For example, Waiguan (S.J.5) is used with reducing method for acute elbow pain and an excessive condition of the collaterals of the Shaoyang meridians; Tongli (H.5) is applied with reinforcing method for difficult speech and aphonia due to weakness of qi, or a deficient condition of the collaterals of the Shaoyin meridians. Luo (connecting) points are often applied in the treatment of various chronic diseases involving the internal impairment or accumulation of pathological substances such as stagnant qi, coagulation of blood, phlegm, damp, etc. Pathogenic qi may reach a collateral through a meridian, because "meridians are involved at the onset of diseases whilst collaterals are involved in the chronic cases."

### Distribution & Indications of the Fifteen Luo (Connecting) Points

| Luo (Connecting) Points | Connected Meridians | Indications: Excess | Indications: Deficiency |
|---|---|---|---|
| Lieque (Lu.7) | large intestine meridian | feverish palm and wrist frequent urination | shortness of breath, |
| Tongli (H.5) | small intestine meridian | fullness in the chest | difficult speech |
| Neiguan (P.6) | Sanjiao meridian | cardiac pain | restlessness |
| Zhizheng (S.I.7) | heart meridian | motor impairment | warts |
| Pianli (L.I.6) | lung meridian | toothache. Deafness | cold in teeth, chest fullness |
| Weiguan (S.J.5) | pericardium meridian | spasm of elbow | motor impairment of the elbow |
| Feiyang (U.B.58) | kidney meridian | nasal obstruction, pain in back and head | epistaxis |
| Guanming (G.B.37) | liver meridian | syncope | Wei syndrome |
| Fenglong (St.40) | spleen meridian | sore throat, aphonia, mania | foot drop |
| Gongsun (Sp.4) | stomach meridian | sudden abdominal pain, diarrhea | edema |
| Dazhong (K.4) | urinary bladder meridian | restlessness, dysuria | lumbar pain |
| Ligou (Liv.5) | Gall bladder meridian | prolapse of uterus, hernia | itching genitalia |
| Jiuwei (Ren 15) | connecting with abdomen | abdominal pain | itching in abdominal region |
| Changqiang (Du 1) | connecting with head | spinal rigidity | dizziness, heavy head |
| Dabao (Sp.21) | connecting with hypochondrium | | |

**The Sixten Xi Points:**

The Xi (cleft) Points are the places where the qi of the meridian is deeply converged. Each of the 12 regular meridians has a Xi (cleft) Point on the extremity, as do the Yinwei, Yangwei, Yinqiao and Yangqiao Meridians, 16 in all. Xi (cleft) Points are located below the elbows and knees except for Liangqiu (St.34) which is superior to the knee. They constitute another group of important points apart from the Five-shu Points.

Early records of Xi (cleft) Points date back to Zhenjiu Jiayi Jing (A Classic of Acupuncture and Moxibustion). Xi (cleft) Points are used for treating acute disorders of their related internal organs as well as of the areas supplied by the meridians. Needling these points can regulate the circulation of qi and blood in the diseased areas.

| The Sixteen Xi (Cleft) Points | Indications |
|---|---|
| Kongzui (Lu.6) | hemorrhoid bleeding, hemoptysis, shortness of breath |
| Wenliu (L.I.7) | toothache, common cold, hemorrhoids |
| Liangqiu (St.34) | epigastric pain |
| Diji (Sp.8) | acute diarrhea |
| Yinxi (H.6) | cardiac pain, insomnia and mental mania |
| Yanglao (S.I.6) | blurring of vision and tinnitus |
| Jinmen (U.B.63) | infantile convulsions and systrema |
| Shuiquan (K.5) | dysmenorrhea, prolapse of uterus |
| Ximen (P.4) | cardiac pain, palpitation, hypochondriac pain |
| Huizong (S.J.7) | pain in the heart area, enteritis |
| Waiqiu (G.B.36) | mania with emotional excitement and insanity with emotional depression |
| Foot-Zhongdu (Liv.6) | hernia, uterine bleeding |
| Fuyang (U.B.59) | acute diarrhea. sciatica, numbness, lumbar pain |

| | |
|---|---|
| Jiaoxin (K.8) | orchialgia. amenorrhea, night sweating |
| Yangiiao (G.B.35) | chest pain, numbness of the lower extremities |
| Zhubin (K.9) | relieving pathogenic qi, hernia and beriberi |

They also have the function to alleviate acute pain of the internal organs. For example, puncturing Liangqiu (St.34) for acute gastric pain; Kongzui (Lu.6) for acute bronchial hemoptysis; Shuiquan (K.5) for dysmenorrhea; Ximen (P.4) for cardiac pain and furuncle; Foot-Linqi (Liv.6) for swelling and pain of the testis, etc. The Xi (cleft) Points can also be used to treat acute sprain, points being selected from meridians passing through the injured area.

Clinically, combination of the Xi (cleft) Points and the Eight Influential Points can often enhance the therapeutic effect of the acupuncture treatment, e.g. Liangqiu (St.34) and Zhongwan (Ren 12) for severe epigastric pain; Kongzui (Lu.6) and Shanzhong (Ren 17) for cough and hiccup with difficult breathing.

Observation of Xi (cleft) Points can sometimes be of help in diagnosing acute disorders. Often there is a reactive spot at a Xi (cleft) Point when a particular organ or meridian is affected, e.g. tenderness can be felt at Ximen (P.4) in case of acute pleurisy; or at Liangqiu (St.34) in case of acute mastitis.

**The Back-shu and Front-mu Points:**

The Back-shu (shu) are the points on the back where qi of the respective zangfu organs is infused. They are located on either side of the vertebral column, in close proximity to the spinal ganglia and their respective zangfu organs, hence the name Back-shu points. Each of the zangfu organs has a Back-shu point, as does the Sanjiao, a total of twelve.

Front-mu Points (mu) are the points on the chest and abdomen where qi of the respective zangfu organs is infused. They are located on the chest and abdomen in close proximity to their respectively related zangfu organs, hence the name Front-mu points. Each of the zangfu organs and the Sanjiao has the Front-mu point, twelve in all.

In the application of the Back-shu and Front-mu points, consideration is given to their respective Yang and Yin characteristics. Front-mu points are located on the ventral Yin aspect of the body while the Back-shu points are on the dorsal Yang aspect. The qi of the Back-shu and Front-mu points communicates directly with their related zangfu organs. Clearly, the Back-shu and Front-mu points constitute an important group of specific points. A feature in the distribution of these points is that the level of the Front-mu points on the abdomen corresponds to that of the Back-shu points on the back, both Front-mu and Back-shu points being located at almost the same level as their respectively related zangfu organs. As well as being the points at which the qi of the respective zangfu organs is infused, they are also the places where the pathogenic factors can lodge, causing diseases of either the zangfu organs or of the body surface. In the light of the above, it can be seen that the Front-mu and Back-shu points'are of great significance in the physiology, pathology, diagnosis and treatment of diseases.

The Back-shu points are located on the first line of the Urinary Bladder Meridian of Foot-Taiyang on the back, 1.5 cun lateral to the Du Meridian. They are the places through which the qi of the Du Meridian communicates with the urinary bladder meridian and then infuses into the specific internal organs. Points on the first and second lines of the Urinary Bladder Meridian of Foot-Taiyang have similar indications to those points of the Du Meridian and Huatuo Jiaji points located at the same level. This demonstrates a close relationship between the Back-shu points and the spinal ganglia.

Further, as regards location, the more superior an internal organ is, the higher the corresponding Back-shu point will be; and vice versa. For example, the lung is the most superior organ among the zangfu; consequently, its related point, Feishu (U.B. 13), is the highest among the Back-shu points. The urinary bladder is the most inferior organ, its related point Pangguangshu (U.B.28) is also the lowest among the Back-shu points.

The Front-mu points are also in close proximity to their corresponding internal organs. For example, the Front-mu point of the lung Zhongfu (Lu.l) is the highest whilst Zhongji (Ren 3), the Front-mu point of the urinary bladder, is the lowest. Front-mu and Back-shu points are not necessarily points from their corresponding meridians. Their special influence is due to their close proximity to their corresponding internal organs, rather than their location on specific meridians. Among the Front-mu points, only three are situated on their corresponding meridians, namely Zhongfu (Lu.1), Riyue (G.B.24) and Qimen (Liv.14). None of the Back-shu points is from its corresponding meridian except Pangguangshu (U.B.28), the Back-shu point of the urinary bladder. Therefore, the distribution of the Back-shu and Front-mu points is another unique characteristic.

Back-shu and Front-mu points are not only important in the treatment of the diseases of the internal organs, but are also of clinical significance in the diagnosis of zangfu disorders. When any of the zangfu organs malfunctions, positive reactions such as sensitivity or tenderness will be manifested at the corresponding Back-shu or Front-mu points. Palpation of the sensitive points can be a useful aid to diagnosis. Stimulating techniques such as acupuncture, moxibustion or massage may be applied to these points to relieve disorders of their corresponding organs. For instance, injection of streptomycin in a small dosage at Feishu (U.B.13) or Zhongfu (Lu.1), the Back-shu and Front-mu points of the lung, may help patients suffering from active tuberculosis to build up resistance against the diseases. Puncturing Dachangshu (U.B.25) and Tianshu (St.25), the Back-shu and Front-mu points of the large intestine, may help alleviate the symptoms and signs of acute bacillary dysentery, repeated treatments resulting in a negative stool culture. Puncturing or applying moxa to the corresponding Front-mu points is especially effective in dealing with lingering disorders of the internal organs.

Disorders of both Yin meridians and the five zang organs are sometimes manifested at the Back-shu points on the Yang aspect of the body, and disorders of the Yang meridians and the six fu organs are sometimes manifested at the Front-mu points on the Yin aspect of the body. When Yang is diseased, Yin is also involved, and vice versa. So Back-shu points are often prescribed for disorders of the zang organs, while the Front-mu points are often prescribed for disorders of the fu organs in the clinic. Such an application of Back-shu and Front-mu points is also known as "expelling Yin disorders from Yang meridians, and expelling Yang disorders from Yin meridians".

The chapter Genjiepian of the book Lingshu states, "The key to applying acupuncture therapy is to master the method of regulating Yin and Yang." Puncturing the corresponding Back-shu and Front-mu points simply regulates the balance between Yin and Yang, so as to either force the pathogenic factors out of the body or treat internal disorders of the zangfu organs. For example, the Lung Meridian of Hand-Taiyin is a Yin meridian. When it is affected, Feishu (U.B.13) can be applied. The Stomach Meridian of Foot-Yangming is a Yang meridian. When it is affected, Zhongwan (Ren 12) can be used.

Besides, Back-shu points can also be applied for dealing with disorders of the five sense organs. For example, Ganshu (U.B.18) is often used for eye disorders because the liver opens into the eye; Shenshu (U.B.23) for disorders of the ear because the kidney opens into the ear; Feishu (U.B.13) for nasal disorders, because the lung opens into the nose; and Xinshu (U.B. 15) for oral or tongue ulceration because the heart opens into the tongue and the tongue is the mirror of the heart, etc.

**I. Selection of acupuncture points.**

Local Point selection

Distal Point Selection

Symptomatic Point Selection

Specific Point Usage

Points Based on Western Medical Theory

**II. Combining Points**

Combining points on the front (Yin aspect of torso) with points on the back( Yang aspect of torso)

Combining Yang channel points with Yin Channel points

Combining point on the left with points on the right

Combining points above with points below

Combining local with distal points

## III Specific Points Usage

*Five Transporting points*

Back-Shu

Front-Mu

Yuan-Source

Luo-Connecting

*Eight confluent points of extra meridians*

Xi-Cleft

Lower He-Sea

Crossing Points

## Selection of Acupuncture Points:

Acupuncture treatment is administered at specific points or sites on the body. For this reason, the selection and combination of points in an acupuncture prescription is most important. At the same time, the physician must be able to choose flexibly between one or more acupuncture methods, depending upon the characteristics of the disease. Below, is a summary of point selection and combination strategies. Together with clinical applications.

## Principles of Point Selection

Point selection may be divided into three broad groupings:

local points chosen in the vicinity of the disease,

distal points chosen away from the disease,

points chosen for particular symptoms,

specific point usage,

points chosen based on Western medical knowledge.

In practice, each may be used in combination with, or independent of the others.

## Local Point Selection

Local refers to the vicinity of the pain. Thus, pain the head, neck forearm, low abdomen, knee, foot, etc. can be treated via points in the same locality.

Diseases of the limbs and superficial diseases of the body are commonly treated by this method.

**Examples:** Pain of the knee can be treated at local points GB 34, Sp9, Sp 10, St 34, Xi Yan (St 35 with other side of patella). GB 34 is the influential points of the tendons.

Pain of the wrist is needled at SJ 4, Sj 5, or LI 5, SI 6.

Many diseases of the head and body may also be treated through local points.

Eye diseases can be treated at UB 1, GB 1,

Ear diseases at SJ 21, SI 19, GB 2,

Asthma at Ren 22, UB 13,

Stomachache at Ren 12, St 21 UB 21.

The efficacy of needling local points to treat disease can be explained not only on the basis of traditional channel theory, but more recently by neural segment theory as well. For example in acupuncture anesthesia, the point SI 18 is used for surgery on the cranium, and the point LI 18 for operations on the thyroid.

Similarly in the clinical treatment of diseases of the Viscera, it is common to select a vertebral point on the same horizontal plane as the affected organ. Choosing a point in the same or neighboring neural segment as that of the pain or disease is also compatible with the rules of traditional local point selection.

**Distal Point Selection**

Distal refers to a location far from the site of the pain, usually a point below the elbow or knee. The method is commonly used to treat diseases of internal organs.

**Examples:** Lung 6 for coughing blood.

PC 6 for chest pain.

ST 36 for abdominal pain.

This method may also be used for diseases of the head and trunk.

**Examples:** LI4, ST 44 for toothache, the LI channel enters the lower gums and can stop toothaches on the lower jaw. The

Stomach channel enters the upper gums, St 44 can stop toothaches on the upper jaw.

SI 3 for stiff neck. because SI 3 is one of the Eight Confluent Points, intersecting with the Du Channel. Du Channel runs through the neck.

UB 54 for lower back pain. Because the UB channel runs through the lower back.

The technique of needling distal points is related to the channel theory of root and branch, whereby a disease above is treated by a point below, and vice versa.

In addition to selecting distal points according to traditional theory, they may also be selected on the basis of nerve distribution. Generally, this is most useful for treatment of disorders on the limb, whereby a point located on a nerve trunk or root above the diseases is selected for needling.

**Examples:** Diseases of the fingers may be treated via points on related nerves. PC6 on the median nerve near the wrist and LI 11 on the radial nerve near the elbow as well as point on the more distant brachial plexus.

Diseases of the lower limb may be treated at GB34 on the peroneal nerve and more distally at points along the sciatic nerve or sacral plexus.

## Symptomatic Point Selection

Local and distal points selections are based upon the distance of the points from the site of the diseases. However, some diseases are not local but systemic in nature, and can be treated at points long associated with relieving a particular diseases. Prominent among such points are the meetings points first mentioned in the "Classic of Difficulties":

UB 17 for diseases affecting the blood (the influential point of blood)

Ren 17 for diseases of the Qi. (influential point of Qi)

Lu 9 for diseases of the vessels. (influential point of vessels)

GB 34 for diseases of the tendons. (influential point of tendons)

GB 39 for diseases of the marrow. (influential point of marrow)

UB11 for diseases of the bones. (influential point of bones)

Liver 13 for diseases of the Yin Organs, Lung, Spleen, Heart, Kidney, and Liver.

Ren 12 for diseases of the Yang organs, stomach, large and small intestine, urinary bladder, San Jiao and G.B.

Stimulation of these points has proven effective in relieving the disorders with which each is associated. The same is true of the other special point groups. Certain individual points have also traditional been useful in treating specific symptoms:

Du 14 for reducing fever, (because Du 14 is the crossing point of the 6 yang channels and Du Mai)

Du 26, for reviving patients form unconsciousness. (Du channel enters the brain.)

Pricking and Bleeding Lu 11 and SI 1 for sore throat.

LI11, Sp 10, Sp 6 for pruritus. (Itching) LI11 cleans wind and heat, Sp 10 and Sp 6 to nourish blood and expel wind evil.

Ren 4, St 36, for general weakness. Ren 4 tonifies Yuan source Qi, and Stomach 36 tonifies digestive function hence increasing Gu Qi.

**Points Chosen Based on Western Medical Theory**

The efficacy of needling local points to treat disease can be explained not only on the basis of traditional channel theory, but more recently by neural segment theory as well. For example in acupuncture anesthesia, the point SI 18 is used for surgery on the cranium, and the point LI 18 for operations on the thyroid.

Similarly in the clinical treatment of diseases of the Viscera, it is common to select a vertebral point on the same horizontal plane as the affected organ. Choosing a point in the same or neighboring neural segment as that of the pain or disease is also compatible with the rules of traditional local point selection.

Hua Tou Jia Ji Points treated consistant with spinal nerve distribution

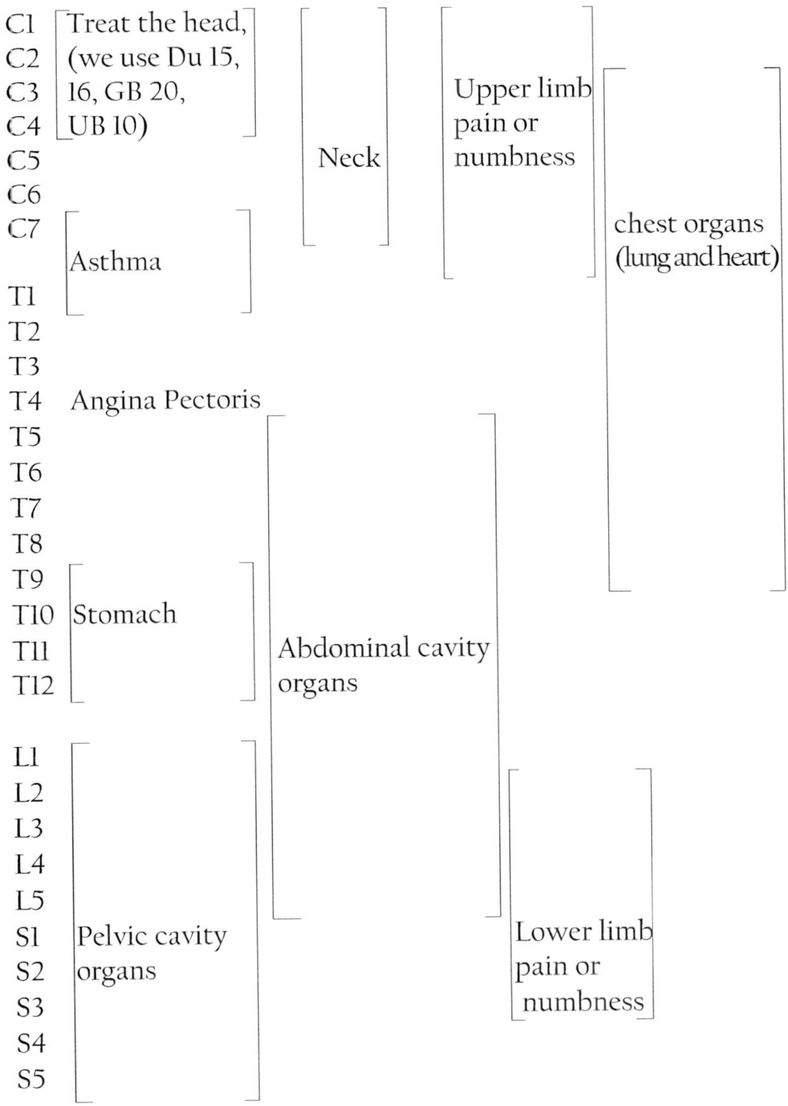


In addition to selecting distal points according to traditional theory, they may also be selected on the basis of nerve distribution. Generally, this is most useful for treatment of disorders on the limb, whereby a point located on a nerve trunk or root above the diseases is selected for needling.

Diseases of the fingers may be treated via points on related nerves. PC6 on the median nerve near the wrist and LI 11 on the radial nerve near the elbow as well as point on the more distant brachial plexus.

Diseases of the lower limb may be treated at GB34 on the peroneal nerve and more distally at points along the sciatic nerve or sacral plexus.

## II Combining Points

In addition to the methods of individual point selection outlined above, there are several traditional methods of combining one point with others in an acupuncture prescription. These techniques are flexible, permitting many variations according to the particular needs of the case.

### Combining Points on the Front (Yin aspect of torso) with Points on the Back(Yang aspect of torso)

This method is also known as the combination of abdomen-yin points and the back-yang points. Points on the front and back appropriate to a particular disease can be used in combination.

**Example:** Stomach disease, both St 21 on the abdomen and UB 50 on the back could be needled in tandem.

Among the most commonly used front-back combinations are two special point groups. The Back-shu points and the front-mu points. Because these points are closely related to diseases of the Zang-fu organs.

**Example:** Ren 12 (St Front Mu) and UB 21 (Stomach Back-Shu) for Stomach diseases.

### Combining Yang Channel Points with Yin Channel Points

As we know, the primary yang channels are connected with the primary Yin channels in a yin/yang relationship. By combining a point on a yang channel with another on its paired yin channel, the cumulative effect is greater than needling either point separately.

**Examples:** Combining Stomach 36 on the yang channel with Sp 4 on the yin channel for stomach diseases.

Lung 9 with LI 11, on the paired Yang channel, for coughing.

The most well-known combinations of this kind are between the Yuan-Source points on the first channel, primarily affected by a disease, and the Luo-Connecting point on the paired channel. In this combination the source point is called the "host," Example:Diseases affecting the Lung channel may be treated through that channel's source point (Lu 9) in combination with the Luo-connecting point (LI 6) of its paired Yang partner, the Large Intestine channel.

Conversely, a disease affecting the Large intestine channel could be treated by that channel's source point, (LI 4,) together with the connecting point, (Lu 7) of its Yin partner, the lung channel.

The method would also encompass the use of a single point, the Luo connecting point of the paired channel.

**Example:** For a disease associated with the kidney channel, UB 58, the Luo-connecting point of the Kidney's paired meridian would be chosen. Conversely, diseases of the UB can be treated by Kidney 4, the Kidney's Luo-Connecting point.

### Combining Point on the Left with Points on the Right

Because channel points are bilateral, it is common to treat diseases of the internal organs by manipulating the same point on both sides in order to strengthen the effect.

**Example:** UB 21 on both left and right sides of the spine, or St 36 on both legs can be needled to treat diseases of the stomach.

Further, because of the intersection of the channels on the right side with those on the left, a point on the right may be chose to treat a disease of pain on the left side of the body, and vice versa.

**Example:** In the case of "stroke," not only may a point on the side affected by the paralysis be selected, but the same point on the healthy side may be used as well.

### Combining Points above with Points below

Above refers to point on the arms and above the waist, (Ren 8). Below refers to points on the legs or below the waist (Ren 8). This method of point combination is most commonly practiced on the limbs.

**Example:** In the case of stomach diseases, PC 6 on the arm maybe combined with St 36 on the leg.

For toothache, LI 4 of the hand can be combined with St 44 on the foot.

Traditionally, a distinctive use of the above-below combination was made with respect to the confluent points of the eight extraordinary channels. A confluent point on an extraordinary channel affected by a disease above, would be combined in an acupuncture prescription with a meeting point on a extraordinary channel below.

**Example:** For diseases of the heart, chest, abdomen, PC 6 on the arm may be combined with Sp 4 on the foot.

For ear ringing, SJ 5, on the arm can be combined with GB 41 on the foot.

### Combining Local with Distal Points

**Example:** When there is stomach problems, the local points Ren 12 and UB 21 or the distal points St 36, PC 6 and Sp4, could be used separately. The combination method, however, uses both the local and distal points together.

### Specific Points Usage

Specific points are those on the fourteen meridians with specific therapeutic significance. Since specific points have different distributions and effects, they bare different names. The following represents a brief description of their applications.

### The Five Transporting points. (Five-Shu)

These are five points on the twelve regular channels, namely the Jing-well, Ying-spring, Shu-stream, Jing-river, and He-sea.

The five transporting points may be selected according to their therapeutic properties.

Jing-well points are selected for fullness in the epigastrium. (Liver/wood element disharmony)

Ying-spring points are for febrile diseases. (Heart/fire element Difficulties)

Shu-stream points are for a heavy sensation of the body and/or painful joints. (Spleen/earth element problems)

Jing-river points are for cough and asthma due to pathogenic cold or heat. (Lung/metal element ailments)

He-sea points are for diarrhea due to rebellious Qi or Zang organ disharmony. (Kidney/water element afflictions)

Jing-well points on the Yin channels belong to the wood element. Jing-well points on the Yang channels belong to the metal element. Because metal controls wood, tonifying the Jing-well points on the Yang channels well result in the sedation of liver energy which is often the needed treatment. Also, you can sedate the Jing-well points on the Yin channels for a similar effect.

Another way to use the Jing-well points that treat more than just the Wood element, can be found in using Pc-9 with Kid-1. This technique makes use of the above/below combination which, in this case, has the effect of balancing fire (Pericardium) and water (Kidney) which balances above and below along with fire and water. Connecting the Qi of these two opposing elemental forces calms the Shen.

Ying-spring for Febrile diseases and Heart disharmony.

Heart belongs to fire. Febrile diseases are "fiery."

Signs and symptoms include: Irritability and sleeplessness, sores on the tongue and the lips, flushed face, thirst, painful and dark colored urine, dry stool, hematemesis (vomiting blood), nosebleeds, delirium or mania in severe cases, red tongue with yellow coat, rapid pulse.

Thus, tonifying the grandmother of fire, (water) which is found at the Ying-spring points of the Yang channels will sedate the fire element's fire. Sedating the Yin channel's Ying-spring (fire) points will help to turn down the fire in the heart or elsewhere.

Shu-stream points for spleen diseases and/or a heavy sensation of the body and/or painful joints.

Shu-stream points are for heavy sensations in the body and painful joints due to spleen Qi deficiency. This Qi Xu will also diminish the efficiency of the Spleen's function of transportation and transformation. With this hypofunction, dampness will be stored up within the body, or lead to a Splenic disorder due to cold-damp retention within the Spleen proper.

Signs and symptoms include: sensation of fullness in the abdomen, anorexia, nausea and vomiting, weakened limbs, loose stool, pale tongue with white greasy coat, and slow, soft pulse.

Sedating the grandmother of earth (wood) which is found at the Shu-stream points of the Yang channels will serve to tonify earth. Tonifying the Shu-stream points on the Yin channels will help to build up the strength of the earth element and the end of Splenic disharmony.

Jing-river for lung diseases and/or cough and asthma due to pathogenic cold or heat.

Jing-river points are for cough and asthma due to pathogenic cold or heat. Lungs belongs to metal, when lungs are attacked by pathogenic wind-cold or wind-heat, obstruction of the Lung Qi results.

Signs and Symptoms include: Cough, asthma, dry throat, sore throat hoarseness, and nasal obstruction.

Sedating the grandmother of metal (fire) which is found at the Jing-river points of the Yang channels will serve to tonify metal. Tonifying the Jing-river points on the Yin channels will help to build up the strength of the metal element and the end of Metal disharmonies.

He-sea for Kidney diseases and/or diarrhea due to rebellious Qi.

When the Kidney Qi is deficient, it is unable to grasp the Da Qi of the lungs. Signs and symptoms include: Shortness of breath, dyspnea, and difficult inhalation (normal exhalation).

Another area affected by Kidney Qi deficiency is its reinforcement and astringent functions.

Signs and symptoms include: enuresis (withholding of urine), spermatorrhea, diarrhea, pale tongue with white fur, and a deep and weak pulse. Sedating the grandmother of water (earth) which is found at the He-sea points of the Yang channels will serve to tonify water. Tonifying the Jing-river points on the Yin channels will help to build up the strength of the water element and the end of water disharmonies.

| Channel | Jing-Well | Ying-Spring | Shu-Stream | Jing-River | Sea He- |
|---|---|---|---|---|---|
| Lung | Lu 11 | Lu 10 | Lu 9 | Lu 8 | Lu 5 |
| Pericardium | P 9 | P 8 | P 7 | P 5 | P 3 |
| Heart | H 9 | H 8 | H 7 | H 4 | H 3 |
| Spleen (Pancreas) | Sp 1 | Sp 2 | Sp 3 | Sp 5 | Sp 9 |
| Liver | Liv 1 | Liv 2 | Liv 3 | Liv 4 | Liv 8 |
| Kidney | K 1 | K 2 | K 3 | K 7 | K 10 |
| Large Intestine | L.I. 1 | L.I. 2 | L.I. 3 | L.I. 5 | L.I. 11 |
| San Jiao | SJ 1 | SJ 2 | SJ 3 | SJ 6 | SJ 10 |
| Small Intestine | S.I. 1 | S.I. 2 | S.I. 3 | S.I. 5 | S.I. 8 |
| Stomach | St 45 | St 44 | St 43 | St 41 | St 36 |
| Gall Bladder | GB 44 | GB 43 | GB 41 | GB 38 | GB 34 |
| Urinary Bladder | UB 67 | UB 66 | UB 65 | UB 60 | UB 40 |

Use of transportation points in a mother/son combination for tonifying and sedating.

As mentioned earlier, the Jing-well, Ying-spring, Shu-stream, Jing-river and He-sea points of the channels are attributed to the five elements.

On the Yin channels, the order, from the Jing-well point upward from distal to proximal, is wood, fire, earth, metal, and water.

On the Yang channels, the order, from the Jing-well point upward from distal to proximal, is metal, water, wood, fire, earth.

One way in which these points can be therapeutically utilized is by selecting them according to their relationships in the five element model.

Inter-promoting (mother to son), interacting (grandmother to grandson), overacting (too much grandmother to grandson), and counteracting (grandson pushing back to grandmother).

Beginning with the interpromoting relationship of the five elements, each channel has a "mother" point and a "son" point. The "mother point" of a channel has a reinforcing effect on that channel, while the "son point" has a reducing effect. In the case of an excess condition, one can reinforce the mother and reduce the son on the affected channel.

In clinical practice, the two needle method as was just described can be used on the mother and son points of the affected channel, or on the points along the mother and son channels.

### Mother-Son Treatment with both Points on the Affected Channel

The Liver channel pertains to wood. An excess syndrome of the Liver channel can be treated by sedating Liver 2, the fire point on the Liver channel. Fire is the son of wood and Liver 2 is the fire point on the Liver channel, hence sedating the son will give the mother a chance to settle down from her excess state.

The deficiency state of the Liver channel can be treated by tonifying Liver 8, because this is the water point on the Liver channel, and water is the mother of wood, so when mom feels good, she can better nourish her son. Liver 8 is the mother point of the Liver channel. This is using the principle of "tonifying the mother for deficiency syndrome."

Then there is the technique of using the same principle, but on the mother and son channels, rather than the mother and son points on the same channel

### Mother-son Treatment with Points on the Mother or Son Channel

For an excess syndrome of the Liver channel, one would treat the Ying-spring point on the Heart channel (Heart 8), because the Heart is the Fire channel. That makes it Liver's son. Ht 8 is the horary (fire) point on Liver's son channel, hence you are "sedating the son for excess syndromes."

Deficiency syndromes of the Liver channel can be treated by tonifying the horary point on the mother channel which is the kidney. Kidney 10 is the horary point (water point on the water channel). This technique is based on the principle of "tonifying the mother for deficiency syndromes."

Mother-son treatments with points based on the interior/ exterior relationship.

For a deficiency syndrome of the Liver channel, reinforcing GB 43, the mother point of the GB channel will tonify wood because GB 43 is the mother point on the Yang wood channel.

Excess syndromes of the Liver channel can be treated by reducing GB 38, the son point of the GB channel. Because GB 38 is the fire point and hence the son point on the Yang wood channel.

### Back-shu and Front-Mu Points

The Back-Shu and Front-Mu points are closely related to diseases of the Zang-Fu organs. When there is the pathogenic change in the Zang-Fu organ, a palpitated reaction to this change, in the form of tenderness or sensitivity, can be detected in the corresponding Back-Shu or Front-Mu point. Thus, whenever an internal organ is affected, the Back-Shu point and the Front-Mu points pertaining to that organ may be prescribed either independently or in combination with other specific points as will be demonstrated later.

Yin diseases of the Zang-Fu organs can be treated with Back-Shu points. Yin diseases (this includes Zang organ syndromes, deficiency syndromes and cold syndromes) can all be treated with the Back-shu points. Yin diseases reach Yang. The Evil Qi of the Yin diseases may reach the back-shu points. This is called "Treating Yang for Yin diseases." Another deep thought is "Lead Yin evil out through Yang points." So, needling the Back-shu points to treat Yin diseases leads the evil Qi out through the Back-shu points.

**For example:** UB 13 on the back is needled to treat productive cough, fullness in the chest, etc. due to Yin-type diseases of the lung, in this case, Wind cold.

Yang diseases can be treated with the front-Mu points. Yang diseases may include Fu organ syndromes, excess syndromes, or heat syndromes. "Yang diseases reach Yin." The Qi of Yang diseases may reach the Front-Mu points. The treatment principle is then called "Treating Yin for Yang diseases". Utilizing the therapeutics of "leading Yang evil out through the Yin points." Thus, needling the front-Mu points to treat Yang diseases is leading the evil Qi out through the front-Mu points.

**For example:** Ren 3 (the Front-Mu of the U.B.) is needled to treat copious, frequent urination, burning pain in the urethra, dark yellow urine, etc. due to damp or heat in the U.B..

The Back-Shu points above (and including) UB 17 can, in addition to the Yin diseases described above, treat Yang diseases such as Exterior cold or heat, chest or back pain (due to Lung heat, or wind heat or cold). UB 13 can treat common cold expelling wind heat or wind cold evil. Which explains why the Lung Shu point is so versatile for Lung or exterior disharmonies.

The Front-Mu under the level of Ren 8 can treat Yin diseases as well as Yang in the same way as the Back-Shu points above UB 17 can treat Yang. For example, Ren 4 can treat leanness due to consumption; Qi, Yang, Yin, or Jing collapse; or stroke associated with extreme Qi, Yin, Yang, or Jing Xu. It's a strong point.

The reason Back-Shu points above UB 17 are good for Yang diseases as well as Yin, is because they are situated on the Yang (top half) of the Yang aspect of the torso (the back) . The are like "Yang within Yang" and since "Ultimate Yang becomes Yin", they begin to take on the Yin functions of treating Yang diseases. The same thing applies to the front-Mu points below the level of Ren 8. The are found on the Yin aspect of the body, and the lower, or Yin half of the abdomen, and hence they represent "ultimate Yin" which can begin to take on Yang attributes and thus, treat Yin syndromes.

### Combining Points on the Back-Shu with Points on the Front-Mu

Certain disease syndromes are not simple, they can exhibit signs of both excess and deficiency. In these cases, it is appropriate to use both the front-Mu and back-Shu points.

UB 13 + Lu 1 = treatment of Lung diseases.

UB 18 + Liv 14 = treatment of Liver diseases.

UB 19 + GB 24 = treatment of Gall Bladder diseases.

UB 21 + Ren 12 = treatment of Stomach diseases.

UB 25 + St 25 = treatment of Large Intestine diseases.

UB 28 + Ren 3 = treatment of Urinary Bladder diseases.

Combining Front-Mu points with lower He-sea points on the Yang channels, treats Yang diseases (Fu organ syndromes, excess syndromes, heat syndromes)

**Note:** Lower He-sea implies the three extra He-sea points from the hand Yang channels as well as the three He-sea points on the foot yang channels as was discussed earlier.

**For Example:**

St 25 (L.I. Front-Mu) + St 37 (L.I. Lower He-sea) = treatment of Damp-Heat in the Large Intestine.

According to the Nei Jing. it is written that "Lower He-sea points treat Fu organ diseases."

Combining Back-shu ooints with Yuan-source points treats yin diseases (Zang organ syndromes, deficiency syndromes, cold syndromes).

**For Example:**

UB 13 (Lung back-Shu) + Lu 9 (Lung Yuan-source point) = treatment of asthma due to Lung Qi deficiency.

UB 23 (Kidney back-Shu) + Kid 3 (Kidney Yuan-source point) = treatment of spermatorrhea due to Kidney Qi deficiency.

Back-Shu points and Yuan-source points can both treated deficiency diseases. Together, their effects are enhanced.

**Yuan Source Points**

The Yuan-source points are located on the six Yang channels, and arranged behind the Shu-Stream points of the Five Transporting points. On the six Yin channels, you'll find the Yuan-source points conveniently located smack-dab on the Shu-stream points.

The Yuan-source points are closely related to San Jiao. Acupuncture on the Yuan-source points can dredge the source Qi in the San Jiao and regulate the functions of the internal organs. Hence, Yuan-source points can treat diseases of both the Zang and Fu organs.

### Combining Yuan-source Points of Zang Organs with Yuan-source Points of Fu organs

Yuan-source points of Yang channels on the hand combined with the Yuan-source points of the Yin channels on the foot. (OR) The Yuan-source points of Yin channels on the hand combined with Yuan-source points of Yang channels on the foot.

This technique is beneficial when treating diseases that effect the entire body. Using the hand and foot Yuan-source points together, circulates the Qi's therapeutic action throughout the entire body.

**Example:**

Liver 3, (Yuan-source point of the Liver meridian of foot Jue Yin) combines with L.I. 4, (Yuan-source point of L.I. meridian of hand Yang Ming) for dizziness, tinnitus, numb limbs and tight tendons due to Liver yin deficiency.

### Yuan-source Points Combining with the Luo-connecting Points (connecting internally, externally related channels)

Most beneficial when internally/externally related pairs of channels have a disease together.

### Yuan-source Points combined with Back-Shu Points

Back-Shu points and Yuan-source points can both treated deficiency diseases. Together, their effects are enhanced. What, you didn't get it last time this came up?

### Yuan-source Points combined with He-sea Points or Lower He-sea Points

Interior/Exterior channel relationships. Yuan-source points of Yin channels combined with He-sea or lower He-sea points of Yang channels.

**Example:**

Sp 3 (Yuan-source point of Spleen channel) combined with St 36 (He-sea point of Stomach channel) for abdominal pain, diarrhea, nausea, and vomiting.

Liv 3 (Yuan-source point of Liver channel) combined with GB 34 (He-sea point of GB channel) for dizziness, bitter taste or dryness in the mouth, burning pain in the chest and hypochondrium due to Liver or G.B. fire.

This combination of points (Yuan + He-Sea) is used when the etiology of the disease is a disharmony between the internally/externally related organs.

**Same Channel. Yuan-source Point Combined with He-sea Point on the Same Channel**

L.I. 4 (Yuan-source point of L.I. channel) combined with L.I. 11 (He-sea point of L.I. channel) for headache, toothache, sore throat, dry mouth all due to wind-heat evil.

Liver 3 (Yuan-source) combined with Liver 8 (He-sea) for distention. Cramping and cold pain in the perineum and lower abdomen, or pain from contraction of the scrotum due to accumulation of cold in the Liver channel.

**Different Channels, not internally/externally Related**

L.I. 4 combined with St. 36. Regulates Stomach and L.I. for treatment of dry stool.

LI 4 to tonify Jin (as in Jin/Ye) and St. 36 tonifies the stomach to push the fecal matter out the intestines.

Liver 3 combined with St. 36. Disperses stagnated Liver Qi, regulates Stomach Qi, for treatment of stomachache due to Liver Qi stagnation. Regulates liver qi and tonifies earth that has been attacked by wood.

**Luo-Connecting Points**

The Luo-connecting points are closely related to collaterals. A Luo-connecting point connects with its partner in the Interior/Exterior relationship. That's why the Luo-connecting points are indicated in the syndromes of their partners in the Interior/Exterior relationship.

For instance, Spleen 4, the Luo-connecting points of the spleen channel of foot tai yin, can treat not only the diseases of the Spleen channel, but also those of teh Stomach channel. Lu-7, the Luo-connecting point of the LUng channel of Hand Tai Yin can treat not only the diseases of the Lung channel (cough, asthma), but also those of the L.I. channel (toothache, head and neck diseases).

As for Du 1, Ren 15, and Sp 21 (The Luo-connecting point of the so-called "Greater Collateral of the Spleen, rules collaterals and blood vessels), they are mainly selected to treat their respective diseased parts and disorders of the internal organs.

**Eight Confluent Points of the Extra Meridians**

"Yi Xue Ru Men" (Introduction to Medicine) says that "among the 360 points on the whole body, 66 points are located at the four extremities are important, and among these 66 points, the Eight Confluent points are considered the most important."

The Eight Confluent points are the points where the extra meridians connect to the 12 primary meridians.

There are four Luo-connecting points among the eight confluent points. They are Pc-6, Sp-4, SJ-5, Lu-7, and two Shu-Stream points which are SI-3 and GB-41. (UB-62, Kid 6 have no function other than their connections to the Eight Extras-Yin Qiao Mai and Yang Qiao Mai.)

In practice, the eight confluent points of extra meridians may be used independently.

Sp-4 for diseases of the Spleen, Stomach, and Chong Mai.

Pc-6 for diseases of the P.C., Heart, San Jiao, and Yin Wei Mai.

Lu-7 for diseases of the Lung, L.I., and Ren Mai.

Ki-6 for diseases of the Kidney and Yin Qiao Mai.

SJ-5 for diseases of the San Jiao, Pericardium and Yang Wei Mai.

GB-41 for diseases of the Gall Bladder, and Dai Mai.

SI-3 for diseases of the Small Intestine and Du Mai.

UB 62 for diseases of the U.B. and Yang Qiao Mai.

The confluent points on the upper limb can be combined with the confluent points on the lower limb.

Sp-4 is combined with PC-6 to specifically treat diseases of the Heart, Chest, and Stomach. (The curative effect is wonderful!)

Lu-7 is combined with Ki-6 to specifically treat diseases of the Lung, chest, throat and diaphragm.

SJ-5 is combined with GB-41 to specifically treat diseases of the outer canthus, ear, shoulder, neck or cheek.

SI-3 is combined with UB 62 to specifically treat diseases of the inner canthus, nape, shoulder.

**Xi-Cleft Points**

Each of the 12 regular channels has one Xi-Cleft point. In addition one Xi-Cleft point can be found on each of Yin Wei, Yang Wei, Yin Qiao, Yang Qiao Channels. There are 16 Xi-Cleft points in all. The Xi-Cleft points are used primarily in treatment of the acute pain and diseases appearing in their corresponding channels and organs can stop pain and/or bleeding.

Xi-Cleft on the Yin channels can stop bleeding.

Example:

Lu 6 for hemoptysis.

Sp 8 for Menorrhagia

Xi-Cleft on the Yang channels can stop pain ,

Example:

L.I. 7 for toothache, sort throat, headache.

St. 34 for Stomachache

Lower He-Sea Points

"The Disorders of the Six Fu organs can be treated by the He-Sea points" (Miraculous Pivot-Ling Shu) According to this theory, the lower He-sea points are selected to treat diseases of their respective Fu organs.

**For instance:**

Dysentery and appendicitis is treated by St-37, because St 37 is the lower He-sea point of the L.I. channel.

UB 39 is used for retention of Urine due to dysfunction of San Jiao.

### Crossing Points

These are points located at the intersection of two or more channels. The channels that cross can be primary, extraordinary, or both. They can be used to treat disorders of each of their pertaining channels. They are often used to treat the diseases simultaneously in meridians intersecting each other.

**For Example:** Sp-6, a crossing point for the three foot yin channels, used for diseases of the liver, spleen and kidney channels.

*Chapter Four*

# Five Elements Theory

According to ancient chinese philosophy this universe as well as it's living creatures are composed of five basic elements, such as wood, fire, earth, metal and water, these also specifically relate to various visceras of the body either of yin or yang mode, the life force flows from one to another of these visceras and influence the bodily physiological functions, likewise for any malfunction of physiological activities the concerned viscera is to be treated to bring normalcy, as balance in percentage of the five elements in the body is essential for normal functioning of the body.Deficiency or excess presence of any of the five elements is also considered to be the basic cause of ailments, which could be ascertained through examination of the tongue for the colour of its coating. Green,black and yellow coating respectively features wood, water and earth deficiency, while a red tongue shows excess fire.In traditional Chinese philosophy, natural phenomena can be classified into the Five Elements (Chinese: pinyin: wÔxíng): wood, fire, earth, metal, and water (mù, huÒ, tÔ, jîn, shÔi). These elements were used for describing interactions and relationships between phenomena. Five phases is another way of translating wÔxíng — literally, "five goings". Traditional Taijiquan schools relate them to footwork and refer to them as five "steps".

The doctrine of five phases describes both a generating (shçng) cycle and an overcoming (kè) cycle of interactions between the phases. In the generating cycle, wood generates fire; fire generates earth; earth generates metal; metal generates water; water generates wood. In the overcoming cycle, wood overcomes earth; earth overcomes water; water overcomes fire; fire overcomes metal; metal overcomes wood.

TCM uses different perspectives to analyze health problems - the 8 Principal Patterns (Exterior/Interior, Excess/Deficiency, Hot/ Cold, Yang/Yin), Pernicious Evils (Wind, Heat, Dampness, Dryness, Cold, and Fire), etc. The 5 Elements is another of those approaches.

Central to understanding the 5 Elements is to realize that Chinese medical therminology often is at the same time very poetic and very literal. For example Wind Cold imbalances are those in which wind and cold do play a role. The Chinese worldview is far more integrated than the typical Western viewpoint. The Western perspective tends to be linear; the Chinese perspective tends to be holistic or weblike. The title of a very famous book on TCM is The Web That Has No Weaver. Pull on any strand in a web, and it will affect all parts of the web. Whereas Western thought tends to look at just what is happening along one strand (linear), holistic thought considers all parts of the web.

The 5 Elements can sound very esoteric to Westerners, and there are some esoteric aspects to it. One way to look at the 5 Elements are they are descriptions of different aspects of energy. But these descriptions of aspects of energy go beyond the Western idea of kinetic-potential energy. And these descriptions are at once both symbolic and literal, and the symbolism grew out of a culture very close to nature.

Think for a movement about what happens in the spring. The weather is starting to WARM. Plants are PUSHING UPWARD out of the soil. Trees are leafing OUT. There is a lot of BIRTH and NEW LIFE in the animal kingdom. ENERGY levels are RISING (in contrast to the winter when people were withdrawn, sleepy, gathered in, slow, etc.). There are new beginings in the spring. There is an explosion of newfound energy released in new growth. This is the element Wood. The spring is the time of increasing Yang (warm, upward, outward, rapid) in contrast to the winter which is the most Yin (cold, downward, inward, slow) time of the year.

The predominate atmospheric energy in the spring, the Wood time of year, is Wind. The summer is the most Yang time of the year. In fact, Yang energy gets so intense at this time of year that it starts to change into its opposite. Whereas people (and animals) tend to be bursting with energy and activity in the spring, at the height of summer the Heat is so much that people start to wear

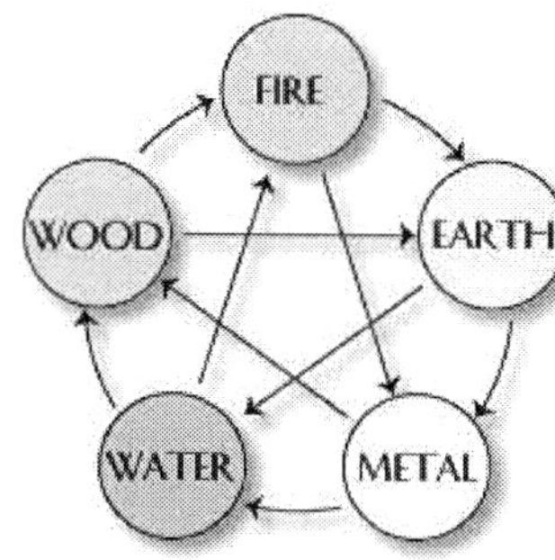


out and slow down. The fall is the time of waning Yang and increasing Yin. People start to slow down, gather inward for the approaching winter. Winter is the most Yin time of year, but after several weeks of being restricted indoors, people begin to long for increased activity and letting loose and getting out. Cabin fever as it's called in the West. Get me out of this house!!!!! I want to go somewhere, do something. Yin begins to decrease and Yang increases in the spring.

If this were just a description of the seasons of the year and their effects on people and animals, there wouldn't be a 5 Elements theory in TCM. As it is, thinking in terms of the 5 Elements has some very practical applications - in terms of understanding some imbalances and in terms of being able to fine-tune treatment. There are relationships between the 5 Elements which can be used in healing.

The 5 Elements are Wood, Fire, Earth, Metal, and Water. Wood is linked to the spring, the Liver (Yin Wood), the Gall Bladder (Yang Wood), the East, and Wind. Fire is linked to the summer, the Heart (Yin Fire), the Small Intestine (Yang Fire), the South, and Heat. Earth is linked to late summer, the Spleen (Yin Earth), the Stomach (Yang Earth), the center, and Dampness. Metal is linked to the fall, the Lungs (Yin Metal), the Large Intestine (Yang Metal), the West, and Dryness. Water is linked to the winter, the Kidneys (Yin Water), the Bladder (Yang Water), the north, and Cold.

This is not just an artificial system of correspondences that sounds nice and poetic. The Kidneys do tend to be very vulnerable to Cold. The Liver does tend to be particularly vulnerable to Wind, the Spleen to Dampness, the Heart to Heat, and the Lungs to Dryness. In many places in the world the spring does tend to be the most windy time of the year, the summer the hottest, the late summer the most humid, the fall dry, and the winter cold. One thing one learns quickly to do in TCM is to pay attention to the weather especially very extreme weather (like an unusually windy spring) and unseasonable weather (like cold snaps in the summer or warm spells in the winter). Extreme and/or unseasonable weather will tend to trigger health imbalances in many people. There will tend to be an increase in certain problems during or immediately following certain seasons. For example, the Liver is the Yin Wood Organ, and cases of infectious hepatitis and cases of pink eye do tend to be more numerous in the spring than at other times of the year. (In TCM the Liver is said to "open into the eyes".) Some people do tend to have kidney and bladder problems more often and more severe in the winter than at other times of the year. Some people do tend to have more digestive system problems when it's very humid.etc.

But this is not all there is to the 5 Element Theory. The 5 Element Theory also maps relationships between Elements which have practical applications both in diagnosis and treatment.

One of the best known of these 5 Element relationships is the Mother-Son rule. This states that if one tonifies the Mother, the Son automatically is tonified. If one sedates the Mother, the Son automatically is sedated. Wood is the Mother of Fire, Fire is the Mother of Earth, Earth is the Mother of Metal, Metal is the Mother of Water, and Water is the Mother of Wood. A good way to remember part of this sequence is that when one burns Wood with Fire, ash (Earth) results. Metal is found within Earth - Earth is the Mother of Metal. Water makes possible the growth of Wood. Water is the Mother of Wood.

Now, let's take this from the realm of the merely poetic to the realm of the practical. Let's look a little closer at Water is the Mother of Wood. The Kidneys is the Yin Water Organ; the Liver is the Yin Wood Organ. There is a condition in TCM called Liver Yin Deficiency. There also is a condtion called Liver and Kidney Yin Deficiency. In some cases of Liver Yin Deficiency, the Deficiency of Yin is just in the Liver, and treatment is directed toward increasing Liver Yin. Simple, straightforward. But what about those cases where both Liver and Kidney Yin Deficiency are present? What happens if one just tonifies Liver Yin? You have to keep on and keep on and keep on tonifying Liver Yin because the Root of the problem is that there's not enough Yin in the Kidneys for the Kidneys (the Mother) to pass onto the Liver (the Son). The Kidneys supply the

Yin for the Liver (and for the entire body for that matter). The Liver and Gall Bladder may be weak and prone to problems because the Kidneys are weak and not supplying what the Liver needs. The Organ Theory in TCM states that the Liver and Gall Bladder almost never are Qi Deficient. (Maciocia, Foundations, p. 303) But in the real world, one will run into cases where weak Kidneys appear to be dragging down Liver function. The Organ Theory doesn't account for many of these cases, but the 5 Elements Theory does, and what is more important, the 5 Elements Theory gives general guidelines for treatment. Tonify/ sedate the Mother in order to tonify/ sedate the Son. When one starts to look at some findings from Western medicine from a TCM 5 Elements perspective, the 5 Elements Theory starts to look even more valid. For example, certain liver problems can be traced to problems in the kidneys and urinary system. One role of the liver recognized by Western physiology is to detoxify certain things in the body. The kidneys get rid of certain waste products. If the kidneys are not doing their job of waste excretion properly, this can cause an overload on the liver and lead to some liver problems. Likewise, a poorly functioning liver can overburden the kidneys. Sometimes, a big part of effective healing is knowing which problem(s) to start with, to concentrate on first, and the 5 Elements Theory can give extra insight into this.

There are other guidelines in the 5 Elements Theory, but I won't go into those today. I recommend learning the basics of 5 Elements Theory, and starting to consider this perspective when analyzing and correcting imblances. Being able to use this theory can add that little extra understanding that can make a great deal of difference in proper treatment, especially when faced with "knotty" (complicated) problems that aren't responding satisfactory to treatment. The 5 Elements Theory is used primarily in acupuncture, but being aware of certain relationships and general treatment guidelines per the 5 Elements Theory can give herbalists that little extra insight that can make the difference between satisfactory and unsatifactory outcomes.

Because Traditional Chinese Medicine is holistic, each organ cannot be explained fully unless the TCM relationship/ homeostasis with the other organs is understood. TCM also looks at the functions of the organs rather than fixed areas and, therefore, describes different organs that are not actually physical, like the San Jiao. This also leads to controversy about the validity of TCM, which comes a lot from the difficulty of translating and lack knowledge about TCM concepts and Chinese culture. So, to avoid conflict and to keep an open mind, please realize that these notions evolved in a different culture and are a different way of viewing the human body.

Zang-Fu theory translates roughly into "theory about solid organ-hollow organ". It is a concept within traditional Chinese medicine and part of the TCM model of the body. There are five zang and six fu . The association between the zangfu and particular souls or spirits is a later accretion and has been largely absent from the discourse of traditional Chinese medicine for at least the past 200 years.

This theory treats each of the Zang organs as organs that nourish the body. The Zang systems include organs, senses, emotions, and the musculoskeletal system—essentially, the entire person divided into five categorical systems. Zang organs are also known as yin organs, and each has a Fu partner, a yang organ (see Yin Yang). Fu organs can be viewed as hollow organs that aid in digestion. In addition to bodily functions, each Zang organ is the home of an aspect of the spirit.

With a thorough understanding of the Zang Fu organs, practitioners can achieve therapeutic results accordingly. The theory is always in service of practical, therapeutic application, with the goal of an "elegant" treatment. An elegant treatment uses the least amount of force for the greatest therapeutic benefit, and requires true mastery of the art of traditional Chinese Medicine.

The five elements are associated energetically with the following Zang-Fu organs:

Wood: Liver, home of the Hun (Ethereal Soul), paired with the Gall Bladder

Fire: Heart, home of the Shen (Aggregate Soul) paired with the Small intestine (and secondarily, the San Jiao or Triple burner and Pericardium)

Earth: Spleen, home of the Yi (Intellect), paired with the Stomach

Water: Kidney, home of the Zhi (Will), paired with the Bladder
Metal: Lung, home of the Po (Corporeal Soul), paired with the Large Intestine

The doctrine of five phases was employed in many fields of early Chinese philosophy, including seemingly disparate fields such as music, medicine, and military strategy.

Correlations between the five elements and other categories:

The Yuèlìng chapter of the Lîjì and the Huáinánzî make the following correlations:

| Element | Direction | Color | Musical Note |
|---|---|---|---|
| Wood | east | blue/green | jué (mi) |
| Fire | south | red | zhî (sol) |
| Earth | center | yellow | gông (do) |
| Metal | west | white | shâng (re) |
| Water | north | black | yû (la) |

| Element | Heavenly creature | Season | Direction | Planet | Tastes | Sense | Viscera | Finger |
|---|---|---|---|---|---|---|---|---|
| Wood | Qîng-lóng the Green Dragon | Spring | east | Jupiter | sour | sight | liver | ring finger |
| Fire | Zhû-què the Red Phoenix | Summer | south | Mars | bitter | sound | heart | middle finger |
| Earth | Huáng-lóng the yellow Dragon | Change of seasons | center | Saturn | sweet | smell | spleen | index finger |
| Metal | **Bái-hû** the White Tiger | Autumn | west | Venus | hot | taste | lung | thumb |
| Water | **Xuán-wû** the Black Tortoise-Serpent | Winter | north | Mercury | salty | touch | kidney | little finger |

Some other correspondences are shown below:

The elements have also been correlated to the eight trigrams of the I Ching:

| Element | I Ching | Trigrams |
|---|---|---|
| Wood | Wind, thunder | :\|\| (xùn) \|:: (zhèn) |
| Fire | Fire | \|:\| (lí) |
| Earth | Earth, mountain | ::: (kûn) ::\| (gèn) |
| Metal | Sky, lake | \|\|\| (qián) \|\|: (duì) |
| Water | Water | :\|: (kǎn) |

Acupuncture treats the human body as a whole that involves several "systems of function" that are in many cases associated with (but not identified on a one-to-one basis with) physical organs. Some systems of function, such as the "triple heater" (San Jiao, also called the "triple burner") have no corresponding physical organ. Disease is understood as a loss of homeostasis among the several systems of function, and treatment of disease is attempted by modifying the activity of one or more systems of function through the activity of needles, pressure, heat, etc. on sensitive parts of the body of small volume traditionally called "acupuncture points" in English, or "xue" (cavities).

There are twelve primary channels, called meridians, which run vertically, bilaterally, and symmetrically and every channel corresponds to and connects internally with one of the twelve Zang Fu ("organs"). This means that there are six yin and six yang channels. There are three yin and three yang channels on each arm, and three yin and three yang on each leg.

The three yin channels of the hand (Lung, Pericardium, and Heart) begin on the chest and travel along the inner surface (mostly the anterior portion) of the arm to the hand.

The three yang channels of the hand (Large Intestine, San Jiao and Small Intestine) begin on the hand and travel along the outer surface (mostly the posterior portion) of the arm to the head.

The three yang channels of the foot (Stomach, Gallbladder, and Bladder) begin on the face, in the region of the eye, and travels down the body and along the outer surface (mostly the anterior and lateral portion) of the leg to the foot.

The three yin channels of the foot (Spleen, Liver and Kidney) begin of the foot and travel along the inner surface (mostly posterior and medial portion) of the leg to the chest or flank.

The flow of qi through each of the twelve channels is comprised of an internal and an external pathway. The external pathway is what is normally shown on an acupuncture chart and it is relatively superficial. All the acupuncture points of a channel lie on its external pathway. The internal pathways are the deep course of the channel where it enters the body cavities and related Zang-Fu organs. The superficial pathways of the twelve channels describe three complete circuits of the body.

The flow of energy through the meridians is as follows: Lung channel of hand taiyin to Large Intestine channel of hand yangming to Stomach channel of foot yangming to Spleen channel of foot taiyin to Heart channel of hand shaoyin to Small Intestine channel of hand taiyang to Bladder channel of foot taiyang to Kidney channel of foot shaoyin to Pericardium channel of hand jueyin to San Jiao channel of hand shaoyang to Gallbladder channel of foot shaoyang to Liver channel of foot jueyin then back to the Lung channel of hand taiyin →

| **(Zang)** | | **(Fu)** |
|---|---|---|
| Lungs | ← | Large Intestine |
| Spleen | → | Stomach |
| Heart | ← | Small Intestine |
| Kidneys | → | Bladder |
| Pericardium | ← | San Jiao |
| Liver | | Gallbladder |

Traditional Chinese medical theory holds that acupuncture works by normalizing the "flow" of qi "vital energy" in the body. Pain or illnesses are treated by attempting to remedy local or systemic accumulations or deficiencies of qi. Pain is considered to indicate blockage or stagnation of the flow of qi, and an axiom of the medical literature of acupuncture is "no pain, no blockage; no blockage, no pain".

While it is claimed by some that there is no physical evidence for the existence of qi or for its claimed effects, and that acupuncture is therefore a pseudoscience or metaphysical belief, many patients experience the sensations of stimulus known in Chinese as "deqi" (得氣obtaining the qi") This kind of sensation was historically considered to be evidence of effective treatment. Often deqi takes the form of a propagation of sensation along the trajectory of the so-called acupuncture "channels" or meridians. Research into the phenomena of "deqi" has mostly been conducted in China and Japan.

Treatment of acupuncture points may be performed along the 12 main or 8 extra meridians located throughout the body. 10 of the main meridians are named after organs of the body (Heart, Liver etc.) two after so called body functions (Heart Protector or Pericardium, and San Jiao, "triple heater"). The two most important of the eight "extra" meridians are situated on the midline of the anterior and posterior aspects of the trunk and head.

The acupuncturist will decide which points to treat by thoroughly questioning the patient, and utilizing the diagnostic skills of traditional Chinese medicine such as observation of the left and right radial pulses at three levels of imposed pressure.

As illustrated above, according to ancient chinese philosophy the universe as well as it's living creatures are composed of these five basic elements, such as wood, fire, earth, metal and water, and these elements specifically  connected to various visceras of either yin or yang, the life force flows from one to another of the visceras and influence the bodily physiological functions, as balance in percentage of these five elements of the body is essential for normal functioning, likewise for any malfunction of physiological functions the concerned viscera is to be treated to bring back normalcy.

Deficiency or excess presence of any of the five elements is also considered to be the basic cause of ailments, which could be ascertained through examination of tongue for the colour of it's coating. Green, black and yellow coatings respectively feature wood, water and earth deficiency, while a red tongue shows excess fire.

**Chinese Body Clock:**

East and West have independently discovered repeating patterns of changes occurring in our bodies throughout the day. These are known as the Chinese Body-Clock and chronotherapy.

The Chinese Body-Clock is a system that describes how energy peaks in each meridian (or organ function) for two hours in every 24-hour period. This concept is also known as the Law of Midday-Midnight.

As an example, the Stomach meridian energy peaks from 7 am to 9 am, so this is the optimal time to take nourishment. Western Medicine also places importance on eating a good breakfast.

To help diagnosis and treatment planning, acupuncturists note the time of day when a symptom appears. If a patient wakes at a certain time, the practitioner may look at the corresponding meridian (line of energy that relates to organ function) to see if it is disturbed or blocked.

In contrast,according to ancient chinese belief the regular twelve channels which correspond to the twelve visceras have specific time of treatment when according to ancient believe the visceras work in their full vigour.

The clock or time table is as under:

| Hours | Organ |
|---|---|
| 3 AM- 5 AM | Lung |
| 5 AM- 7 AM | Large Intestine |
| 7 AM- 9 AM | Stomach |
| 9 AM-11 AM | Spleen |
| 11 AM-1 PM | Heart |
| 1 PM- 3 PM | Small Intestine |
| 3 PM- 5 PM | Urinary Bladder |
| 5 PM- 7 PM | Kidney |
| 7 PM- 9 PM | Pericardium |

| | |
|---|---|
| 9 PM-11 PM | San Jiao |
| 11 PM-1 AM | Gall Bladder |
| 1 AM- 3 AM | Liver |

While the Chinese Body-Clock has been around for thousands of years, Western medicine recently developed the concept of Chronotherapy, using the same ideas. Chronotherapy is the concept of taking drugs at the time they are most needed by the body. Both the Chinese Body-Clock and chronotherapy fit a 24-hour body cycle called the circadian rhythm.

Western medicine reports that circadian changes are seen in normal lung function, which reaches a low point in the early morning hours. This dip is especially pronounced in people with asthma. Lung meridian time is 3am to 5am. Here again, East and West say the same thing.

Another time of interest is Large Intestine time (from 5am to 7am). It is recommended that if you have a problem with "elimination" that you use this time to establish a normal bowel pattern.

*Chapter Five*

# Diagnosis in Traditional Chinese Medicine

When people tell about diagnosis they take it to imply that what specific symptoms are related to the person. In reality the manifestation of any given symptom indicates by its presence on a prior constitutional weakness that allowed it to be expressed. In other words, the patient had either a genetic and/or karmic predisposition that allowed this symptom to become manifest. The inner tradition focuses on constitutional issues which comprise that aspect of self that can never fundamentally be changed because it comprises one's inborn nature. Medicine can help compensate for our constitutional weaknesses but cannot ultimately change what has been present from conception. Hence the inner tradition does not focus on achieving a cure as an end point of treatment. Rather, the focus is placed on guiding the patient through the process of healing. A condition is considered to be healed when it no longer limits a patient's self-expression or hinders quality of life.

Even after substantial improvement, all symptoms, like habits, have a tendency to return. After all, the constitutional basis that allowed them to manifest in the first place is still present, and all people tend to fall back into their old patterns of behavior. When a patient initially comes for treatment, he or she may be suffering from migraine headaches four days a week. The condition may be so debilitating that the patient is virtually unable to function. After a successful course of treatment, the patient may have only one or two migraine headaches a year. The patient whose quality of life is now greatly improved may tell friends that the headaches have been cured. It is clear, however, that the patient still has the same inner disposition that created the headaches in the first place.

Ultimately, symptoms are warning signs of deeper imbalance. Patients must learn to recognize their symptoms in their early stages before they become fully manifest. They may then learn to make the appropriate internal shifts necessary to avoid becoming ill. As people heal, they must be encouraged to think of their symptoms as signs that some internal matter needs attending to. By taking responsibility for maintaining their own health, patients are less dependent on the healer and should need treatment with decreasing frequency.

In TCM it is vitally importantly that one listens to what the client has to say. This is vitally important in all systems of healing, but TCM recognizes how critical it is. The weakest link in any healing system is always analysis/ diagnosis. Proper treatment depends on the proper analysis of the underlying root.

TCM healers not only listen to what clients say, they listen and observe the way clients say thing. For example, if speech is rapid, this suggests a problem with Heat. Heat speeds things up (the speech, the pulse, the body movements). If the speech is slow, this suggests a problem with Cold because Cold slows things down (the speech, the pulse, the movements).

There will be variations based on other factors. For example, in the U.S., people raised in the North, in particular in New York City will tend to speak a lot more rapidly than people raised in the South. These are regional differences that need to be taken into account. But in general, when things are speeded up (speech, pulse, movements) suspect and rule in or rule out a Heat problem. When things are slowed, suspect and rule in or rule out a Cold problem. (One important exception to Cold slowing things down is that well-conditioned athletes will have slower than normal pulses.)

The loudness and the force of the voice tends to be important clues too though not as exact as the fast-slow thing indicating possible Heat-Cold problems. In general, loud voices and a forceful manner of speaking will point to Excess conditions (problems caused by there being too much of something). In general, a low, quiet voice and a lack of forcefulness in speaking (or moving) will point to Deficiency conditions (problems caused by there not being enough of something). I say "in general" because there are a lot of exceptions to this one. For example, a person with severe Excess Cold problems probably won't be very loud or very forceful.

One area of Western medicine that is all but neglected is that people with a given medical condition will tend to say certain things which are typical of that condition. For example, some of the typical comments made by a person with CFIDS are "exercise makes me sicker, alcohal makes me feel worse, I have to rest up for special activities and then rest up afterwards to recover, I never know how I'm going to feel from day to day or hour to hour or even minute to minute," etc. Diabetics may talk about "nervous energy", and may make comments like "I feel like I have to keep busy and do something, but I'm too tired to be keeping busy." (BTW, this is a comment that also is typical of Yin Deficiency. Yin Deficiency frequently is a factor in diabetes, BUT Yin Deficiency doesn't always manifest as diabetes. Yin Deficiency may be marked by both agitation and fatigue. As far as I know it's the only TCM syndrome which is marked by both fatigue and agitation. There are a lot of TCM syndromes that can manifest as fatigue, and there are several which can manifest as agitation, but Yin Deficiency is the one which can manifest as both agitation and fatigue. So when you hear someone talk about having "nervous energy" even though they're tired, automatically consider the possibility of Yin Deficiency and rule in or rule out. You'll need to rule in/ rule out because it also is possible that a person may be suffering from more than one TCM syndrome - one that accounts for fatigue and another that manifests as agitation.)

What I'm talking about here goes beyond the usual noting of symptom profiles in Western medicine (i.e., fatigue, thrist, increased urination, etc). It involves learning to watch out for specific comments (as well as manner of saying things things) that people with a specific problem typically will say.

Western doctors used to pay a lot more attention to learning typical comments than they do today. This practice has all but died out in Western medicine. However, it never died out in TCM and has remained a mainstay of analysis in TCM. In TCM, typical comments frequently are listed in the profiles for TCM syndromes.

One of the most well-known of the typical comments in TCM is "plum pit in the throat." People in cultures beside China may talk about a feeling of a "stone in the throat". People in the U.S. may talk about "having a lump in the throat". The central idea in these descriptions is the feeling of an obstruction in the throat. This points very, very strongly to Liver Qi Stagnation. So when you hear someone talk about a plum pit, a stone, a lump, or some other obstruction in the throat (when there is no actual obstruction like a tumor in the throat), automatically think about the possibility of Liver Qi Stagnation and rule in or rule out.)

The feeling of an obstruction in the throat (when there's not an actual physical obstruction) is very, very suggestive of Liver Qi Stagnation in particular. However, there are other comments that can suggest Qi Stagnation in general. For example, if a person comes in and complains of feeling "tight" or "things needing to loosen up" or "things not moving very smoothly", suspect Qi Stagnation problems. Note: Some people with Qi Stagnation problems will actually report after taking herbs to move Qi or after acupuncture or after starting Qi Gong exercises that "it feels like things are loosening up on the inside". They may also talk about feeling more relaxed.

If someone talks about hating winter, automatically consider the possibility of Cold problems. It may be an abnormal sensitivity to Exterior Cold invading to the Interior or Deficiency Cold (Yang Deficiency - not enough Yang energy in the body to warm the body properly). If someone talks about hating the summer and having more problems in the summer than at other times of the year, automatically consider Heat problems

The Three Levels: Body, Mind, and Spirit

Using the language of classical Chinese medicine it is impossible to talk of the separation implied by the English words body, mind, and spirit. Hence the character xin refers to the physical, emotional, and spiritual heart. The Chinese language uses one term, xin, that has a multitude of meanings implicit within it. On the other hand, the English language uses three terms, body, mind, and spirit, to address what is implicitly thought to represent a unified whole, namely, the human being. Think of each of the five elements as comprised of spiritual, emotional, and physical realms of being. For example, the spiritual aspect of the wood element corresponds to the hun and its ability to be in contact with jing in a way that informs one of his or her life plan. The mental aspect of wood involves the decision-making faculties of the gallbladder which transmit the potential of that plan into the world. The physical aspects of wood are comprised by the actual organs of the liver and gallbladder, as well as all material aspects of being associated with these officials such as the tendons, ligaments, eyes, and the course of the liver and gallbladder meridians.

The functional basis of disharmony may emanate primarily from the physical, emotional, or the deeper realms of spiritual being. For example, a lack of benevolence and the presence of belligerence indicate dysfunction in the spiritual and emotional realms of the wood element. It is quite possible, however, that at the time of the assessment the patient exhibits no physical symptomatology in the wood element. A patient diagnosed with hepatitis C, a severe physical illness of the liver, however, may be perfectly healthy in the spiritual and emotional domains of liver function. Hence the patient may be tranquilly benevolent and possess healthy self-esteem. Identifying the level of being that perpetuates dysfunction in each patient is a primary task for the practitioner of the inner tradition.

Of the three depths, the spirit possesses the capacity to move most quickly. In just one moment, the spirit may heal in a way that binds one again to true self and one's life purpose. Healing in this way is signaled by increased experience of the virtues associated with one's constitutional type. Hence a person who is wood constitutionally will be better able to experience the virtue of benevolence as it exists at his or her core. Increased contact with one's source of virtue corresponds to a restitution of the basis of one's capacity for intuition.

The mind's capacity to heal is somewhat slower than the spirit's. Although profound insight may occur in a moment, the tendency of the mind is to continually fall back into habituated patterns of thought and belief. Only commitment to manifesting innate virtues paired with conscious vigilance can prevent the mind from seizing control and motivating one's attitudes and actions. Healing of the mind is signaled by an increase of behaviors that reflect one's constitutional virtues. While the spirit may know virtue, it is the mind that governs the movement of qi and wills actions that are consistent with fulfilling destiny.

Of the three depths, the body takes the longest to heal. Once a functional imbalance has manifested physically, it is relatively more concrete and harder to influence through treatment. Spirit is that which allows us to be in contact with virtue, and mind is that which allows our actions to reflect virtue. After original nature is lost and one is separated from the source of virtue, it takes many years of dysfunctional thought and behavior for illness to become embodied. Although spirit and mind may move toward healing relatively quickly, it will again take years for correct thought and action to be once again embodied as physical health.

This last assertion may contradict what some believe to be true about acupuncture. After all, many people experience long-lasting relief from chronic pain with just a few acupuncture treatments. One such example is John discussed in Chapter 10, whose pain associated with eight years of polyneuropathy disappeared after only one session. However, immediate relief of this nature is predicated in large part on movement of spirit and mind and often does not reflect a true physical healing at all. Despite his decrease of pain and renewed positive outlook, any objective measure such as a test of nerve conduction velocity would have revealed that my patient still had polyneuropathy. Imbalances of spirit and mind take years to become embodied as physical illness. Rectification of the spirit and mind may lead a person to feel better long before the physical embodiment of dysfunction is actually healed. It is therefore imperative to guide people to live in a healthier way so that true healing is promoted and the tendency to recreate one's illness is mitigated.

This preceding discussion illustrates an important premise in the inner tradition: Therapeutic measures administered with the intention of promoting healing will be received by the deepest aspects of self that perpetuate dysfunction. Of course, the focus of constitutional diagnosis is to direct healing toward the deepest aspects of the patient's being. One's constitutional dynamics are the basis for all expressions of true self in life. In directing treatment to this depth, the practitioner lays a foundation for subsequent healing by attending primarily to the most essential aspects of being. These principles are also present physiologically. Functional imbalances often begin with excessive physical and/or emotional work and then proceed to qi, blood, yin, yang, and ultimately jing deficiency. Deficiency of jing signifies the physiological depth of an imbalance. If a patient is jing deficient one must tonify this root of the imbalance to promote substantial healing.

If the symptoms of dysfunction are suppressed, illness will be driven deeper into the level of being that perpetuates imbalance and subsequently increase dysfunction in the other levels of being. If an imbalance of spirit is treated in a way that suppresses its expression, then the root of the imbalance will continue to perpetuate dysfunction as the patient becomes increasingly distanced from original nature. Eventually what began as a spirit-level dysfunction may become embodied as physical illness. For example, a patient who has been physically abused and subsequently experiences rage and depression may be given antidepressants as a long-term intervention. These drugs do not address the root cause of the problem, however, that may be located in the spiritual depth of the liver official. In time, the spiritual dysfunction that has been unattended to will undermine the functioning of the mind and body, ultimately leading to physical illness.

In contrast, illness may begin in the physical realm with the invasion of an external wind/cold pathogen. In this case antibiotics may be administered that eliminate the bacterial source of the infection but do nothing to eliminate the wind/cold. Excess heat generated as the body attempts to move the stagnation of cold will, over time, consume fluids. Depletion of fluids, in turn, will predictably lead to the more serious state of lung yin deficiency. By the time the yin of the lungs is injured, the imbalance is likely to have entered the spirit and emotional realms and the patient may evidence grief, longing, and difficulty receiving quality in life. Note that the suppression of symptoms is not limited to the inappropriate use of Western medical interventions. Treatment in any modality that eliminates pain but does not educate the patient has the potential to perpetuate ignorance and drive illness deeper.

There are numerous methods by which a practitioner of TCM will obtain diagnostic information by viewing the face. The system represented on this page is one of many. This one most closely represents the system presented in the classic Chinese text: "Simple Questions." It was further modified by Dr. Tian De Yang.

Any colors inappropriate to the normal color of the area would suggest a pathology. Most often we look for the five colors in the face. For instance, if we were to see the color green in the forehead region we might look for further confirmations of pathology associated with "wood overacting on earth." Or the Liver's function causing problems in the digestive system.

It is interesting to note that even with the wide varieties of colors represented by different races, there is still a superficial color that can arise atop the "host" color which, would then be useful for diagnostic purposes.

**Color in Diagnosis**

People's complexions are different because their physical constitutions are different. Even for the same person, the complexion constantly changes according to the fluctuation of the emotions and the difference in the state of health. The complexion turns bluish when extremely angry, reddish when happy, blackish when fearful, whitish when worrying and yellowish when overthinking. The proverbs that say, "The face is turning like black ink" and "The face is becoming black and blue" imply sudden emotional changes such as fear, shock or rage. The face of a teenager coming out after being interrogated for charges of theft is whitish and the face of a student coming out of an examination hall is yellowish. Also, a person who thinks too much usually has digestive problems and a person with digestive problems has a yellowish complexion. A person who laughs a lot has vigorous activity of the Heart and a reddish complexion and a person who worries a lot sighs constantly and has a whitish complexion. Accordingly, the conditions of the internal organs can be observed with the colors that show on the surface of the body. These colors are not just manifested on the face, but there are also differences in the pigment of feces, urine, menstrual blood, vaginal discharge, tongue coating, lips, eyes, phlegm, etc.

### Color and its Related Organ

Red is related to the Heart, white to the Lungs, yellow to the Spleen, blue/green to the Liver and black to the Kidneys.

### Red and the Heart

Red is the color of the Fire Element, so red light is a light that is related to the Heart. A face turns reddish when the activity of the Heart is exuberant, thus joyful emotion, fever or even drinking alcoholic beverages turns the face reddish. All of them definitely arise from the exuberant activity of the Heart. However, the health of the Heart should not be inferred from the appearance of the color red. There are both healthy and unhealthy shades of red. Red is the color with the longest wavelength so it is a Yang color. In bull fighting, shaking a red object in front of the bull's eyes makes him even more fierce. In cardiac edema, the face color becomes reddish purple or brownish.

### White and the Lungs

White is a color related to the Lungs. A person who worries a lot constantly sighs and has a whitish complexion. Also, a person with constitutionally weak Lungs generally has a whitish complexion. This person can maintain his or her health as long as he or she does not get a reddish glow. However, if he or she does get a reddish glow, like the color of a peach blossom, it is an indication that a lung disease is in progress. A person who has a white complexion with luster is magnanimous with profound thoughts, so there are many who have the character of a big time politician - the so-called noble type - with this complexion.

### Yellow and the Spleen

Yellow is the color of the Earth Element, so the Spleen and the Stomach are like the Earth. The Spleen produces Blood and the Stomach ingests nutrients in order to produce the flesh, similar to the Earth nurturing all things in nature. A person with strong digestive organs has a yellowish complexion with luster and a person with a disease of the digestive organs has a sallow complexion and is emaciated, fatigued or has a diseased color that is hard to describe with words.

### Blue and the Liver

A red color is due to the congestion of arterial blood. As the result of strong heart activity, a large amount of arterial blood flows too quickly and the duration in which the blood is in contact with the tissues is too short. Accordingly, a fresh red color shows up because there are large quantities of oxygen within the blood since a small amount of oxygen is transferred to the tissues. A blue color occurs as a result of the stagnation of venous blood in the tissues (or dark purplish or blackish color). The stagnation of venous blood is a phenomenon that appears when the activity of the heart is weak. The organ that regulates the activity of the Heart is the Liver. Perhaps the liver secretes a blue colored substance.

Blue is a color with a short wavelength so it settles and calms. One gets excited when looking at the color red, but settles down when looking at the color blue. Having transcendental or sentimental feelings without particular reasons when looking at blue/green mountains or going into the forest is largely due to receiving the influence of that color. It is said that shaking a blue cloth in front of fierce cattle and in front of a horse calms them down.

What is the necessity of the Liver to manifest the color blue? It can be explained by the following reasons. The color blue is a light that settles and calms, thus impeding activities. Recall that the Liver is an organ in charge of combat and a motive for combat is anger. As such, the emotion of anger belongs to the Liver and in times of anger the color blue appears. The color blue has two functions that are needed in combat. One is to internally curtail the activity of the Heart. In other words, it saves and accumulates energy then lets it out forcefully all at once in order to fight fiercely. Another is to show the color blue externally toward an opponent to settle and suppress his activity and at the same time to give him feelings of fear. This is why a person who normally has a bluish complexion becomes highly sensitive, angers easily and often has indigestion. This indigestion arises from the opposing relationship between Liver and Spleen, that is Wood and Earth.

## Black and the Kidneys

Black is the color of Water and Yin-Coldness. Also, nighttime is dark. The com-plexion becomes dark when one is cold and also when one is feeling great fear. A person who normally has a black complexion, like a frightened person, is very weak sexually and has little courage. A healthy person with a black complexion is said in a proverb to have "Iron black color," so he is extremely strong sexually and has boundless energy. The color of the skin changes as a sign of pregnancy and there is a black color like freckles and blotches on the forehead, on the bridge of the nose, around the eyes, around the mouth, etc. In the center line of the abdominal wall, namely the "Conception channel,"13 a colored pigment settles in which is black and a dark brown color settles in the external genital region and vagina.

In general, the black color can be seen in Basedow's disease, which is seen as the result of hyperthyroidism or in acromegaly (a disease with the enlargement of nose, mandible, ends of extremities and the whole body), which is seen as the result of the hyperfunction of the frontal lobe of the pituitary gland. The relationship of black to the Kidneys can be recognized if a certain amount of attention is paid. Edema due to a kidney disease can be distinguished by the complexion being a dark white color, as opposed to a reddish purple color of edema due to heart disease. The color white belongs to the Lungs and dark color belongs to the Kidneys, so the Lungs and Kidneys are: "Metal and Water Zang organs of mutual generation."

## Healthy Color and Unhealthy Color (Techniques of Observing Color)

It is extremely difficult to explain this healthy and unhealthy color in words. There is no other way than to train the power of observation by paying attention to the color of the complexion of as many people as possible. It is the same as the teller of a bank being able to easily discern counterfeit notes but not being able to explain their method of discovery to anyone else. There will be no other words than merely, "somehow it feels different." The colors of the complexions of people are difficult to explain, but there is something on which to judge whether it is healthy or unhealthy by observation. This judgement of health and sickness on the basis of color has great importance in Oriental medicine: "Observing the shape and watching the color"14 reflects this. In reality, "Observing the shape and watching the color" is not only necessary in Oriental medicine, but also in Western medicine and in observing the emotions of other people in our daily lives. It is hard to avoid getting blamed for being ambiguous regarding this observation of color, but I am going to state a few essential points.

### Method of Observing Color (Presence of Qi; Absence of Qi; Presence of Spirit; Absence of Spirit)

When observing the complexion of a person, one must be careful about the existence or absence of Qi and Spirit. In everyday conversation, terms such as "Color of Qi looks bad" or "Color of the Spirit is good" are frequently used. "Qi" and "Spirit" are abstract expressions of the movement of life which we can sense. When they are further differen-tiated, Qi is an abstract expression of the emotion and Spirit is an abstract expression of the life force or the state of health. The "color of Qi not being so good" means that there is emotional trouble and the "color of Spirit not being so good" implies that it looks as though there is a disease.

Complexion, regardless of the type of its color, must have vitality. As long as there is vitality, the color of Spirit will be good even if one is emaciated and as long as there is no vitality, the color of Spirit will be bad even if one is plump. A person has a particular complexion according to individual characteristics and that complexion changes according to living conditions. A farmer who constantly gets sunlight has dark skin and a scholar who constantly studies indoors has fair skin. However, receiving the same degree of sunlight still results in all different complexions and studying indoors in the same degree also results in different complexions; these are all due to individual characteristics. The skin is a healthy color especially when there is vitality. When there is vitality in a reddish complexion, the Heart is strong and when there is no vitality, the Heart has become fatigued by excessive activity.

**Red Color**

Presence of Spirit - Exuberant Heart Qi

Absence of Spirit - Decline in Heart Qi

**White Color**

Presence of Spirit - Exuberant Lung Qi

Absence of Spirit - Decline in Lung Qi

**Yellow Color**

Presence of Spirit - Exuberant Spleen Qi

Absence of Spirit - Decline in Spleen Qi

**Blue Color**

Presence of Spirit - Exuberant Liver Qi

Absence of Spirit - Decline in Liver Qi

**Black Color**

Presence of Spirit - Exuberant Kidney Qi

Absence of Spirit - Decline in Kidney Qi

### Mutual Generating and Controlling Cycles in Complex Colors

The color of a person's complexion does not simply appear in one color among the five colors, but the five colors appear in small amounts, thus a so-called red or blue implies the strongest color among them. Accordingly, to observe color in practice is extraordinarily complicated, but it is generally enough to diagnose health or illness entirely through the presence or absence of vitality. Yet there are times when only one type of color shows up strongly or at times two, three, four or five types of colors appear strongly, all individually following the channels. When all five colors appear together, it is a sign that the time of death is drawing near. A color of an autumn leaf showing up on the complexion of a sick person is said to be inauspicious because an autumn leaf has red, yellow, blue, white and black colors.

When many colors are combined, observation under the following standards will generally be very helpful:

The colors of Zang organs in a mutual generating relationship are good. For example, a combination of yellow and white (Earth generates Metal), white and black (Metal generates Water), black and blue (Water generates Wood), blue and red (Wood generates Fire), and red and yellow (Fire generates Earth) reflect no problems in general.

When the colors of Zang organs in the mutual controlling relationship are combined, it is generally unhealthy. For example:

### Red and White (Fire controls Metal)

Since this is a color of peach-blossoms, it is the most brilliant color, but it is an extremely bad color when observed from the point of view of health and longevity. This color shows up mostly among patients under 30 years old with a lung disease. The following statements illustrate why this color is unhealthy: "A young man with brilliance, easily acquiring wealth and fame, is a sign of early withering," "A young man with a blossomed flower complexion dies young" and "Men of talent and beauty all die young."

### White and Blue (Metal controls Wood)

This means having a bluish pale complexion. It is a color commonly seen in older women who were widowed at a young age. This is the complexion of a person weakened by a long time of continued strong resentment (Liver) and grief (Lung). Yin-type lung disease patients generally possess this complexion.

### Blue and Yellow (Wood controls Earth)

A green color results when these two colors are combined; jaundice seems to belong here. Other than the green color in the pigment of bile, I have not been able to find examples to clearly explain this color, but I believe that this complexion will be found if many patients are observed.

### Yellow and Black (Earth controls Water)

This color can be seen frequently in chronic diseases of the stomach, especially in gastric atony.

### Black and Red (Water controls Fire)

This complexion has a black color with a red flush, so it seems to look slightly excited: A patient with a lung disease who had a strong constitution prior to the disease generally has such a complexion.

At this point, I would like to caution my readers that these examples must not be over interpreted and presumed as facts. Just because a lung disease patient has the color of (e) above, one must not come to a hasty conclusion that a person having this color has a lung disease. A person with a weak body, searching through the pages of a pathology and symptomatology book, can easily believe that they are suffering from each disease in the book. One should not look at the mirror while reading this and say, "black and red color, blue and yellow color - oh no! I have this disease."

There are mirrors which have a yellow, blue or white tinge, so there are no correct mirrors. Colors look different depending on their relationship to surrounding light rays. There are also some people who have a slight defect in the optic nerves and there also exists a relationship between visual perception and the emotional activity of the moment. There is no need to foolishly be afraid just because something looks a certain way at a quick glance. Therefore, since there is a concern that the main point will be missed in ascertaining the constitution and disease with the observation of color only, the signs and symptoms of Yin-Yang should be observed through other methods including: pulse diagnosis, channels, observation of color, food preferences, Deficiency-Excess, Exterior- Interior, Above-Below, etc.

## Practical Diagnosis (Locating Acupuncture Points)

Locating acupuncture points requires an understanding of anatomical landmarks. Once these landmarks are located, the space between these landmarks are described in "cun" which is a chinese word that translates to "anatomical inch". There are always three cun from the eyebrow to the forehead hairline. However, on a large headed person, those "cun" will be longer than on a child. But because acupuncture points are located on the patient according to the patient's unique anatomy, the ruler length between different people will vary widely.The distance between the grooves in the skin of middle phalanx in folded position of the middle finger of the person to be treated is one cun of the person, likewise the width of the thumb of the person to be treated is one cun of the person, also four finger breadths is three cun of the person, one of the ten parts of one cun is called one fen.

### Head & Neck Cun Division

| *Body Part* | *Cun* | *Between* |
|---|---|---|
| Top midline | 12 | The forehead hairline and the neck hairline. |
| Top midline | 14 | The glabella or eyebrow, and the occipital protuberance's inferior border. |
| Forehead width | 9 | The two forehead hairline corners. |
| Forehead height | 3 | The glabella (eyebrow) and the forehead hairline. |
| Throat height | 3 | The clavicle medial end and the mandible angle, or between the hyoid and the manubrium's superior border (when the head is straight). |
| Neck width | 9 | The inferior ends of the two mastoid bones. |
| Neck height | 3 | The neck hairline and the seventh cervical (C7) spinous process. |

### Torso Cun Division

| *Body Part* (head & limb) | *Cun* | *Between* |
|---|---|---|
| Front width | 8 | The two nipples. |
| Chest width | 8 | The front midline and the armpit (axillary) anterior end (when the arms lie straight alongside the body). |
| Chest width | 8 | The front midline and the acromial tip. |
| Abdomen width | 4 | The front midline and the rectus abdominis muscle's lateral border. |
| Upper abdomen height | 8 | The umbilicus center and the xiphisternal joint. |
| Lower abdominal height | 5 | The umbilicus center and the pubic symphysis superior border. |

| | | |
|---|---|---|
| Back width | 3 | The back midline and the scapular spine's medial end (when the arms lie straight alongside the body). |
| Lower back width | 3 | The two PSIS (posterior superior iliac spines). |

**Arm Cun Division**

| *Body Part* | *Cun* | *Between* |
|---|---|---|
| Upper arm length | 9 | The front end midline and the armpit axillary anterior end and the elbow (cubital) fold. |
| Lower arm length | 12 | The elbow (cubital fold and the wrist (carpal) crease. |
| Back shoulder length | 3 | The acromion and the armpit (axilla) posterior end (when the arms lie straight alongside the body). |

**Leg Cun Division**

| Body Part | Cun | Between |
|---|---|---|
| Thigh lateral length | 19 | The femur greater trochanter superior border and the knee (popliteal) fold and joint. |
| Thigh lateral length | 18 | The femur greater trochanter peak and the knee (popliteal) fold and joint. |
| Thigh medial length | 18 | The pubic symphysis superior border and the femur medial epicondyle superior border. |
| Knee length | 2 | The patella superior and the inferior borders. |
| Lower leg lateral | 16 | The lateral ma tip and the knee length (popliteal) fold and joint. |
| Lower leg medial length | 13 | The medial malleolus and the tibial medial condyle inferior border. |
| Foot lateral height | 3 | The lateral malleolus tip and the sole. |
| Foot medial height | 3 | The medial malleolus tip and the sole. |

## Use of Fingers to Measure Cun

| Cun | Between |
|---|---|
| 3 | The two sides of the 4 fingers (at the level of the proximal interphalangeal joints, when the fingers are held together. |
| 2 | The index finger's tip and the proximal interphalangeal joint (and fold). |
| 1.5 | The two sides of the index and middle fingers when they are held together at the level of the proximal interphalangeal joints. |
| 1 | The two sides of the thumb at the proximal interphalangeal joint. |

### The Relationship between Local and Distal Points

Symptoms occurring locally can be treated distally. The following is a guide to the relationship between local and distal points.

| Diseased area | Local Points | Distal Points |
|---|---|---|
| Head | | |
| Forehead | St 8, Du 23, GB 14, Yin Tang | L.I. 4, St 41, St 44 |
| Temple | Tai Yang, GB 8, GB 20 | SJ 5, GB 41 |
| Nape | UB 9, UB 10, Du 14, Du 16 | SI 3, SI 6, UB 60, UB 63, UB 65, UB 67 |
| Vertex | Du 20 | Liv 3 |
| Eyes | UB 1, UB 2, GB 1, GB 20, Qiu Hou | Liv 3, GB 37 |
| Nose | L.I. 20, Du 23, Bi Tong | Lu 7 L.I. 4 |
| Teeth | St 6, St 7, St 5, Ren 24 | L.I. 4, St 44 |
| Ears | SJ 21, SI 19, GB 2, SJ 17, GB 20 | SJ 5, GB 41, SJ 3, GB 43, Kid 3 |
| Tongue | Ren 23, Du 15 | Ht 5, Pc 7, Sp 5, Kid 6 |
| Throat | SI 17, Ren 23 | L.I. 1, Lu 7, Lu 10, Lu 11, Kid 6, St 44 |
| Trunk | | |

| | | |
|---|---|---|
| Chest | Ren 17, Ub 13, Lu 1 | Pc 6, Lu 5 |
| Upper Abdomen | Ren 12, St 21, UB 21 | St 36, Sp 4, Pc 6 |
| Middle Abdomen | St 25, Ren 6, UB 25, UB 27 | St 36, St 37, St 39 |
| Lower Abdomen | Ren 3, Ren 4 | UB 40, Sp 6 |
| Costal region | Liv 13, Liv 14, GB 24, UB 18, UB 19 | SJ 6, GB 34, Liv 3 |
| Lumbar region | UB 23, UB 25, UB 52 | UB 40 |

**Starting Acupuncture Treatment**

*Acupuncture Needles*

Generally filfiform needles made of stainless steel are used of length measuring from 15 to 150 mm and having diameter of 0.45mm to 0.26mm.

*Methods of Puncture*

The actual practice of acupuncture consists of inserting needles into any of hundreds of points located over the 12 basic meridians and over a number of specialized meridians. The needles usedmay be slightly arrowheaded or may have extremely fine points. The typical insertion is 3 to 10 mm (0.1 to 0.4 inch) in depth; some procedurescall for insertions up to almost 25 cm (10 inches). Once inserted, a needle may be twisted, twirled, or connected to a low-voltage alternating current for the duration of its use. The physician frequently inserts needles at a considerable distance from thepoint on which they are to act; for example, a needle inserted into the pad of the thumb is expected to produce analgesia in the abdomen. Similarly, successive points on a specific meridian may affect widely different areas or conditions; e.g.,the first six points of the yin lung meridian deal primarily with swollen joints, excessive heat in joints, bleeding of the nose, heart pains, mental depression, and inability to stretch the arms abovethe head. The location of the points is mastered by the use of innumerable diagrams and models.

Puncture consists of three stages insertion, retention and withdrawal.

Insertion is carried out in three directions according to need, perpendicular(90 degree to the skin), oblique(45 degree to the skin) and horizontal (15 degree to the skin).

The direction and depth of insertion depends on type and condition of the ailment but it is measured taking into account the position of vital organs and veins or arteries of the body. In chronic ailments the needles are usually kept for 10-15 minutes and for acute ailments from one to several hours, however for patients who are not able to tolerate retention, such as infants, children and audults who are inclined to faint , on imparting deqi* the needles the needles are withdrawn immediately.

Stimulation is usually given by lifting and thrusting or rotation of the needle or by combination of the two methods.

Scraping and vibration are also used, whereas, electrical stimulation is the most convenient way.

Deqi is the local sensation of acupuncture comprising of heaviness, numbness,tingling like mild electric shock, burning and swelling, which is felt by the patient during treatment. Pain is usually not a sensation.

Acupuncture originated in China almost four thousand years ago. The oldest continuously practiced health care, it is used by one-third of the world's population for primary treatment. Acupuncture is endorsed by the World Health Organization as an effective means of medical therapy. Acupuncture is based on the flow of energy through the body in topical pathways, called meridians or channels, that were mapped out on the body thousands of years ago. There is no Western anatomical equivalent for these energetic pathways, yet recent medical studies suggest they do exist. Energy flows through these meridians which are located just below the surface of the skin. When this energy is moving well and freely, we enjoy good health. If the energy becomes low, obstructed or cannot move well, then we begin to exhibit symptoms, such as headaches, pain in joints and muscles, and even inappropriate emotions. Acupuncture treats the symptom by addressing the deeper, underlying causes. By helping move the body's energy, it allows both physical and emotional balance to be regained and natural healing to occur. Acupuncture is one of the oldest medical practices. It balances the vital life energy called Qi (pronounced *chee*). Qi moves along meridians in the body. In a healthy person, the Qi circulates freely, in a natural state of balance. However, when Qi is blocked (which happens for a variety of reasons), health problems or serious diseases can occur.

Meridian therapy is a modern form of acupuncture that moves Qi past the blockages to restore health. The acupuncture techniques and needles used in meridian therapy are different than in traditional acupuncture. In meridian therapy, the practitioner uses only a few hair-thin needles and, in many cases, will not even insert the needles into the body. The result is a stress-free, pain-free session.

The most important diagnostic tool the meridian therapist has is the pulse. There are 12 pulses felt at multiple locations on both wrists, each align with a meridian in your body. I check the pulses repeatedly throughout your treatment to measure the effect of each step in the therapy.

During the acupuncture session I will also ask questions and take notes. Sometimes a casual word or phrase can give me the information I needs to understand how the Qi is moving in your body.

Meridian therapy sessions usually last from 30 to 45 minutes. Treatments are once or twice a week until the Qi has been restored to its proper balance (and related symptoms have been reduced or eliminated). After that, treatments are spaced to help maintain good health.The initial session will be from sixty to ninety minutes and will include an in-depth interview, reviews of health history and personal history to mutually determine if one may be helped by acupuncture. Needles may or may not be used during the first session. When the acupuncturist does needle, she or he will place needles in carefully preselected points on certain meridians. These disposable needles are the highest quality sterilized stainless steel, and about the width of a human hair. When the needles are placed, a person may have a sensation ranging from no feeling at all, a tingling, a dull ache, or a slight stinging sensation. Sensations that are felt when the needle is placed generally last a few seconds.

The number of needles used vary, depending on one's needs. A typical treatment consists of four to eight needle placements. The needles are left in for ten to twenty minutes, then removed and disposed of. Follow up treatments are one hour and include a review of the results of the previous treatment. One is able to resume normal activities immediately after a session.

When starting treatment, it is best to receive acupuncture once weekly. Within four to six sessions one will know if acupuncture will help. Sessions will be spaced farther apart as one progressively responds to treatment. Very often, people who become "symptom free" continue to receive maintenance treatments every three to four months.

## The Benefits of Acupuncture

Acupuncture is helpful in dealing with stress, insomnia, arthritis, chronic fatigue syndrome, high blood pressure, migraine, fibromyalgia, TMJ, gynecological problems, back pain, joint problems, tendonitis, and other physical issues. Because acupuncture is a holistic therapy, it may also be used to address problems such as depression and other emotional problems. Acupuncture is widely used to ease withdrawal from substance abuse.

## Acupuncture and Conventional Medical Care

Acupuncture blends well with conventional medical care. Acupuncture practitioners cooperate fully with other health care practitioners and recommend that you consult your physician or primary health care provider before starting any complementary health care modality. Physicians are aware of the use of acupuncture for pain management and many recommend its use for their patients.

The primary use of acupuncture in China today is for surgical analgesia. Chinese surgeons estimate that 30 percent of surgical patients obtain adequate analgesia with acupuncture, which is now performed by sending electrical current through the needles rather than by twirling them. American physicians who have observed surgery performed while the patient is under acupuncture have verified that it is effective in some patients, but put the figure closer to 10 percent. Brain surgery is especially amenable to this form of analgesia. Chinese surgeons claim that acupuncture is superior to Western, drug-induced analgesia in that it does not disturb normal body physiology and therefore does not make the patient vulnerable to shock.

Chinese doctors also treat some forms of heart disease with acupuncture. As part of an attempt to put the practice on a more scientific basis, one Chinese study tested the effects of acupuncture treatment on more than 600 people with chest pain caused by reduced blood flow to the heart. Results showed that almost all the patients greatly reduced their use of medicine and that most were able to resume work. Other physiological conditions treated with acupuncture are ulcer, hypertension (high blood pressure), appendicitis, and asthma.

In the United States, scientists have begun to investigate the use of acupuncture to treat a variety of medical conditions. In 1998 a National Institutes of Health (NIH) panel reviewed scientific studies of acupuncture and concluded that the technique effectively relieves nausea and vomiting caused by chemotherapy and surgical anesthesia. Good evidence also suggests that acupuncture relieves nausea during pregnancy and pain after dental surgery. Controlled studies of acupuncture for other medical conditions have not yet produced conclusive results.

The human body is an organic entity, so local pathological changes may affect the whole body. Moreover, the pathological changes of the internal organs may reflect on the body surface.

Diagnostic methods in traditional Chinese medicine include four basic methods: inspection, auscultation and olfaction, inquiry and palpation. The case history, symptoms, and signs gained through those four diagnostic methods are analyzed and generalized to find the causes, nature, and interrelations of the disease, and to provide evidence for the further differentiation of syndromes. The four diagnostic methods are therefore indispensable and important steps in the differentiation and treatment of syndromes.

Inspection is a method to examine the patient by observation of the expression, appearance, color, and abnormal changes of secretion and excretion, etc.

*1. Observation of the Mind*

This is to observe the patient's spirit, clearness of consciousness, coordination and vigour of movements, and keenness of response in order to judge the excess or deficiency of yin, yang, qi, and blood in the zang-fu organs and make a prognosis of the disease condition. Strength of Spirit: The patient is in good spirits, the body resistance and functions of the zang-fu organs are normal, therefore the patient has a good prognosis. Generally speaking, the patient is in good spirits, behaves normally with a sparkle in the eye, and has a keen response. Loss of Spirit: The patient is spiritless, indifferent in expression, has dull eyes and a sluggish response, or may even be unconscious or have a mental disturbance. This shows damage to the body resistance, a severe disease condition, and a poor prognosis.

*2. Observation of the Complexion*

Observe the color and luster of the facial region. Generally, a lustrous complexion with normal color indicates ample qi and blood, and a mild disease with a good prognosis. If the complexion is deep in color and withered, this indicates a serious disease condition with damage to the qi and essence, and a difficult treatment with poor prognosis.

**White Color:** A white color is the sign of a qi and blood deficiency. A pale complexion indicates a yin excess with yang deficiency. A qi deficiency manifests a lusterless and pale complexion and is accompanied by swelling. A pale emaciated face indicates a blood deficiency. A sudden pale complexion with cold sweat is the sign of sudden prostration of yang qi due to febrile diseases caused by exogenous pathogenic wind-cold.

**Yellowish Color:** a yellowish color is the sign of spleen deficiency and damp accumulation. A complexion that is yellowish, withered and lusterless indicates a qi deficiency of the spleen and stomach. A yellowish, flabby complexion is the sign of damp accumulation due to spleen dysfunction of transportation and transformation. The yellow color of the face, eyes, and skin indicates jaundice. In traditional Chinese medicine a bright orange yellow is diagnosed as yang jaundice caused by pathogenic damp-heat; dark yellow in yin jaundice due to pathogenic cold-damp.

**Red Color:** Redness indicates excessively full blood vessels due to excessive heat. A red complexion is mostly due to the fever of a common cold, or may be a heat syndrome due to excessive yang in the zang-fu organs. Malar flush with bright red color indicates xu heat syndromes due to yin deficiency and yang preponderance.

**Bluish Color:** Bluish color indicates syndromes of cold, pain, and blood stasis or convulsion, and is the manifestation of qi and blood obstruction in the channels. Pathogenic cold causes stagnation of qi and blood leading to pain. Children's high fever also shows a bluish complexion, the symptoms of acute convulsion.

**Black Color:** Black color indicates kidney deficiency, humor accumulation, and blood stasis. This is the manifestation of excessive cold and water, or stagnation of qi and blood. If the complexion is as black as bronze, it is mostly due to an extreme weakness of kidney yang and cold accumulation manifesting as xu-cold syndromes. A dark dray color around the eyes denotes phlegm-humor syndrome due to kidney deficiency. This leads to a dysfunction of the water metabolism or leukorrhea, due to the downward flowing of kidney essence. A dark gray malar can be seen in patients with frequent urination due to kidney deficiency. A dark gray complexion indicates prolonged stagnation of blood such as a consumptive disease with blood deficiency accompanied by menoplania or amenia.

*3. Observation of the Tongue*

**Tongue Proper Pale Tongue:**

Indicates xu and cold syndromes or symptoms due to yang qi deficiency and insufficiency of qi and blood.

**Red Tongue:** Indicates heat syndromes, mostly shi types of disease caused by interior heat, or symptoms of fire preponderance due to yin deficiency.

**Deep Red Tongue:** Denotes the excessive heat seen in febrile disease due to invasion of exogenous pathogenic heat which as been transmitted from the exterior to the interior of the body. It also can be seen in miscellaneous diseases due to a preponderance of fire caused by yin deficiency, or seen in diseases of accumulated fire in the liver channel.

**Purplish Tongue:** Shows the syndrome of blood stagnation. A tongue with purplish spots or petechiae also indicates blood stagnation.

**Tongue Appearance Flabby Tongue:** A flabby tongue body with teeth marks on the margin and pale in color indicates a yang deficiency of the spleen and kidney leading to accumulation and obstruction of phlegm-dampness.

A flabby tongue with a deep red color indicates excessive pathogenic heat attacking the heart and spleen.

**Thin and Small Tongue:** This indicates consumption and deficiency of blood and yin. A thin and small tongue with a pale color denotes deficiency of both qi and blood. A thin dry tongue with a deep red color is mainly due to a preponderance of fire and great exhaustion of body fluids.

**Rigid Tongue:** Seen in febrile diseases due to the invasion of exogenous pathogenic heat transmitted into the pericardium or due to an obstruction of pathogenic phlegm. It may also be seen in high fever leading to consumption of body fluids and preponderance of pathogenic heat. It is a prodrome of wind-stroke (cerebral stroke).

**Deviated Tongue:** This is a prodrome of wind-stroke.

**Cracked Tongue:** Cracks on the tongue with deep red color indicate excessive heat. A cracked pale tongue indicates insufficiency of yin and blood. However, a cracked tongueof long term duration without any other symptoms can be considered normal.

*Tongue Coating*

In the first place, the properties of tongue coating should be examined.

**Thinness and Thickness:** Generally, if substantial pathogenic factors such as damp, phlegm or food accumulation occur and cause obstruction, they further affect the spleen and stomach leading to the ascent of turbid qi and forming of a thick tongue coating. A white thin tongue coating is formed if nonsubstantial pathogenic factors such as wind, heat, dryness, or cold attack the body; or if the pathogenic factors stay on the body surface; or if body resistance is weak during the disease development.

**Moistness and Dryness:** The normal tongue coating is moist, which indicates that plenty of body fluid is flowing upward. If the tongue coating is dry, it is due to body fluids failing to moisten the tongue. A dry tongue coating may also be present in some febrile diseases where pathogenic heat consumes the body fluid. A slippery tongue coating may be due to pathogenic damp-humor floating over the tongue surface.

**Sticky and Curdled Tongue Coating:** A sticky coating is due to hyperactivity of endogenous pathogenic phlegm and damp rising tot he tongue, and is mostly seen in diseases caused by pathogenic damp-heat or phlegm-humor. A curdled tongue coating is the outcome of food accumulation in the stomach leading to the ascent of turbid qi to the tongue surface. It is also seen in disease caused by phlegm-damp.

**Peeled Tongue Coating:** Mostly due to deficiency of qi and yin. If peeled tongue is accompanied by a sticky coating, it indicates a complicated disease condition to which the body resistance is weakened.

**No Tongue Coating:** Changes in the tongue coating indicate fluctuation in the disease condition. For example, if a qi deficiency of the stomach is manifested by no tongue coating at an early stage, the tongue coating will reappear after the stomach qi is recovered. If a disease has no tongue coating, then suddenly appears, this indicates a perversive flow of stomach qi, or excessive pathogenic heat. If a disease has a tongue coating at the beginning which disappears abruptly, this indicates stomach yin fluid has decreased. If a thick coating gradually turns into a thin white coating, this indicates that pathogenic qi is being gradually weakened, and the disease condition is becoming milder.

Generally, an observation of the thinness and thickness of the tongue coating will indicate the depth of pathogenic qi. The tongue's moistness or dryness shows the body fluid condition. The degree of curdling and stickiness of the tongue coating indicates the dampness of the stomach and spleen. The appearance or disappearance of tongue coating signified the cure or worsening of the disease condition.

*Color of Tongue Coating*

**White Coating:** Indicates exterior-cold syndromes. A white and thin coating is seen mostly in exterior syndromes, while a white and thick coating appears in interior-cold syndromes. If there is a powder-like whitish coating covering the tongue surface, it is caused by the internal accumulation of summer-humid heat and is usually seen at the onset of pestilential diseases.

**Yellow Coating:** Indicates interior and heat syndromes. A light yellow tongue coating is seen in cases of slight fever. A deep yellow color indicates high fever.

Brownish tongue coatings represent an accumulation of pathogenic heat.

**Grayish Coating:** Denotes interior-heat syndrome or interior-cold syndrome.

A grayish black and slippery coating on the tongue usually indicates symptom-complex due to cold-damp in the interior. A grayish, yellow, and sticky tongue coating usually indicates the accumulation of damp-heat. Grayish and dry tongue coatings are usually due to the consumption of body fluid by excessive heat.

**Black Coating:** This is often seen at the serious and dangerous stage of disease, and indicates extreme heat or cold. A black, yellow, and dry coating with thorns on the tongue surface usually denotes consumption of body fluid by extreme heat. A black and slippery tongue coating shows excessive cold due to yang deficiency.

Auscultation (listening) and olfaction (smelling) are two methods used to diagnose a disease.

*1. Listening*

**Listening to the Voice**

**Speaking Voice:** Generally, speaking in a loud and sonorous voice indicates syndromes of heat or shi type, while a feeble, low voice indicates syndromes of the cold or xu type.

**Disordered Speaking:** Speaking incoherently and loudly or deliriously indicates shi syndrome. Speaking verbosely, feebly, and intermittently indicates syndromes of the xu type. Muttering to oneself denotes qi deficiency of the heart. Stuttering speech suggests upward disturbance of wind-phlegm.

**Listening to the Respiration**

**Feeble Breathing:** Feeble breathing accompanied by shortness of breath usually indicates xu syndromes.

**Coarse Breathing:** Forceful breathing with a coarse voice belongs to the shi heat type syndromes. Asthma with feeble, short breathing is a category of xu type asthma.

*Listening to the Cough*

Course coughing usually indicates shi type syndromes. A low cough with weak breathing indicates xu syndromes.

*2. Smelling*

Foul breath is due to pathogenic heat in the stomach, indigestion, caries, and an unclean mouth. Sour breath indicates food accumulation in the stomach. The offensive smell of a secretion or excretion including stool, urine, sputum, pus, leukorrhea, etc., usually indicates heat syndromes of the shi type. A stinking smell usually indicates cold syndromes of the xu type.

*3. Inquiring*

Inquiring involves asking the patient or the patient's companion about the disease condition to assist diagnosis. Because the chief complaint of the patient is of primary importance, the main information dealing with the problem must be carefully solicited. It is necessary to grasp the important clinical data as well as to get a general understanding of the patient's disease condition. The main categories of concern are:

**Chills and Fever Aversion to Cold and Fever**

At the beginning of a disease, aversion to cold and Fever occurs simultaneously. This indicates exterior syndromes due to invasion by exogenous pathogenic factors. The exterior syndromes due to invasion by exogenous pathogenic cold and wind are characterized by severe aversion to cold, mild fever accompanied by an absence of thirst, no sweat, headache, general pain, superficial and tense pulse, etc. The exterior syndromes due to invasion by exogenous pathogenic wind-heat are characterized by severe fever, mild aversion to cold accompanied by thirst, sweating, sore throat, superficial and rapid pulse, etc.

### Alternating Chills and Fever

This particular symptoms occurs when exogenous pathogenic factors are in between the exterior and interior of the body, accompanied by a bitter taste in the mouth, dry throat, fullness of the chest, hypochondrium, etc. If a high fever follows the first occurrence of chills and is complicated with a severe headache which subsides after the fever is gone, this indicates malaria.

### Fever Occurring Without Chills High fever

This is usually due to the transmission of exogenous pathogenic cold from the exterior to the interior, which then changes into heat; or the transmission of exogenous pathogenic heat from exterior to interior resulting in shi type interior-heat syndrome accompanied byprofuse sweating, thirst, forceful pulse, etc.

### Tidal Fever

This is one of the main characteristics of yin deficiency or shi heat syndrome of the Yangming channel. Tidal fever due to yin deficiency often occurs at noon or night, accompanied by a dry red tongue. Tidal fever usually appears at dusk associated with constipation, abdominal distension, penis pain, etc.

### Perspiration

Sweat is transformed from evaporated body fluid by the function of yang qi. So perspiration has a certain clinical significance in reflecting the status of yang qi and body fluid. On should first ask whether the patient has sweat or not. If the patient is sweating, further questioning should be concerned with the characteristics and accompanied symptoms of perspiration.

### Sweating of No Sweating

Exterior syndromes without sweating are caused by exogenous pathogenic factors. Exterior syndromes with sweating are mostly exterior heat syndromes due to the invasion by exogenous pathogenic wind heat; or they may be exterior xu syndromes due to exogenous pathogenic wind.

### Night Sweating

Is usually the manifestation of yin deficiency, accompanied by tidal fever, flushed malar, red tongue proper with scanty coating, thready and rapid pulse.

### Spontaneous Sweating

This is a sign of qi or yang deficiency associated with fear of cold, lassitude, etc.

### Profuse Sweating

Excessive sweating together with high fever, thirst with desire for cold drinks, forceful pulse, etc. belong to interior shi heat syndrome. This is the outcome of excessive yang and heat compelling the outward flow of sweat. Dripping with sweat accompanied by lassitude, feckless breathing, cold extremities, and feeble pulse indicates the total prolapse of yang qi, also known as "sweating from exhaustion."

### Sweating of the Head

Caused by heat in the upper jiao or damp heat in the middle jiao. It is caused by the heat in the upper jiao, it will be accompanied by irritability, thirst, yellow tongue coating, superficial and rapid pulse. if it is the result of damp heat accumulation, it will be associated with heaviness and tiredness of the body, dysuria, yellowish and sticky tongue coating, etc.

### Food and Drink Appetite, and Taste No Appetite

This is a symptom caused by the dysfunction of transformation and transportation of the spleen. Symptoms are emaciation due to chronic disease, poor appetite, loose stool, lassitude, and pale tongue proper with a thin white coating. If anorexia is associated with fullness of the chest, abdominal distension, thick and sticky tongue coating, then it is caused by the obstruction of pathogenic damp in the spleen.

### Food Repulsion

This is usually due to the accumulation of food in the stomach and intestines. It is often accompanied by distension and fullness of the epigastrium and abdomen, acid regurgitation, and a thick and sticky tongue coating.

### Quick Hunger

This is due to strong stomach fire and causes fast digestion.

Hunger and Anorexia Combined: This is due to injury of stomach yin and disturbance of xu heat.

### Craving for Dirt Due to Intestinal Parasites

This is common in children, and is a sign of parasitosis accompanied by emaciation, abdominal distension and pain, etc.

### Thirst

Whether the patient is thirsty or not often reflects the condition of body fluids. During the process of disease development, if there is no thirst, then the body fluid has not yet been damaged and it indicates a cold syndrome. If the patient is thirsty, it indicates a consumption or stagnation of the body fluid failing to nourish the upper body.

Generally, thirst with a desire for excessive drinking is commonly seen in heat syndromes. Severe thirst with a preference for hot drinks indicates a phlegm-humor obstruction which prevents the upward flow of body fluids. The upward flow of water usually causes vomiting after drinking due to thirst. If the patient is thirsty, but doesn't want to drink, this indicates acute febrile diseases where the pathogenic factors have invaded the nutrient (ying) and blood (xue) systems of the body. If excessive drinking does not relieve the symptoms of thirst and then excessive urination follows, this suggests diabetes.

### Taste

Clinically, a bitter taste in the mouth is caused by pathogenic heat, especially the overflowing of heat from the liver and gall bladder. A sweet taste in the mouth is usually due to damp heat in the spleen and stomach. A sour taste is due to the accumulation of heat in the liver and stomach. A sour taste similar to spoiled food indicates injury by the accumulation of food. Tastelessness in the mouth is usually due to the dysfunction of transportation and transformation.

### Defecation and Urination Shape of the Stool

Dry stools shaped like sheep-dung are due to stagnation of heat or exhaustion of body fluid. A mucous stool is a sign of excessive damp caused by spleen deficiency. Loose bowels following dry stool are due to a dysfunction of the spleen and stomach, and an imbalance between dryness and dampness. Stools which are sometimes dry and sometimes loose are usually due to liver qi stagnation and spleen deficiency. Liquid stools with undigested food are due to the yang deficiency of the spleen and kidney. Diarrhea with yellow watery stool and burning of the anus is caused by damp heat in the stomach and intestines. Formed stools with undigested food and foul smell are the result of food accumulation.

### The Color of the Stool

Tarry stools are the symptoms of hemorrhaging in the spleen and stomach. Bloody and pussy stools are a sign of dysentery.

### The Smell of the Stool

Sour stinking stools are due to the accumulation of heat. A rotten egg stink is due to food accumulation.

### The Sensation of Defecation

A burning sensation in the anus during defecation is due to pathogenic heat in the rectum. Mild prolapse of the anus during bowel movements is the outcome of chronic diarrhea due to the sinking of qi and spleen deficiency. Tenesmus is a sign of dysentery due to qi stagnation in the intestines. Fragmentary defection is a manifestation of the liver failing to cause a free condition for qi. Diarrhea occurring soon after abdominal pain, and pain relieved after bowel movements, are signs of food accumulation. Pain not relieved after bowel movements is a sign of spleen deficiency and liver preponderance resulting in "liver-wood subjugating the spleen-earth."

### The Color of Urine

Deep yellow urine indicates heat, while clear and profuse urine indicates cold. Turbid urine or a mixture of urine with sperm denotes the downward flowing of damp heat. Brownish urine indicates that pathogenic heat has injured the blood vessels.

### The Amount of Urine

An increased amount of urine indicates kidney qi deficiency. A decreased volume of urine is caused by the consumption of body fluid or by dysfunction of qi activities causing failure to transform body fluids into urine. Dribbling of urine or retention of urine indicates the exhaustion of kidney qi or the downward flowing of damp heat.

### The Sensation of Urination

A stabbing pain during urination, accompanied by an urgent and burning feeling, is caused by damp heat. Pain after urination mostly indicates the declining of kidney qi. Dribbling urination is due to the non-consolidation of kidney qi. Nocturnal enuresis is caused by the deficiency of kidney qi. Unconsciousness accompanied by incontinence of urine indicates that the heart has failed to control the mind and the urinary bladder has lost its restrictive capacity.

*Pain*

### Headache

Occipital headache, referring to the nape and the upper back, is a disease of the Taiyang channel. Frontal headache, referring to the supraorbital ridge, indicates a disease of the Yangming channel. Headaches of the temporal region are diseases of the Shaoyang channel. Vertex headache is a pain of the Jueyin channel. headache related to the teeth is a pain of the Shaoyin channel due to invasion by cold.

### Pain of the Chest

This is mostly due to the obstruction of phlegm or blood stasis, leading to qi stagnation.

### Pain in the Hypochondriac Region

Is caused by obstruction in the liver and gall bladder channel, or by malnutrition of these channels.

### Epigastric Pain

Is caused by disorders of the stomach.

### Abdominal Pain

Lower lateral abdominal pain is caused by qi stagnation of the liver, obstruction of the liver channel, or appendicitis or hernia. Pain around the umbilicus is seen in parasitosis, food accumulation, constipation, etc. Lower abdominal pain and distension is caused by dysuria and/or retention of urine. If there are no complicated urination symptoms, the usual cause is retention of blood in the lower jiao.

### Low Back Pain

Is mostly due to a deficiency of the kidney, invasion by cold damp, or blood stagnation in the channels.

### Pain of the Limbs

Pain may appear in joints, muscles, or channels and collaterals due to the invasion of exogenous pathogenic factors.

### The Nature of Pain

A wandering pain associated with numbness or itching is due to invasion by pathogenic wind. Pain associated with heaviness and soreness is most often caused by pathogenic damp. Severe pain with a cold feeling or fear of cold is caused by pathogenic cold. Pain accompanied by redness, swelling, and heat or fear of heat is due to pathogenic fire (heat). Distending pain or referred pain is caused by qi stagnation. Pain which is aggravated by pressure relates to the shi type of symptoms complex. Pain which is alleviated by pressure is related to the xu type of symptom complex.

### Sleep

Insomnia associated with palpitation, dreams and nervousness is usually caused by the insufficiency of blood nourishing the heart. Insomnia accompanied by restlessness in the mind and difficulty in falling asleep indicates yin deficiency leading to preponderance of fire. Insomnia complicated by bitter taste, vomiting saliva, palpitation, irritability, and an inability to fall asleep indicates the internal disturbance of phlegm-fire. Insomnia due to the disharmony of the stomach indicates a derangement of stomach qi leading to restlessness in the mind during sleep.

Hypersomnia is commonly seen in febrile diseases caused by exogenous pathogenic factors; in qi deficiency caused by chronic diseases; in failure of the spleen yang to ascend due to the obstruction of damp; or in the condition of yang deficiency leading to excessive yin.

*Menses and Leukorrhea*

### Antedated Menstruation

Red color and an excessive amount indicates heat syndrome. Light color, post-menstrual pain in the lower abdomen is most often due to a deficiency of both qi and blood.

### Postdated Menstruation

Dark purple menstrual flow with clots, and premenstrual abdominal pain, most often indicates cold syndromes or blood stasis. Postdate menstruation with a scanty light-coloured flow indicates blood deficiency.

### Indefinite Menstruation

If it is associated with dysmenorrhea or distension of the breasts before menstruation, it is caused by the stagnation of liver qi.

### Amenorrhea

Many factors may cause amenorrhea, such as pregnancy, blood stasis, blood exhaustion, consumptive diseases, qi stagnation in the liver, etc.

### Incessant Menstrual Flow

If it is dark purple color with clots and abdominal pain, this indicates deficiency of the chong and ren channels, or failure of blood control by the spleen due to the sinking qi of the middle jiao.

### Leucorrhoea

Thin and whitish leucorrhoea with little odor indicates deficiency of the spleen and kidney. Excessive yellowish and thick leucorrhoea with offensive smell indicates the downward flow of damp heat.

*4. Palpation*

Palpation is a method of diagnosis using the hand to touch, feel, and press certain areas of the body to ascertain the patient's disease condition. Generally there are two types: pulse feeling and body palpation.

**Pulse Feeling**

In traditional Chinese medicine the pulse is considered as having three divisions: cun, guan, and chi. A normal pulse is neither superficial nor deep, neither quick no slow, and it beats in medium frequency, i.e., 4-5 beats per breath, with a regular rhythm.

To feel the pulse correctly, place the patients hand comfortably on a cushion with the palm facing upward. First, the practitioner should put their middle finger on the guan division, then the index and ring fingers should naturally fall on the cun and chi divisions. Finger force should at first be light, then moderate and finally heavy to get a general picture of the depth, rhythm, strength, and form of the pulse. An even force should be applied on the three regions. Through comparisons of the three regions, the practitioner can gain a correct impression of the pulse as a whole. A normal pulse is of moderate frequency, i.e., 4-5 beats per breath, regular rhythm, even and forceful.

The following are abnormal pulses commonly seen in the clinic:

**Floating Pulse (fumai):** When the pulse is pressed lightly it appears under the finger, and when pressed heavily it becomes weak. It often occurs in the early stages of diseases caused by exogenous pathogenic wind cold and heat, i.e., exterior syndromes. If it is seen in patients who are suffering from prolonged chronic diseases, it indicates a dangerous site where the yang qi of the body flows outward.

**Deep Pulse (chimai):** No clear pulse is felt by superficial pressure, only by heavy pressure. This indicates an interior syndrome.

**Rapid Pulse (sumai):** The pulse beats rapidly at a rate higher than the normal 5 beats per breath (i.e., more than 90 times per minute). This indicates a heat syndrome.

**Xu Type Pulse (xumai):** If the pulses of the three regions are weak and forceless, this indicates xu type syndromes. These are mostly caused by both qi and blood deficiencies and are seen during the process of chronic diseases.

**Shi Type Pulse (shimai):** If the pulses of the three regions are forceful with both light and heavy pressure, shi type syndromes are present.

**Slippery pulse (huamai):** If the pulse is smooth and flowing, like a pearl rolling on a plate, this indicates excessive phlegm, retention of food, or shi heat type syndromes.

**Rough Pulse (semai):** This pulse is uneven and has a roughness similar to scraping bamboo with a knife. It indicates a deficiency of blood and essence, qi stagnation, and blood stasis.

**Fine Pulse (ximai):** This pulse is as fine as a silk thread, and indicates exhaustion of qi and blood.

**Full Pulse (hongmai):** This pulse beats like a dashing wave, with one rising wave following another. It indicates excessive heat.

**Wiry Pulse (xuanmai):** This pulse is straight and long, like a tremulous music string, seen usually in diseases of liver, gall bladder, pain, or phlegm-humor.

**Tense Pulse (jinmai):** The pulse is taut and forceful, like a tightly stretched cord, and occurs in diseases caused by cold, pain, or retention of food.

**Hollow Pulse (koumai):** This pulse is floating, large, and empty inside, feeling like a scallion stalk. It indicates a massive loss of blood and essence.

**Hesitant Pulse (cumai):** This pulse is rapid with irregular intermittent beats. It indicates excessive yang and shi heat, qi stagnation, pathogenic phlegm mixture with cold, blood stasis, etc.

**Knotted Pulse (jiemai):** This pulse is slow and uneven with irregular intervals. It indicates excessive yin, qi stagnation, pathogenic phlegm mixture with cold, blood stasis, etc.

**Intermittent Pulse (daimai):** This pulse is slow with regular intervals. it indicates qi exhaustion of the zang organs, or

syndromes of wind and pain caused by emotional pathogenic fright and fear.

*Body Palpation*

This is a diagnostic method to ascertain abnormal changes in the body and to determine the location and nature of the disease through palpation and finger pressure.

**Palpating the Skin and Muscle:** Generally, if there is excessive pathogenic heat in the body, the patient will usually have heat on the body surface. Yang qi deficiency has a cold body surface on palpation. If the surface feels hot on first palpation becoming slightly hotter when you palpate longer, this indicates that the pathogenic heat has proceeded from the exterior to the interior of the body. Body palpation showing moist and smooth skin demonstrates that the body fluid is not yet damaged. If the skin and nails are very dry, this indicates consumption of the body fluids. If body palpation shows swelling and further pressure makes a depression, this indicates edema. If a depression appears on pressure and disappears after taking the hand away, this indicates qi distension. Palpating the skin can also indicate the patient's sweat condition.

**Palpating Hands and Feet:** Coldness of the four extremities is mostly due to yang deficiency and excessive pathogenic cold. An overheating of the four extremities indicates excessive heat. Coldness of the four extremities with heat in the chest and abdomen is due to the retention of internal heat preventing the flow of yang qi outward. Heat in the dorsum of the hand is a sign of disease caused by exogenous pathogenic factors.

**Palpating the Epigastrium and Abdomen:** If the patient has fullness and distention of the hypochondrium, palpation may demonstrate hardness and pain in this region. This is known as an accumulation of excessive pathogenic factors in the chest of the xu type. If the hardness extends over a large area in the chest, it is due to phlegm-humor. Palpation of the abdomen showing abdominal distention with a tympanitic note on percussion, but with normal urination, indicates qi tympanites. Abdominal distension with a splashing sound like water, and accompanying dysuria indicates was tympanites or ascites. If hand pressure relieves the abdominal pain, it is considered to be a xu type; if the pain is made worse by pressure, it is a shi type. Immovable hard masses in the abdomen with pain fixed in a certain area are due to blood stasis. However, if the patient feels that lumps sometimes appear and disappear with unfixed pain, and palpation of the abdomen shows they do not exist, then this is due to qi stagnation.

**Palpating Channels and Points:** Clinical practice proves that in some diseases there may occur tenderness or abnormal reactions along the courses of the affected channels or at certain points. These signs have significance in diagnosis by palpation, especially in acupuncture treatment. For example, there may be tenderness at Pt. Zhongfu (Lu. 1) or Pt. Shufu (K. 27), which are closely related to the disorders of the lung and trachea. In diseases of the heart and stomach, tenderness may occur at Pt. Jugue (Ren 14), Pt. Zhongwan (Ren 12), Pt. Burong (St. 19), or Pt. Liangmen (St. 21). In disorders of the liver and gall bladder, tenderness may be at Pt. Qimen (Liv. 14) and Pt. Riye (G.B. 24). In diseases of the spleen, tenderness may occur at Pt. Zhangmen (Liv. 13) and Pt. Huangmen (U.B. 51). In disorders of the kidney, Pt. Jingmen (G.B. 25) and Pt. Zhishi (U.B. 52) may have tenderness. Tenderness at Pt. Tianshu (St. 25). Pt. Daji (St. 27) and Pt. Fujie (Sp. 14) may be closely related to disorders of the intestines. Tenderness at Pt. Guanyan (Ren 4), Pt. Qihai (Ren 6) and Pt. Zhongji (Ren 3) may have a close relation with disorders of the urinogenital system. When there are abnormal reactions appearing at the above points, they may reflect pathological changes of the related zang or fu organs.

## *Chapter Six*

# Evaluation and Diagnosis

Acupuncture is based on the flow of energy through the body in topical pathways, called meridians or channels, that were mapped out on the body thousands of years ago. There is no Western anatomical equivalent for these energetic pathways, yet recent medical studies suggest they do exist. Energy flows through these meridians which are located just below the surface of the skin. When this energy is moving well and freely, we enjoy good health. If the energy becomes low, obstructed or cannot move well, then we begin to exhibit symptoms, such as headaches, pain in joints and muscles, and even inappropriate emotions. Acupuncture treats the symptom by addressing the deeper, underlying causes. By helping move the body's energy, it allows both physical and emotional balance to be regained and natural healing to occur. Acupuncture is one of the oldest medical practices. It balances the vital life energy called Qi (pronounced *chee*). Qi moves along meridians in the body. In a healthy person, the Qi circulates freely, in a natural state of balance. However, when Qi is blocked (which happens for a variety of reasons), health problems or serious diseases can occur.

### Acupuncture and TCM

The teachings of the religious sects forbade the mutilation of the dead human body; hence traditional anatomy rests on no sure scientific foundation. One of the most important writers on anatomy, Wang Ch'ing-jen, gained his knowledge from the inspection of dog-torn children who had died in a plague epidemic in AD 1798. Traditional Chinese anatomy is based onthe cosmic system, which postulates the presence of such hypothetical structures as the 12 channels and the three so-called burning spaces. The body contains five organs (heart, lungs, liver, spleen, and kidneys), which store up but do not eliminate; and five viscera (such as the stomach, intestines, gallbladder, and bladder), which eliminate but do not store up. Each organ is associated with one of the planets,colours, tones, smells, and tastes. There are 365 bones and 365 joints in the body.

According to the physiology of traditional Chinese medicine, the blood vessels contain blood and air, in proportions varyingwith those of the yin and the yang. These two cosmic principles circulate in the 12 channels and control the blood vessels and hence the pulse. The Nei ching says that "the blood current flows continuously in a circle and never stops. Itmay be compared to a circle without beginning or end." On this insubstantial evidence it has been claimed that the Chinese anticipated Harvey's discovery of the circulation of the blood. Traditional Chinese pathology is also dependent on the theory of the yin and the yang; this led to an elaborate classification of diseases in which most of the types listed are without scientific foundation.

In diagnosis, detailed questions are asked about the history ofthe illness and about such things as the patient's taste, smell, and dreams. Conclusions are drawn from the quality of the voice, and note is made of the colour of the face and of the tongue. The most important part of the investigation, however, is the examination of the pulse. Wang Shu-ho, who wrote the "Pulse Classic," lived in the 3rd century BC, and innumerable commentaries were written on his work. The pulse is examined in several places, at different times, and with varying degrees of pressure. The operation may take as long as three hours. It is often the only examination made, and it is used both for diagnosis and for prognosis. Not only are the diseased organs ascertained but the time of death or recovery may be foretold.

The Chinese materia medica has always been extensive and consists of vegetable, animal (including human), and mineral remedies. There were famous herbals from ancient times; but all these, to the number of about 1,000, were embodied by LiShih-chen in the compilation of Pen-ts'ao kang-mu (the "Great Pharmacopoeia") in the 16th century AD. This work, in 52 volumes, has been frequently revised and reprinted and is still authoritative. The use of drugs is mainly to restore the harmony of the yin and the yang and is also related to such matters as the five organs, the five planets, and the five colours. The art of prescribing is therefore complex.

Among the drugs taken over by Western medicine from the Chinese are rhubarb, iron (for anemia), castor oil, kaolin, aconite, camphor, and Cannabis sativa (Indian hemp). Chaulmoogra oil was used by the Chinese for leprosy from at least the 14th century, and about a century ago it began to be used for this purpose by Western physicians. The herb mahuang (Ephedra vulgaris) has been used in China for at least 4,000 years, and the isolation of the alkaloid ephedrine from it has greatly improved the Western treatment of asthma and similar conditions.

The most famous and expensive of Chinese remedies is ginseng. Western analysis has shown that it has diuretic and other properties but is of doubtful value. In recent years reserpine, the active principle of the Chinese plant Rauwolfia , has been isolated; it is now effectively used in the treatment of high blood pressure and some emotional and mental conditions.

Another treatment is moxibustion, which consists in making a small, moistened cone (moxa) of powdered leaves of mugwort, or wormwood (Artemisia species), applying it to the skin, igniting it, and then crushing it into the blister so formed. Other substances are also used for the moxa. Dozens of these are sometimes applied at one sitting. The practice is often associated with acupuncture.

## Acupuncture and Conventional Medical Care

Acupuncture blends well with conventional medical care. Acupuncture practitioners cooperate fully with other health care practitioners and recommend that you consult your physician or primary health care provider before starting any complementary health care modality. Physicians are aware of the use of acupuncture for pain management and many recommend its use for their patients.

When you go to a Chinese medicine practitioner, whether for treatment of an illness, acute pain, or to begin a program of preventive care, the doctor will follow a system of evaluation and diagnosis that depends on observation and questioning. In accordance with the philosophy of the Tao, diagnosis is a process of perceiving signs and symptoms and relating them to one another to reveal how they form patterns of harmony or disharmony. Each symptom or sign has meaning only in relationship to other signs and symptoms and to the whole of your mind/body/ spirit.

### The Four Examinations

In order to begin to develop an accurate picture of your whole being, the Chinese medicine practitioner examines you, using the traditional Chinese method, called the Four Examinations: inquiring, looking, listening/smelling (these two seemingly different acts are grouped together—in Chinese they are the same word) and touching. This process of examination reveals which of the Eight Fundamental Patterns of disharmony are at work and what type of disharmony of the Essential Substances, Organ Systems and channels you may have.

The Four Examinations are sometimes done formally, but often the practitioner uses intuition and casual observation to create a vivid profile of a patient. Every gesture, word and attribute provides clues to a person's health and well-being.

Let's look at each step in the diagnostic process in more detail, breaking down the Four Examinations into their components, so you'll know what to expect.

### Inquiring

The Chinese medicine doctor takes a great deal of time to ask you about yourself. Your answers allow the practitioner to benefit from the knowledge that you have, for no one can know your body as well as you do. Questioning allows the practitioner to observe your emotions, voice and self-presentation. Basic questions focus on:

Your reaction to heat and cold

Your patterns of perspiration

If and when you experience headaches or dizziness

What type of pain, if any, you may have

Your bowel and bladder function

Your thirst, appetite, and tastes

Sleep patterns

Your sexual functioning, sexual activity, and reproductive history

General medical history

General physical activity

Emotions

Looking

### Evaluation of the Tongue

The tongue is the mirror of the body. Harmony and disharmony are reflected in the tongue's color, moisture, size, coating and the location of abnormalities.

Healthy Organ Systems and a lack of External Pernicious Influences produce a healthy tongue, which is pinkish red, neither dry nor too wet, fits perfectly within the mouth, moves freely and has a thin white coating.

Imbalances in the Organ Systems and/or invasion by Pernicious Influences produce an unhealthy tongue. External Pernicious Influences produce changes in the tongue coating. Interior problems, such as Organ System or Essential Substance disharmonies, produce changes in the tongue body.

When examining the tongue, the Chinese medicine doctor looks at the color of the tongue body, its size and shape, the color and thickness of its coating or fur, locations of abnormalities, and moistness or dryness of the tongue body and fur. These signs reveal not only overall states of health but correlate to specific organ functions and disharmonies, especially in the digestive system. To evaluate the tongue accurately, always do the examination in natural light.

### Tongue Body

The tongue body is a fleshy mass and has color, texture, and shape independent from the apparent qualities ofthe tongue coating. A pale tongue body indicates deficient Xue, Qi, or Yang or Excess Cold. An overly red tongue body indicates Excess Heat. A purple tongue indicates that Qi and/or Xue are not moving harmoniously and are stagnant. Pale purple means the Stagnation is related to Cold. Reddish purple is related to Stagnation of Heat. When the tongue is black or gray, it indicates extreme Stagnation; if black and dry, that indicates extreme Heat Stagnation; if black and wet, that indicates extreme Cold Stagnation. Bright red indicates Deficient Yin or Excess Heat. Dark red indicates Excess Heat. Cracks in a red tongue indicate Deficient Yin or Heat Injuring the Fluids. If the tongue is pale and cracked, there is Deficient Qi or Xue. Thorny eruptions of the buds on the tongue alert the doctor to Heat or Stagnant Xue.

### Tongue Fur

The tongue's coating is best described as moss or fur. It arises when the Spleen causes tiny amounts of impure substances to drift upward to the tongue. When the Spleen and stomach are in balance, there is a uniform density of fur, with a slightly thicker area in the center of the tongue. Thick fur indicates excess. Thin fur is related to deficiency during illness, but is normal if you are well. Fur that is wet indicates Excess Jin-Ye (fluids) and/or a Deficient Yang. Dry fur is a sign of Excess Yang or Deficient Jin-Ye. A greasy fur is a sign of mucus or dampness in the body. If the fur looks peeled off or missing, it reveals Deficient Spleen or Yin or fluids. White, moist fur indicates Cold. Yellow fur means Heat. However, white fur, resembling cottage cheese, points to heat in the Stomach. Gray/black fur with a red body is associated with extreme Heat; gray/black fur with a pale body is a sign of extreme Cold.

### Size and Shape

The healthy tongue rests comfortably in the mouth. It is neither too small nor too large. If a tongue is enlarged and flabby, it indicates Deficient Qi. If, in addition to being enlarged and flabby, the tongue has scalloped (or tooth marked) edges, then it indicates dampness due to Deficient Qi or stagnation of fluids. If the tongue is enlarged and hard, it is a sign of Excess. If it swells so that it fills the mouth and is deep red, that means Excess Heat in Heart and Spleen are a problem. A small, thin tongue can indicate Deficient Yin or Xue.

## Movement

A trembling, pale tongue indicates Deficient Qi. A flaccid tongue that is pale often reveals extreme Qi or Xue Deficiency. A flaccid tongue that is deep red reveals severe Yin Deficiency. A trembling, red tongue indicates interior Wind. If the tongue sits off-center in the mouth, early or full-blown Wind stroke may be present. A rigid tongue accompanies an Exterior Pernicious Influence and fever. This may indicate the invasion of the Pericardium by Heat and Mucus Obstructing the Heart Qi.

## Location of Abnormalities

The location of disturbances on the tongue are vivid indications of where disharmonies in the mind/body/spirit are located. Certain organs are associated with the Upper, Middle and Lower Triple Burner, which are in turn associated with the front, middle and back sections of the tongue. For example, if there are red spots on the front third of the tongue, which is associated with the Upper Burner, this indicates that there is Heat in the Lungs. If the tip of the tongue is red, that indicates Heat in the Heart. Menstrual cramps, when associated with Stagnant Xue, are often accompanied by purple spots on the edges of the tongue in the Liver/Gallbladder area.

## The Role of Tongue Diagnosis

Not all tongue irregularities are indications of disharmony, however. Food and drugs may change the coating or color of the body of the tongue. For example, coffee yellows the coating and Pepto-Bismol turns the tongue black.

Furthermore, some people have minor, unchanging cracks on their tongue, which are considered normal. Others are born with what is called a geographic tongue, which is covered with severe cracks and covered with hills and valleys. This is considered normal by some practitioners, but a sign of congenital disharmony by others.

The way a tongue appears is not an absolute indicator of the location of the disharmony, but when taken as part of an overall pattern that includes a complete evaluation, it offers strong clues to the location of disharmony.

## Evaluation of Body Language:Styles of Movement, Posture and Self-Presentation

Seeking clues to possible Pernicious Influences, the practitioner looks for signs of heat or Cold influences, Excess or Deficiency, Yin or Yang disharmonies. If a person has a heavy-footed walk, loud voice and sits in a sloppy, spread-out posture, that may indicate Excess. If a person acts frail and weak, sits with shoulders slumped and is shy and receding, that may indicate a Deficiency. On the other hand, fast, jerky, impulsive movement and an outgoing personality indicate Heat. If combined with a full, red face, high energy and a loud voice, then both Heat and Excess may be at work. Cold, as you might suspect, is associated with slow but not sloppy movements and a pale face. When coupled with a low voice, shortness of breath, or passivity, Cold and Deficiency may be at work.

## Evaluation of Facial Color

When you are feeling off-balance or have a specific disharmony, facial colors offer clues to the nature and the severity of the imbalance.

There are several different methods of facial diagnosis: Korean, Japanese, Worsley School, even macrobiotic. The following evaluation of facial colors is derived from a combination of Traditional Chinese Medicine and Five Phases principles. I have found this system provides accurate analysis.

TIP In order to obtain a clear idea of what the various facial colors look like, always use natural light when examining your face in a mirror.

## The Significance of Facial Colors

If facial color is bright and fresh, then the disease is called floating and is on a superficial level.

If the color is moist, neither wet nor dry, the disease is not severe and will be easy to treat.

If the color is shallow and scattered over a large area, the number of days of the disease will be short.

If the color is dark and cloudy, then the disease is sinking into the inner organs.

If the color is dark, cloudy and dry, the disease is severe and will be difficult to cure.

If the color is deep and accumulated in one spot, the disease is a long-term one.

Five colors appear on the face: red, green, yellow, white and black. Depending on a person's constitution, a healthy face may have one color that is more predominant than others, but several may be visible. To determine what colors are present in your face, always examine it in natural light. Look for the overall color tone; study the skin to see what tones appear from under the surface; look at any visible veins. For contrast, hold your hand up alongside your face.

Red is the color associated with the Heart Organ System and Xue. If the face is a fresh red, the Xue is Hot. If the face is dark red, the Xue is Stagnant. If it is light red, the Xue is Deficient.

Green is the color associated with the Liver System and circulation of the Xue. If veins on the face appear greenish purple, the Xue is Hot. If the veins appear greenish black, the Xue is Stagnant. If the condition is severe, the veins on the face appear black.

Yellow is the color associated with the Spleen System. If the face appears light yellow, then the Spleen system is Damp and Hot. If the face appears deep yellow, Heat has accumulated. If it is dark yellow, Heat is the result of Xue Stagnation. Withered yellow indicates a Heat Deficiency.

White is the color associated with the Lung System, which regulates Qi, the breathing in of oxygen, and the exhalation of carbon dioxide. If a person is not able to exhale completely-as in emphysema-his or her face will take on a grayish white color. If the person inhales inadequately, then the face will appear pale and lusterless.

Black is the color associated with the Kidney System. If the face is cold and black, the Kidney System is not filtering Xue properly. If the face color is black but bright and moist, the condition can be treated. If the face is not shining, the condition is not good. If the face is withered, the Kidney System Yin is dry. If the face is cloudy and dark, the Kidney System Yang is dying.

Occasionally, there are combinations of colors. This further refines the evalua tion. For example, if the color is red and white, both the Heart and Lung channels are involved.

**Listening and Smelling: Evaluation of Voice**

Listening to the sound of a person's speech, breathing and cough can help identify a disharmony that results from one or more pernicious influence and pattern of disharmony. For example, if the voice is too loud and strident, that indicates Excess, as does the sudden onset of a violent cough. A weak, low voice that doesn't project and a weak cough indicate Deficiency. Losing your voice or hoarseness can indicate either Deficiency or Excess. Wheezing arises from Dampness.

*Evaluation of smell*

According to TCM theory, there are two main odors that clue a doctor to the origin of disharmony. A strong stench from secretions or excretions indicates Excess and Heat. A weaker odor indicates Deficiency and Cold.

Five phases practitioners generally rely on smell more than TCM practitioners do. Each smell is associated with a phase and can indicate disharmony with the associated organ or among organs that are related through the Five Phases cycle. The smells used in Five Phases diagnosis are: goatish, associated with wood; burning, associated with fire; fragrant, associated with earth; rank, associated with metal; and rotten, associated with water.

*Evaluation of Pulses*

There are twenty-eight pulse qualities that are essential to Traditional Chinese Medicine's process of evaluation and diagnosis. Learning to read pulses requires years of study and practice and is not something that can be done at home on yourself. However, your Chinese medicine practitioner will talk to you about your pulse diagnosis, and you will want to have a passing familiarity with the terminology that's used. The most common descriptions are: floating, slippery, choppy, wiry, tight, slow, rapid, thin, big, empty and full.

Pulses are evaluated on a superficial, middle and deep level. The normal pulse resides at the middle level and is usually about four or five beats for each complete inhalation and exhalation of breath.

Disharmonies of the pulses indicate: the condition of Qi, Xue and Fluids; Organ System imbalance(s); the location of the imbalance(s); and the nature (Heat or Cold) of the disease, along with many other qualities.

For example, a wiry pulse may indicate that the Liver System has Stagnant Qi. However, there are no absolute meanings to pulses. They contribute to a diagnosis only when viewed in context with other diagnostic techniques.

*Evaluation of Sensitivity to Touch*

Palpation of acupuncture points and channels can trigger, increase, or reduce pain and indicate disharmony in the associated channels and Organ Systems.

If you have a pain you can't pinpoint, that indicates Stagnant Qi. Stagnant Qi is also indicated by a pain that moves around.

If the pain is fixed, it may indicate Stagnant Xue.

Pain that feels better with pressure is due to Deficiency.

Pain that feels worse with pressure is due to Excess.

Pain that feels better with warmth is associated with Cold.

Palpation of the body does not have to be confined to the twelve channels', fifteen collaterals' or eight extraordinary channels' acupuncture points. Ear acupuncture points are also powerful tools for diagnosis and provide refined clues to the sources of disharmony. They are also useful for self-massage. Reflexology, while not a traditional Chinese method of diagnosis and treatment, is another useful tool at this stage of diagnosis.

## Urine Analysis

Normal urine is pale yellow or straw-colored.

One of the most basic considerations is that scanty dark-colored urine is associated with Heat. This may be Excess Heat or

Yin Deficiency (aka Deficiency Heat). Cloudy urine points to Damp Heat. (Note: If the person is taking a multi-B vitamin, this will cause the urine to be a bright yellow. This is not Heat.)

Large amounts of clear urine often is associated with Cold. If Kidney Yang Deficiency is present, everything the person drinks may go right through him/her.

Large amounts of urine also can be associated with diabetes. Diabetes usually is associated primarily with Yin Deficiency. If the person producing great amounts of urine also complains of feeling thirsty all the time and wanting cold liquids and complains of cravings for sweets, suspect Yin Deficiency and diabetes. Refer clients with possible diabetes to a MD or DO for confirmation. Diabetes is something which is best treated by using both allopathic medicine and TCM as in some cases insulin will be required even if TCM imbalances are identified and corrected.

The fluid intake is going to match the increased urination in most cases of diabetes. The person usually is drinking a lot of water and other liquids. Not so in copious urination with a Root of Yang Deficiency. Yang Deficient (aka Deficiency Cold) people usually do not feel thirsty, drink little, may have to force themselves to drink, and prefer hot liquids, especially soups when they do drink. Also, in Yang Deficiency the tongue and complexion usually are pale; in Yin Deficiency the tongue and complexion usually are red.

**Note:** It's normal for urine to be more concentrated in the summer as people tend to sweat and have less fluid in their bodies. It's normal for people to urinate more in the winter and for urine to be clearer at this time because fluid is not being lost through perspiration.

**Note:** Attack by either Exterior Wind Cold or Exterior Wind Heat can trigger increased urination. Once the Wind Heat penetrates to the Interior, the urine will be dark. But as long as the Wind Heat Evil is in the Exterior, the urine will be clear.

**Summation:** Scanty and dark, think Heat. Copious (great amounts) and clear, think Cold. Cloudy, think Damp Heat. Rule in or rule out.

A strong, foul odor is associated with Dampness. This usually is Damp Heat . This is true not only of urine but feces, semen, and vaginal discharge. If it smells really strong and foul, it's usually Damp Heat. There are exceptions. If there is a fishy odor, suspect Damp Cold. In any event, if it smells foul and strong, suspect Dampness.

Frequent and large amounts of clear urine usually indicates Kidney Yang Deficiency. BUT, frequent trips to the bathroom with little urine each time points to Kidney Qi Deficiency. Remember, one of the functions of Qi is to transport and transform.

Urinary incontinence also points to Kidney and/or Bladder Qi Deficiency. Incontinence in general points to Qi Deficiency. One of the functions of the Kidneys is to "govern opening and closing." When the Kidneys are Deficient, this not only can affect urination with problems like copious amounts of urine (Kidney Yang Deficiency), incontinence of urine and "dribbling" (Kidney Qi Deficiency), it also can play a role in some cases of diarrhea, some cases of chronic nasal drip, leaking seminal fluid, and vaginal discharge. (Note: The opening and closing of skin pores is a Lung function.) If there is incontinence of any kind - urine or feces - suspect Kidney Deficiency and Qi Deficiency as possible Roots and rule in or rule out.

Retention of urine points to Damp Heat. The person has the urge to go to the bathroom but nothing comes out.

**Difficulty in urination** - the person has to push to get the urine out instead of it flowing easily - points to Damp Heat or Kidney Deficiency. Kidney Deficiency is the more likely cause in older people.Swelling of tissues often is associated with Damp Heat, and swelling can be a factor in urination being difficult.

Warner J.W. Fan, M.D., says that Wind Invasion and Heat also can be associated with incontinence.

Maciocia has some words on pain associated with urinating: "Pain before urination indicates stagnation of Qi in the Lower Burner, pain during urination indicates Heat in the Bladder and pain after urination indicates a deficiency of Qi."

When there is pain in the pubic area, and/or physical changes in the area, and/or problems with urination, one also should consider the Liver meridian. The Liver meridian runs right through this area on either side of the front midline of the body. Cold or Heat can lodge in this meridian in this area. There also can be Qi Stagnation problems. In males either Cold or Heat invasion in this area can result in the penis being shrunken. In females Cold or Heat in the Liver meridian can result in some very severe, constant pain associated with the menstrual periods. This pain often will be very localized to the right or left or both of the front midline of the body in the area of the pubic bone.

If urine is reddish yellow or red, suspect and rule in or rule out Liver meridian involvement in the former case and Heat in the Blood in the latter.

Pregnancy sometimes can trigger Qi Stagnation problems in the lower abdomen.

In TCM, sexual desire is associated with the Kidneys. In general, loss of sexual desire or inconstant sexual desire (fades quickly) point to Kidney Yang Deficiency. Some of the Yang tonic herbs, like Epimedium, will increase sexual desire. (P.S.: Herbs like Epimedium are to be used ONLY when Kidney Yang Deficiency is present. This are not herbs to be taken just because a man or a woman wants more sex. Taking Yang tonic herbs (or any other herb) when they are not indicated will result in other problems developing. In the case of Yang tonic herbs, problems like Dryness, agitation, nervousness, Heat, etc.)

Excessive sexual desire and/or wet dreams point to Kidney and Liver Yin Deficiency and/or Liver involvement. The Liver also plays a role in TCM in sexual desire and performance as well as in the health of the urogenital system.

Too much sexual activity can damage the Kidneys, including Kidney Jing. So little also can be injurous.

While selecting an acupuncturist, herbalist, or a chinese medicine doctor, the two most important factors to consider are the doctor's training and your goals.

In order to gain the full benefit of chinese medicine therapy, the practitioner who administers the treatment(s) should have reputable training and a keen sense of the philosophical underpinning of Chinese medicine.

The best way to determine if a practitioner meets those standards is to ask a lot of questions about his or her training, length of practice, scope of practice, specializations, attitudes about wellness and disharmony and understanding of Chinese medicine philosophy.

The Taoist system of belief is not some fancy window dressing that can be cast aside. It is part and parcel of Chinese medicine treatments. No particular Chinese medicine therapy, such as acupuncture or herbal remedies, can deliver its full healing potential if it is separated from the philosophical context of the Tao.

In addition, you want to find a practitioner who is schooled in the chinese medicine therapies that you want to use. There are practitioners who are licensed acupuncturists (L.Ac.) but who do not offer herbal therapy; there are others who are herbalists but provide no acupuncture; there are licensed acupuncturists who also have training as herbalists; and there are doctors of Oriental medicine who provide acupuncture and herbal therapy.

Every acupuncturist should be licensed (in states with licensing requirements) or certified.Your acupuncturist should have either a certificate of training or a long-standing reputation and years of experience. Many schools train people in herbal medicine.

In cases of serious illnesses, you want to select a practitioner who understands Western medical terminology and concepts of the immune system, viruses and cancer, as well as chinese concepts, if you are going for treatment of these problems.

If you have HIV, chronic hepatitis, or CFIDS (chronic fatigue immune deficiency syndrome), be sure that the practitioner's attitude is that you can live with this chronic, manageable viral infection and that acupuncture and herbs may help you be more successful in that process.

When going for treatment, you don't surrender control of your health. Chinese medicine recognizes that we each possess the tools we need to preserve or reclaim good health. The good (or excellent) practitioner simply acts as the guide, helping to coax the body's own defenses to prevent or mend disharmony.

There are four basic healing techniques that the practitioner may suggest as treatments: acupuncture and moxibustion, herbal therapy, dietary therapy, and Qi Gong exercise/meditation. A brief description follows here, and each therapy is discussed in detail in the following chapters.

Diet: Chinese dietary therapy uses foods to strengthen digestion, increase energy and balance the body's energy. Dietary therapy is often used prior to or in conjunction with other therapies to increase the effectiveness of these treatments.

### Acupuncture and Moxibustion

Classic acupuncture is the art of inserting fine, sterile, metal filiform needles into certain points along the channels and collaterals (tributaries of the channels) in order to control the flow of the Qi. These days, practitioners also use electrostimulation of the needles, lasers and even ultrasound to stimulate the points.

Acupuncture is well-known for its effectiveness as a painkiller. Even more powerful is its ability to alter the flow of the Qi so that the body can heal itself when attacked by pathogens that trigger disharmony. Acupressure and massage are subsets of acupuncture.

Moxibustion, the burning of the herb moxa (Chinese mugwort) over channel points and certain areas of the body, is used to warm, tonify and stimulate. It also induces the smooth flow of the Essential Substances, prevents diseases and preserves health. Doing moxa regularly on specific acupuncture points is said to promote strength and longevity. In fact, an old chinese saying is, "Never take a long journey with a person who does not have a Moxa scar on (the acupuncture point called) Stomach 36."

### Chinese Herbal Medicine

Herbal medicine is actually a misnomer. Although the ovenwhelming majority of medicinal substances come from plants, some are derived from minerals and animals. Whatever their origin, they are used to balance the mind/body/spirit as well as to reverse disease processes. Most Chinese herbs should only be taken under the supervision of a trained herbalist.

**Qi Gong Excercise/Meditation:** Qi Gong, the Chinese art of exercise/meditation, uses dynamic movements and still postures in combination with mental and spiritual concentration to influence the flow ofQi. It is a powerful preventive therapy and can help remedy disharmony in the Organ Systems and the channels.

**Diagnosis in respect of Horary Points**

*Step One:*

Determine which organ system is out of balance

*Step Two:*

Determine whether the imbalance is excess (shi) or deficiency (xu)

*Step Three: (for deficiency syndromes)*

Tonify the horary point on the mother organ's channel.

Horary means the point's element and then channels element are the same. i.e. the wood point on the wood channel, or the fire point on the fire channel, the water point on the water channel, the earth point on the earth channel.

Tonify the mother organ's element point on the affected channel.

Sedate the horary point on the "controlling" organ's channel.

Sedate the controlling organ's element point on the affected organ. (for excess syndromes)

Tonify the horary point on the controlling organ's channel.

Tonify the controlling point on the affected channel.

Sedate the horary point on the "son" channel.

Sedate the son point on the affected channel.

## Tonification Prescriptions for Conditions of Deficiency

| | Tonify | | Sedate | |
|---|---|---|---|---|
| Meridian controlling Channel | Horary Pt. on affected Channel | Mother Pt. on Mother | Horary Pt. on affected Channel | Horary Pt. o n Channel |
| Lung | Sp 3 | Lu 9 | Ht 8 | Lu 10 |
| Large Instestine | St 36 | LI 11 | SI 5 | LI 5 |
| Stomach | SI 5 | St 41 | GB 41 | St 43 |
| Spleen | Ht 8 | Sp 2 | Liv 1 | Sp 1 |
| Heart | Liv 1 | Ht 9 | Kid 10 | Ht 3 |
| Small Instestine | GB 41 | SI 3 | UB 66 | SI 2 |
| Urinary Bladder | LI 1 | UB 67 | St 36 | UB 40 |
| Kidney | Lu 8 | Kid 7 | Sp 3 | Kid 3 |
| Pericardium | Liv 1 | P 9 | Kid 10 | P 3 |
| San Jiao | GB 41 | SJ 3 | UB 66 | SJ 2 |
| Gall bladder | UB 66 | GB 43 | LI 1 | GB 44 |

| Liver | Kid 10 | Liv 8 | LU 8 | Liv 4 |
|---|---|---|---|---|

## Sedation Prescriptions for Conditions of Excess

| | Tonify | Sedate | | |
|---|---|---|---|---|
| **Meridian** | **Horary Pt. on controlling Channel** | **Control Pt. on affected Channel** | **Horary Pt. on Son Channel** | **Son Pt. on affected Channel** |
| Lung | Ht 8 | Lu 10 | Kid 10 | Lu 5 |
| Large Instestine | SI 5 | LI 5 | UB 66 | LI 2 |
| Stomach | GB 41 | St 43 | LI 1 | St 45 |
| Spleen | Liv 1 | Sp 1 | LU 8 | Sp 5 |
| Heart | Kid 10 | Ht 3 | Sp 3 | Ht 7 |
| Small Instestine | UB 66 | SI 2 | St 36 | SI 8 |
| Urinary Bladder | St 36 | UB 40 | GB 41 | UB 65 |
| Kidney | Sp 3 | Kid 3 | Liv 1 | Kid 1 |
| Pericardium | Kid 10 | P 3 | Sp 3 | P 7 |
| San Jiao | UB 66 | SJ 2 | St 36 | SJ 10 |
| Gall Bladder | LI 1 | GB 44 | SI 5 | GB 38 |

| | | | | |
|---|---|---|---|---|
| Liver | Lu 8 | Liv 4 | Ht 8 | Liv 2 |

**Horary Points**

| | Shu Point | Well | Spring | Stream | River | Sea |
|---|---|---|---|---|---|---|
| Wood Organs | Liver | 1 | 2 | 3 | 4 | 8 |
| | Gall Bladder | 44 | 43 | 41 | 38 | 34 |
| | Heart | 9 | 8 | 7 | 4 | 3 |
| Fire Organs | Small Intestine | 1 | 2 | 3 | 5 | 8 |
| | Pericardium | 9 | 8 | 7 | 5 | 3 |
| | San Jiao | 1 | 2 | 3 | 6 | 10 |
| Earth Organs | Spleen | 1 | 2 | 3 | 5 | 9 |
| | Stomach | 45 | 44 | 43 | 41 | 36 |
| Metal Organs | Lung | 11 | 10 | 9 | 8 | 5 |
| | Large Intestine | 1 | 2 | 3 | 5 | 11 |
| Water Organs | Kidney | 1 | 2 | 3 | 7 | 10 |
| | Urinary Bladder | 67 | 66 | 65 | 60 | 40 |

**Symptoms Related to Local & Distal Points**

| **Symptoms** | **Points** |
|---|---|
| Fever | Du 14, L.I. 4, L.I. 11, Shi Xuan points, the twelve Jing-well points, Er Jian |
| Coma or Fainting | Du 26, (all ten) Shi Xuan points, the twelve Jing-well points, Kid 1 |
| Loss of Consciousness due to Exhuastion or Shock | Du 20, Ren 4, Ren 8 (moxa), St 36 |
| Spontaneuous Sweating | L.I. 4 |
| Night Sweating | SL 3, Ht 6, Kid 7 |
| Insomnia | Du 24, GB 13, Si Shen Kong, Ht 7, Sp 6, Kid 6 |
| Excessive Dreaming | Ht 7, UB 15, Liv 3, GB 44 |
| Hoarse Voice | L.I. 18, L.I. 4, Pc 5 |
| Lockjaw | St 6, St 7, L.I. 4 |

| | |
|---|---|
| Stiff Tongue | Du 15, Ren 23, Ht 5 |
| Sore Throat | L.I. 4, Lu 11, L.I. 1, L.I. 18 |
| Salivation | Du 26, St 6, L.I. 4 |
| Palpitations | Pc 4, Pc 6 |
| Chest Pain | Ren 17, Pc 4, Pc 6 |
| Cough/Asthma | Lu 7, Ren 22, Ding Chuan, UB 13 |
| Fullness in Chest | Pc 6, Ren 12, Ren 17 |
| Dysphagia | Ren 22, Pc 6 |
| Nausea/Vomiting | Pc 6, St 36 |
| Hiccough | Pc 6, Pc 8, UB 2, UB 17 |
| Abdominal Distension | St 25, Ren 12, Ren 6, Pc 6, St 36 |
| Hypochondriac Pain | SJ6, GB 34 |
| Indigestion | St 36, Sp 5 |
| Malnutrition or Indigestion in Children | Si Feng |
| Insufficient Lactation | SI 1, St 18 |
| Hypertension | St 9 |
| Ben Lou Syndrome | Sp 1, Sp 8, Liv 6 |
| Itching of the External Genitalia | Liv 5 |
| Spermatorrhea, Impotence, Premature Ejaculation | Ren 4, Sp 6 |
| Constipation | St 25, Ren 6, Ren 12, SJ 6, Kid 6 |
| Rectal Prolapse | Du 1, UB 57, Du 20 |
| Spasm of Gastrocnemius Muscle | UB 57, GB 34 |
| Itching | Sp 10, L.I. 11, Sp 6 |
| General Weakness | Ren 4, St 36, Du 4, Ren 6, UB 23 |
| Convulsions | L.I. 4, Liv 3 |
| Epistaxis | Du 23, L.I. 4, Lu 6 |
| Diaorrhea | St 25, Sp 9, St 36, Ren 8 (moxa) |

## Fever

Du 14 is the crossing point of the Du and six Yang channels.

L.I. 4, L.I. 11

The He-sea and Yuan-source point of hand Yang Ming channels. In the Yang Ming channel, Yang Qi develops to its final stages ("The Bright Yang") Tai Yang is greater Yang, Yang Qi is vigorous; Shao Yang is lesser Yang where the Yang Qi is weak. At the He-sea point and Yuan-source points, the Jing QI is lively and at L.I. 4 and L.I. 11, the Yang Qi is liveliest.

## Coma

Du 26:

Ren Zhong (Human Center or Person's Center). The three components of the Chinese universe are Heaven, humanity, and Earth. The nose receives the five Qi from Heaven. The mouth receives the five tastes from Earth. Located between the nose and the mouth, Du 26 can thus be likened unto humankind positioned in the center, between Heaven and Earth. So, Du 26 is called Human Center. It can connect Heaven's Qi and Earth's Qi. The Du channel supervises all the Yang channels of the body just as Heaven supervises the Yang of the universe. The Ren channel takes charge of all the Yin channels of the body. Located between the Du and Ren Channels, Du 26 can regulate Yin and Yang. Coma is considered the prelude to the final separation of Yin and Yang. Additionally, the Du channel enters the brain, which is obviously an important component in the coma state.

Shi Xuan points and the twelve Jing-well points: The Yin channels link with the Yang channels at the twelve Jing-well points. Shi Xuan is located on the tips of the ten fingers, so Shi Xuan points along with the twelve Jing-well points can regulate Yin and Yang thus resuscitating the depleted Yang and rescuing the patient from danger.

## Sweating

1. Heat

2. Wei Yang deficiency: L.I. 4 is the Yuan-source point of the yang Ming channel. It can tonify the Yang.

## Night Sweats (Yin deficiency)

Kidney 7: Jing-river (metal) point of the Kidney (water) channel. Tonifying the mother point for Kidney Yin deficiency.

SI 3: The Shu-stream point of the Small Intestine channel belongs to wood. Sweat is the fluid of the Heart. Tonifying the mother point (wood) of the Heart's (fire) paired channel (S.I.) serves to tonify Heart Yin. Heart 6 is the Xi-cleft point on the Heart channel which will stop bleeding and sweating. Blood and sweat both come from the Heart.

## Stiff Tongue

Du 15, Ren 23:

These two points connect to the root of the tongue. Du 15 is called "Mute's Gate." Heart 5 is the Luo-connecting point of the Heart channel to treat tongue disease. The Heart open into the tongue.

## Insufficient Lactation

S.I. 1: The Small Intestine channel is used for "Ye" (thick fluid) diseases. S.I. 1 is the Jing-well (metal) point for "Ye" deficiency (water) Tonifies metal.

## Hypertension

St 9: Needled Deep, the needle will effect the cervical arterial bulbus which is a part of the coratid artery that monitors and adjusts the blood pressure. Needle even deeper, the acupuncture will effect the sympathetic trunk in such as way that will lower blood pressure.

## Constipation

SJ 6: When constipation is a disorder of Qi, the San Jiao channel is employed for Qi problems in the Zang Fu, especially the inability of the raising of the refined substances and eliminating the "heavy evil."

## General Weakness

Ren 6, St 36, for general weakness. Ren 4 tonifies Yuan source Qi, and Stomach 36 tonifies digestive function hence increasing Gu Qi. Du 4 and Ren 4 tonify Ming Men fire, UB 23 tonifies Kidneys.

## Disorders of Blood

One of the things that strikes the acupuncturist who studies Chinese herbal medicine is the great array of herbs, prescriptions and protocols which treat disorders of blood. By comparison, acupuncture may seem inadequate, and it is sometimes said that there are only three or four acupuncture points which are important in the treatment of blood disorders. A careful examination of the traditional and modern indications of the acupuncture points, traditional commentaries and classical combinations, however, reveals that many acupuncture points are able to nourish blood, dispel blood stasis, clear heat from the blood or stop bleeding. Some of the most important are listed in this article. The indications, discussion and classical combinations for the points given here are concerned only with these actions, and many other important aspects of the use of these points are omitted.

## Tianfu LU-3

*Relevant indications*

Nosebleed, spitting blood, coughing blood, wheezing, dyspnoea, cough, asthma.

## Discussion

According to the Discourse Into the Origins and Development of Medicine "The Lung is the delicate zang, neither heat nor cold is appropriate ... too hot and the fire will melt the metal and the blood will stir". As early as the Spiritual Pivot (Chapter 21: On Hot and Cold Disease) Tianfu LU-3 was indicated for "Severe thirst, internal upsurge, Liver and Lung struggle against each other, blood pours from the mouth and nose". This is a clear reference to the pattern of Liver fire attacking the Lung. Liver fire rushes upwards and scorches the Lung, injuring the blood vessels and giving rise to reckless pouring of blood from the mouth and nose. At the same time there will be coughing, which is characterised in this pattern by bouts of spasmodic coughing with a red face.

*Classical combinations*

Bleeding from the nose: Tianfu LU-3 and Hegu L.I.-4 (Ode to the 100 Patterns).

## CHIZE LU-5

*Relevant indications*

Spitting blood, coughing blood, nosebleed, vomiting blood, Heart pain, Heart agitation.

**Discussion**

Chize LU-5 is the water and he-sea point of the Lung channel. Its principal action is to clear all forms of heat (whether shi or xu) from the Lung. Heat in the Lung may injure the blood vessels and give rise to reckless bleeding, characterised by coughing or spitting of blood or nosebleed.

The Lung channel originates in the middle jiao. As well as being indicated for heat-induced bleeding from the Lung, due to its secondary action of descending Stomach qi, Chize LU-5 may also be used for vomiting blood. The Song of Points for Miscellaneous Diseases states uncompromisingly: "In cases of vomiting blood the action of Chize LU-5 is without comparison".

The Lung and Heart are intimately associated in the upper jiao. Yang Zhao Li says "The Lung and Heart are mutually connected; when there is Lung heat it most easily enters the Heart" and the Spiritual Pivot (Chapter 75) says "If zong qi does not descend, blood will stagnate in the vessels". In the case of Lung heat entering the Heart there will be agitation of the Heart, and in the case of Lung and zong qi deficiency there will be blood stasis giving rise to Heart pain.

*Classical combinations*

Spitting blood, at times hot and at times cold: tonify Chize LU-5 and disperse Yuji LU-10.

**Taiyuan LU-9**

*Relevant indications*

Spitting blood, coughing blood, vomiting blood, agitated Heart with Heart pain and choppy pulse, oppression of the chest, manic raving, pulseless syndrome.

**Discussion**

According to the Plain Questions "The Lung governs the one hundred vessels", and the Classic of Difficulties (45th Difficulty) states "the vessels gather at Taiyuan LU-9". This concept of the hundred vessels was discussed more fully in The Classic of Categories which stated "The flow of the jingmai (channels and vessels) must follow the qi; the qi is dominated by the Lung, therefore it is the meeting of the hundred vessels". These statements refer to the important relationship between the qi and the blood, expressed in the saying "The qi is the commander of the blood", and the statement in The Classic of Categories that "The vessels are the pathways of the blood qi; the movement of the vessels is dependent on qi". In other words, the blood moves through the blood vessels by virtue of the movement of qi, and in the chest and Heart region especially, the circulation of the blood is dependent on the zong qi which is formed from the gu qi and air inhaled by the Lung. Taiyuan LU-9, the Hui-Meeting point of the vessels, is therefore an important point to harmonise the relationship between the zong qi and the blood. When the zong qi is deficient and fails to circulate the blood, it will pool and stagnate in the chest and Heart, giving rise to oppression and fullness, agitation, Heart pain with a choppy pulse, and in severe cases manic raving. Taiyuan LU-9 is further indicated for disorders of the blood vessels in general such as vomiting, spitting or coughing of blood and pulseless syndrome.

*Classical combinations*

Pain of the Lung and Heart: Taiyuan LU-9 and Yuji LU-10 .

Raving speech: Taiyuan LU-9, Yangxi L.I.-5, Xialian L.I.-8 and Kunlun BL-60.

**Yuji LU-10**

*Relevant indications*

Coughing blood, vomiting blood, blood in the urine, genital damp itching, impotence with abdominal distention.

**Discussion**

Yuji LU-10 is the ying-spring and fire point of the Lung. According to the Classic of Difficulties (68th Difficulty), ying-spring points are indicated for "heat in the body", and Yuji LU-10 is effective to clear heat from both the Lung channel and the Lung zang. When heat, a form of yang excess, enters the blood it may lead to excessive and reckless movement, and hence haemorrhage.

Yuji LU-10 is indicated for bleeding disorders affecting all three jiao. Lung heat may injure the vessels of the Lung causing coughing of blood, transmit to the origin of the Lung channel in the Stomach causing vomiting of blood, or transmit to the Heart and thence the Small Intestine and Bladder giving rise to urinary bleeding (which may be accompanied by genital damp itching or impotence).

*Classical combinations*

Vomiting blood: Yuji LU-10, Quze P-3 and Shenmen HE-7 .

Pain of the penis: Yuji LU-10, Taixi KID-3, Zhongji REN-3 and Sanyinjiao SP-6 GUILAI ST-29

*Relevant indications*

Amenorrhoea, irregular menstruation, uterine blood stasis due to cold.

**Discussion**

The name of this point, Guilai ('Return') refers to its ability to restore the menstruation to normal, and its overriding action is to warm the lower jiao, most particularly the uterus in women. The uterus (along with the Stomach and Spleen and the intestines) belongs to that group of the zangfu or extra fu that can suffer from direct attack by exterior pathogenic cold (i.e. without initially giving rise to symptoms and signs of an exterior pattern such as chills and fever, body aches etc.). Injury of the uterus by cold may be due to inadequate clothing or sitting on cold ground, or over-consumption of cold foods and drinks, especially during menstruation or after childbirth. "Qi and blood desire warmth and dislike cold; when cold is encountered they coagulate; when warmth is encountered they disperse and flow", whilst the Spiritual Pivot says "The qi and blood of the human body circulate without stopping, in the same way that the stars do in the upper region and the rivers in the lower region. When a cold pathogen comes to reside in the channels as a guest, the blood will coagulate; when the blood coagulates the channels do not move". Pathogenic cold entering the uterus will cause stagnation of qi and coagulation of blood and disrupt the function of the Ren Mai and Chong Mai, giving rise to disorders such as amenorrhoea, irregular menstruation and abdominal masses. Guilai ST-29 is normally treated with warm needling to warm the uterus and drive out pathogenic cold.

### Yinbai SP-1

*Relevant indications*

Uterine bleeding, menorrhagia, vomiting blood, nosebleed, heat illness with nosebleed, blood in the urine, blood in the stools.

### Discussion

According to the Supplements to Commentaries "The Spleen gathers the blood; when the Spleen is xu it is unable to unite the blood", whilst the Treatise on Disorders of Blood says "When Spleen yang is xu the blood is not gathered". Yinbai SP-1, the jing-well point of the Spleen channel, is one of the foremost acupuncture points for strengthening the Spleen's function of holding blood. This pattern, which is usually chronic in nature, may manifest as bleeding in any part of the body, but most commonly in the lower jiao, whether as uterine bleeding or as bleeding into the urine or stools. In such cases moxibustion at Yinbai SP-1 is frequently employed, and it is particularly helpful to instruct the patient in the daily use of moxibustion at home. The action of Yinbai SP-1 in stopping bleeding, however, is not confined to cases of Spleen deficiency, but may also be applied where shi or xu heat enters the blood level giving rise to reckless bleeding, especially in the upper part of the body (nosebleed, vomiting blood). In these cases, needling is the usual method employed.

*Classical combinations*

Bloody stools: Yinbai SP-1 and Zusanli ST-36.

Bloody dysentery: Yinbai SP-1, Tianshu ST-25, Neiting ST-44, Qihai REN-6, Zhaohai KID-6 and Neiguan P-6.

Vomiting and nosebleed: Yinbai SP-1, Pishu BL-20, Ganshu BL-18 and Shangwan REN-13.

Severe and ceaseless nosebleed: Yinbai SP-1 and Weizhong BL-40.

Hot head and nosebleed: Yinbai SP-1, Feiyang BL-58, Jinggu BL-64, Kunlun BL-60 and Chengshan BL-57 (1000 Ducats).

### Sanyinjiao SP-6

*Relevant indications*

Irregular menstruation, uterine bleeding, uterine bleeding with dizziness, menorrhagia, amenorrhoea, dysmenorrhoea, difficult labour, failure of the lochia to descend, post-partum dizziness, palpitations, blurred vision, insomnia, eczema, urticaria.

### Discussion

Along with Geshu BL-17, Xuehai SP-10 and Diji SP-8, Sanyinjiao SP-6 is considered one of the most important acupuncture points to nourish, harmonise and cool blood and to promote and invigorate its circulation. This action finds its most important application in the treatment of gynaecological disorders, but extends to other disorders where blood disharmony plays an important role such as skin diseases. When Spleen qi or yang is xu there may be: i. inadequate formation of blood (palpitations, blurred vision, amenorrhoea, post-partum dizziness, dizziness associated with uterine bleeding etc.), or ii. failure of the Spleen to hold the blood (uterine bleeding, menorrhagia). By virtue of its ability to tonify the Spleen qi and yang and to strengthen the Spleen's ability to hold the blood, Sanyinjiao SP-6 is an essential point in the treatment of these disorders, especially uterine bleeding and menorrhagia. The further ability of Sanyinjiao SP-6 to regulate the Spleen, Liver and Kidney channels and to treat all disorders of the lower abdomen renders it an important point to treat gynaecological disorders due to blood stasis, Kidney deficiency, phlegm-dampness or Liver stagnation.

*Classical combinations*

Uterine bleeding: Sanyinjiao SP-6, Yinjiao REN-7 and Yangchi SJ-4.

Ceaseless uterine bleeding: Sanyinjiao SP-6, Jiaoxin KID-8, Yingu KID-10 and Taichong LIV-3.

Menorrhagia: Sanyinjiao SP-6, Tongli HE-5 and Xingjian LIV-2.

Disordered menstruation: Sanyinjiao SP-6, Zulinqi GB-41 and Zhongji REN-3.

## Diji SP-8

*Relevant indications*

Irregular menstruation, dysmenorrhoea, abdominal masses in women due to qi and blood stasis.

### Discussion

Diji SP-8 is the xi-cleft point of the Spleen channel. The xi-cleft points are where the qi and blood, which flow relatively superficially along the channels from the jing-well points, gather and plunge more deeply. The xi-cleft points in general are indicated in the treatment of acute conditions and pain, whilst the xi-cleft points of the yin channels have an additional action of treating disorders of blood.

The Spleen controls blood and its channel enters the lower abdomen, joining with the Ren Mai at Zhongji REN-3 and Guanyuan REN-4. Diji SP-8 has a specific and important action on resolving blood stasis in the uterus and lower abdomen, being indicated in the treatment of irregular menstruation, abdominal masses in women and dysmenorrhoea due to this pathology. As the xi-cleft point, Diji SP-8 is especially suited to treating acute dysmenorrhoea, for which purpose it is often combined clinically with Hegu L.I.-4. A specific indication for this point mentioned in the Illustrated Classic of Acupuncture Points on the Bronze Man is a hot flowing sensation spreading down the inner thigh to the knee when pressure is applied to abdominal masses in women.

*Classical combinations*

Irregular menstruation: Diji SP-8 and Xuehai SP-10.

**Xuehai SP-10**

*Relevant indications*

Irregular menstruation, dysmenorrhoea, amenorrhoea, uterine bleeding, clotted uterine bleeding, sudden uterine bleeding, post-partum qi and blood deficiency, urticaria, eczema, erysipelas, herpes zoster, painful hot sores, ulceration and itching of the scrotum, blood lin.

**Discussion**

The name of this point Xuehai SP-10, literally "Sea of Blood", reflects its pre-eminent role in treating various disorders at the blood level. It is generally recognised as having two principal actions: i. invigorating the blood and dispelling stasis, and ii. clearing heat from the blood. These two actions find their expression in its ability to treat a wide range of gynaecological and dermatological disorders due either to blood stasis or heat in the blood.

As far as gynaecology is concerned, normal menstruation depends on a number of factors including the smooth circulation of blood. Impairment of blood circulation and consequent stasis may be due to stagnation or deficiency of qi, traumatic injury, haemorrhage, penetration of cold, blood deficiency, heat, chronic disease or emotional factors, and may give rise to many different disorders of menstruation. These include dysmenorrhoea and uterine bleeding characterised by severe fixed pain and the discharge of dark or clotted blood, and amenorrhoea accompanied by pain and distention, a purple coloured tongue and a choppy pulse. By contrast, if heat enters the blood level, most frequently due to internally generated heat from the Liver or Heart, or due to overconsumption of excessively heating foods, then two principal conditions may arise: i. the movement of blood may become reckless and overflow its bounds leading to uterine bleeding, or the heat may dry the blood leading to amenorrhoea. In both cases there will be signs of heat such as a red dry tongue and a rapid pulse. In fact, both the blood cooling and blood invigorating properties of Xuehai SP-10 come together in its ability to treat uterine bleeding. Blood heat is the most commonly seen pattern of uterine bleeding, and as well as cooling blood, treatment must emphasise resolving stasis, since any pathological bleeding may lead to pooling and stagnation of extravasated blood. This is expressed in the Chinese medicine saying "where there is haemorrhage there is stasis".

Some authorities further attribute blood nourishing properties to Xuehai SP-10 and incorporate it into prescriptions for the treatment of blood deficiency. In the light of Xuehai SP-10's pre-eminence in invigorating blood, this action reflects the saying in Chinese medicine "if blood stasis is not transformed, new blood cannot be generated". This refers to situations either where blood deficiency and consequent poor circulation lead to stasis, or where blood stasis prevents the creation of new blood. Both of these patterns are commonly encountered in post-partum blood deficiency. As far as dermatology is concerned, blood disharmony often plays a central role. The main dermatological patterns treated by Xuehai SP-10 are heat in the blood level characterised by red lesions, and blood stasis characterised by purple lesions. Xuehai SP-10 may also be used for the concomitant blood deficiency and stasis seen for example in eczema with thickening of the skin (lichenif-ication) or post-herpetic neuralgia. Xuehai SP-10 may also be used to treat the manifestations of wind in skin diseases, the most important of which is intolerable itching. This illustrates the Chinese medicine saying "to treat wind first treat the blood; once blood moves wind will be dispelled".

Although the action of Xuehai SP-10 on invigorating and cooling blood is classically confined to the two principal areas of gynaecology and dermatology, its application may be extended to any disorder in the body with these pathologies.

*Classical combinations*

Irregular menstruation: Xuehai SP-10 and Daimai GB-26.

**Dabao SP-21**

*Relevant indications*

Pain of the whole body, weakness of the four limbs, flaccidity of the limbs.

**Discussion**

The name of the point Dabao SP-21 is made up of two characters, 'Da' meaning great, and 'Bao' meaning 'to wrap', or 'to envelop'. According to the Spiritual Pivot "The great luo of the Spleen is known as Dabao ... it spreads in the chest and flanks. When it is shi there is pain of the whole body. When it is xu the hundred joints are flaccid. This channel is like a net embracing the blood of all the luo".

A possible explanation of this statement from the Spiritual Pivot is that one of the functions of the luo-connecting channels in general is to assist in the distribution of qi, and more especially blood, to all the tissues of the body via the network of the minute luo-connecting channels. Since the Spleen controls blood, its great luo-connecting channel dominates this function of blood distribution throughout the body. When blood stagnates "there is pain of the whole body"; when blood is xu and unable to nourish the tissues, "the hundred joints are flaccid".

**Yinxi HE-6**

*Relevant indications*

Heart pain, unbearable stabbing pain of the Heart, fullness of the chest, palpitations, fright palpitations, sudden turmoil disorder with cardiac pain, nosebleed, vomiting blood.

**Discussion**

Yinxi HE-6, the xi-cleft point of the Heart channel (see Diji SP-8 above) is indicated for Heart pain due to blood stasis, and bleeding disorders due to excessive heat agitating the blood. However, in terms of both these actions, Ximen P-4, the xi-cleft point of the Pericardium channel, is clinically more important. Acute severe pain from blood stasis which threatens the survival of the Heart zang is therefore primarily treated by using points of the Pericardium channel, the 'protector' of the Heart This is reflected in the statement in the Spiritual Pivot "The Heart is the great master of the five zang and six fu and the residence of the jing shen ... If the Heart is injured, the shen will depart; if the shen departs, the person will die ... therefore the pathogenic qi that attacks the Heart will be diverted to reside in the Pericardium".

### Xinshu BL-15

*Relevant indications*

Heart pain, oppression of the chest with restlessness, chest pain extending to the back, palpitations, irregular pulse, poor memory, anxiety, weeping with grief, insomnia, excessive dreaming, absent-mindedness as if in a trance, delayed speech development, coughing blood, vomiting blood, nosebleed, night sweating.

**Discussion**

Xinshu BL-15 is the back-shu point of the Heart, where the qi of the Heart emanates from the interior to the body surface, and in common with all the back-shu points (especially those of the yin zang) Xinshu BL-15 has a strong action on regulating and tonifying its corresponding zang at the deepest level. It is used equally to tonify deficiency of Heart blood and to resolve blood stasis.

"Blood is the qi of the shen", and "The Heart is the monarch from which the shen emanates". Since storage is a yin function, it is primarily the Heart blood and yin that have the function of nourishing the Heart and providing the material basis for the Heart to house the shen. Blood and yin deficiency of the Heart may originate from physical causes such as loss of blood, chronic illness and overwork, or from emotional causes. Fei Bo Xiong (1800-1879) said: "The seven emotions injure the five yin organs selectively but they all affect the Heart", whilst "The Heart stores the shen ... when the shen is in excess there is ceaseless laughter, when the shen is insufficient there is sadness". When Heart blood or yin are deficient, the unrooted and unanchored shen loses its harmony and becomes restless and unquiet, resulting in such symptoms as anxiety, poor memory, insomnia and excessive dreaming and weeping with grief.

The Heart controls the pulse, and when Heart qi is deficient and is unable to regulate the blood, there may be palpitations or irregular pulse, especially if the Heart blood is also deficient. In the latter case, palpitations will be more likely to be accompanied by anxiety, in contrast to the palpitations caused purely by qi deficiency which are usually unrelated to emotional changes.

According to essential readings from the medical tradition, "That which is stored by the Heart internally is blood, externally it is emitted as sweat; sweat is the fluid of the Heart". For this reason, Xinshu BL-15 is also indicated for night sweating.

References to the relationship between the Heart, the blood and its vessels abound in the classics. "All blood pertains to the Heart", "The Heart dominates the blood vessels of the entire body" and "The Heart stores the qi of the blood vessels". "The vessels are the pathways of the blood qi, the movement of the vessels is dependent on qi", "When the qi of hand shaoyin channel is exhausted, the vessels will not move, thus the blood will not flow; when the blood does not flow the circulation will eventually stop ... and the blood will die". "In chest bi, pain in the Heart region is caused by yang deficiency and invasion of cold". In Treatment Planning According to Pattern Categories it says "In chest bi, the yang qi of the chest does not move; after a long time, yin takes the place of yang". The above statements all emphasise the close relationship between the circulation of blood in the chest and the qi and yang of the Heart. When Heart yang is deficient and unable to circulate the blood in the chest and Heart, there may be consequential Heart blood stasis giving rise to pain and oppression of the chest. Xinshu BL-15 is an important point for all kinds of Heart and chest pain, whether due to deficiency, stasis of blood, or stagnation of qi or phlegm. The action of Xinshu BL-15 in treating blood stasis as well as blood deficiency, reflects its ability to treat both xu and shi patterns of the Heart with equal effect. According to a number of classics it is an important point to clear heat from the Heart, both shi and xu, but the Illustrated Appendices to the Classic of Categories states "Xinshu BL-15 is indicated for clearing heat of the five zang in combination with the five zang back-shu points". This reflects the application of five phase theory in which the Heart pertains to sovereign fire and plays a role in governing the fire of the whole body. When Heart fire injures the blood vessels of the Lung or Stomach, therefore, there may be coughing or vomiting of blood.

*Classical combinations*

Weeping with grief: Xinshu BL-15, Shenmen HE-7, Jiexi ST-41 and Daling P-7

Melancholy and trance-like absent-mindedness: Xinshu BL-15, Tianjing SJ-10 and Shendao DU-11).

Trance-like mental confusion: Xinshu BL-15, Tianjing SJ-10 and Juque REN-14

Mental stupidity and dull-wittedness: Xinshu BL-15, Shenmen HE-7, Shaoshang LU-11 and Yongquan KID-1.

Agitated Heart: Xinshu BL-15 and Juque REN-14.

Coughing and spitting blood: Xinshu BL-15, Gansh̄u BL-18, Quepen ST-12, Juque REN-14 and Jiuwei REN-15.

**Geshu BL-17**

*Relevant indications*

All blood diseases, epigastric pain, fullness of the abdomen and flank, pain of the whole body, pain of the skin, flesh and bone, stabbing pain of the Heart, Heart pain on eating, tidal fever, night sweating, spontaneous sweating, steaming bone syndrome, fever without sweating, aversion to cold, mania-depression disorder, coughing blood, vomiting blood, spitting blood, blood in the stool, urticaria, bi of the whole body.

**Discussion**

Geshu BL-17 is one of the eight hui-meeting points with a specific action on the blood. Many classics simply state that this point can be used for "all blood diseases". Disorders of blood may be of three main kinds: blood stasis, blood heat and blood deficiency.

Impairment of blood circulation and consequent blood stasis may be due to various causes (see Xuehai SP-10 above). The variety of symptoms that blood stasis can give rise to is extensive, but of these the principal one is pain. Shi pain may be due either to stagnation of qi or stasis of blood, as reflected in the famous adage "when there is no movement there is pain". Pain due to blood stasis is characterised by its fixed and stabbing nature. According to Wang Qingren, the Qing dynasty author of Correcting the Errors of Medicine, "whenever there is pain in the abdomen that does not move, it is blood stasis". Tang Rong Chuan in the Treatise on Disorders of Blood said "... When blood stasis is between the jingluo and the zangfu the whole body is in pain ... when it is in the upper jiao ... there is stabbing obstinate pain of the arm, chest and diaphragm ... when it is in the middle jiao there is pain of the abdomen and flanks". As is clear from its indications, Geshu BL-17 is applicable in all these cases. It should be noted, however, that due to its location and its special action on the diaphragm which intersects the upper and middle jiao, its main sphere of action is on these two areas and it is less used for blood stasis in the lower jiao. Geshu BL-17 is also an important point to treat various kinds of fever due to blood stasis. The Treatise on Disorders of Blood states "when blood stasis is at the level of the pores the ying and wei are not harmonised there is fever accompanied by chills ... when it is half-interior half-exterior ... there is alternating chills and fever ... when it is at the level of the muscles and flesh there will be a burning fever ... when it is in the jingluo and zangfu ... there is necessarily steaming bone consumption fever".

Geshu BL-17 is also indicated for mania-depression disorder, and according to Wang Qingren in Correcting the Errors of Medicine, "In the pattern of insanity, where there is continual crying and laughing, swearing and singing ... then the qi and blood will coagulate in the brain". An alternative explanation for this manifestation is that blood stasis may both transform to heat and obstruct the blood vessels, preventing nourishment from reaching the Heart. This combination of heat and malnourishment may disturb the shen.

Geshu BL-17 is an important point for many kinds of bleeding disorders, primarily due to blood heat or blood stasis. Heat entering the blood level may be due to a number of causes including constitutional heat, exterior pathogenic heat, overconsumption of excessively heating food or drink, or shi or xu heat generated by disharmony of the zangfu. When heat agitates the blood it causes it to move recklessly and burst out of the vessels giving rise to haemorrhage that is usually acute and profuse. Geshu BL-17 is able to cool the blood and stop bleeding, primarily from the upper and middle jiao (Lung and Stomach). Another important cause of haemorrhage is blood stasis. When blood is stagnant and does not move it may be forced out of the vessels giving rise to haemorrhage characterised by its intermittent nature, dark purplish colour and presence of clots. At the same time, haemorrhage of any aetiology is itself in an important cause of blood stasis, as blood that is forced out of the vessels easily pools and stagnates. This is reflected in the saying "where there is haemorrhage there is stasis". The close inter-relationship between blood heat, blood stasis and haemorrhage is further illustrated by the fact that blood heat may condense and dry the blood giving rise to stasis, as stated in the Treatise on Acute Epidemic Febrile Disease by Wu You Ke (1642) "Because latent stagnant fire evaporates the blood's fluid, the blood simmers and forms stasis".

The ability of Geshu BL-17 to nourish blood and yin is clearly overshadowed in the classical indications by its ability to resolve blood stasis and heat. There are three areas, however, that reflect its nourishing and tonifying properties. The first is its ability to treat disorders such as night sweating and steaming bone syndrome due to severe blood and yin xu. The second is the use of Geshu BL-17 with Danshu BL-19 which forms the classical combination of the 'Four Flowers'. The Four Flowers were first mentioned in Secrets of a Frontier Official by Wang Tao (752 AD), who did not specify the points but described rather a complex location method (see below*). The Classic of Supplementing Life with Acupuncture and Moxibustion in the 13th century first defined the Four Flowers as Geshu BL-17 and Danshu BL-19 and said that they dominated blood, being indicated (for treatment by moxibustion) for consumption disorder manifesting as exhaustion with steaming bone syndrome, night sweating cough, asthma, feebleness and emaciation. The third is the special ability of Geshu BL-17 to treat blood deficiency allied to blood stasis. It has long been understood that following haemorrhage, the consequent blood stasis prevents the formation of new blood. This is reflected in the saying: "if blood stasis is not transformed, new blood cannot be generated" and the statement by Tang Rong Chuan "In vomiting blood, nose bleeds and blood in the stool, the blood leaves the channels; any blood that has left the channels is separated and no longer connected with the blood that nourishes the entire body ... this blood is unable to augment with good blood, thus the transformation of new blood is hindered". At the same time, by pooling outside the channels, blood stasis may lead directly to blood deficiency as sufficient blood is no longer available to nourish the body. Thus blood stasis may not only be the cause of, but may be the end result of blood deficiency.

The action of Geshu BL-17 on bi syndrome, commonly referred to as wind-damp in Chinese medicine, which affects the whole body reflects its action of regulating blood. Prolonged bi syndrome may give rise either to blood stasis or blood deficiency. The importance of treating the blood in such cases is reflected in the saying "to treat wind first treat the blood; once blood moves wind will be dispelled".

*The method of locating these points described in the Secrets of a Frontier Official (752 AD) is as follows: a piece of string is tied around the neck, with a knot made at the level of Jiuwei REN-15. When the string is allowed to fall down the back, the knot will then lie on the vertebral column at the crossing point of two diagonal lines the end of each of which leads to one of the four points.

### Weizhong BL-40

*Relevant indications*

Pain and stiffness of the lumbar spine, heaviness of the lumbar region and buttock, nosebleed, clove sore (ding chuang), erysipelas.

#### Discussion

An alternative name for Weizhong BL-40, used in a number of classics, is Xuexi (Blood Xi-Cleft). According to the Inner Classic taiyang channel is abundant in blood. This not only explains the powerful effect of bleeding Weizhong BL-40 to move blood stasis in acute lumbar sprain, but also its ability to cool the blood in cases of nosebleed and a variety of skin disorders, in which case the point may also be bled. Interestingly, the only other channel abundant in blood according to the Inner Classic is the jueyin channel, and this may help to explain certain similarities between Weizhong BL-40 (the he-sea point of the Bladder taiyang channel) and Quze P-3 (the he-sea point of the Pericardium jueyin channel). Both points are bled to clear heat from the blood level and are used in the treatment of injury by summer-heat, sudden turmoil disorder with heat of the four limbs, ceaseless thirst, vomiting and diarrhoea.

*Classical combinations*

Severe and incessant nosebleed: Weizhong BL-40 and Yinbai SP-1.

Carbuncles on the back: needle Weizhong BL-40 and Jianjing GB-21, and place a slice of garlic on the carbuncle and burn moxa. If there is no pain, then moxa until there is pain; if there is pain, moxa until there is no pain, the more moxa the better.

**Shuiquan KID-5**

*Relevant indications*

Amenorrhoea, irregular menstruation, dysmenorrhoea, delayed menstruation with epigastric pain on onset of menstruation, prolapse of the uterus.

**Discussion**

Shuiquan KID-5 is the xi-cleft point of the Kidney channel (see Diji SP-8 above). The Plain Questions (Chapter 1) states: "At the age of fourteen, the Kidney qi of the female is strong, the reproductive function matures, the Ren Mai flows and the Chong Mai fills, the menses come according to their times, and she can bear offspring". Normal development of the uterus and the Ren and Chong Mai, therefore, depend on healthy functioning of the Kidneys. At the same time, harmonious menstruation depends on adequate formation of blood in the body, especially the Liver blood which flows to the Ren and Chong Mai to form menstrual blood. The close relationship between the Kidneys and Liver blood was emphasised in Master Zhang's Medical Encyclopaedia which said "When the jing is not discharged it will return to the Liver and transform into clear blood", whilst the Kidneys themselves play an important role in the formation of blood, stated unequivocally in the Bing Ji Sha Zhuan "The source of blood is the Kidney".

If the Kidneys are deficient, then the function of the Ren and Chong Mai will be disturbed and the formation of blood inadequate. Shuiquan KID-5, the xi-cleft point of the Kidney channel and thus able to treat disorders of blood, regulates the qi and blood in the Kidney, Ren and Chong channels. It is indicated for a variety of menstrual disorders such as amenorrhoea, irregular menstruation, dysmenorrhoea and delayed menstruation, whether characterised by deficiency (of blood or qi) or excess (stasis of blood).

*Classical combinations*

Amenorrhoea with much oppression and pain in the lower Heart (upper epigastrium): Shuiquan KID-5 and Zhaohai KID-6.

Irregular menstruation: Shuiquan KID-5 and Tianshu ST-25 (Ode to the 100 Patterns).

## Jiaoxin KID-8

*Relevant indications*

Uterine bleeding, irregular menstruation, dysmenorrhoea, amenorrhoea, uterine prolapse.

### Discussion

Jiaoxin KID-8 is the xi-cleft point of the Yin Qiao Mai on the Kidney channel. The xi-cleft points of the yin channels have a special action of treating disorders of blood, especially resolving blood stasis, clearing heat from the blood and stopping bleeding. Although the Yin Qiao Mai does not enter the uterus, like all the extraordinary channels, it has a close relationship with the Kidneys and originates at Zhaohai KID-6. Jiaoxin KID-8 is indicated in a variety of menstrual disorders, and most especially uterine bleeding.

According to the Classic of the Central Viscera by the great Han dynasty doctor Hua Tuo, the Kidneys serve the purpose of "wrapping the blood" in women. If the Kidneys are injured by excessively early sexual activity, sexual overindulgence, multiple pregnancies etc, then either the Kidney yin or Kidney yang may become deficient leading to infirmity of the Ren and Chong Mai and hence uterine bleeding. Jiaoxin KID-8 is predominantly indicated in xu patterns of uterine bleeding, particularly in cases of Kidney deficiency, but its status as a xi-cleft point and its secondary action of draining damp-heat renders it suitable in the treatment of uterine bleeding due to blood stasis, reckless movement of hot blood and damp-heat.

*Classical combinations*

Ceaseless uterine bleeding: Jiaoxin KID-8, Yingu KID-10, Taichong LIV-3 and Sanyinjiao SP-6 .

Diminished qi uterine bleeding: Jiaoxin KID-8 and Heyang BL-55 (Ode to the 100 Patterns).

**Siman KID-14**

*Relevant indications*

Abdominal distention, oedema of the abdomen, diarrhoea, constipation, masses below the umbilicus, painful masses, cutting pain below the umbilicus, irregular menstruation, uterine bleeding, blood stasis in the uterus, acute pain due to blood stasis.

**Discussion**

The name of this point, Siman KID-14, is translated as 'Four Fullnesses'. Although there are different interpretations of the meaning of this name, one opinion is that it refers to four kinds of stagnation: qi, water, food and blood. There are clear indications that reflect each of these conditions, for example abdominal distention for qi, abdominal oedema for water, diarrhoea or constipation for food, but overwhelmingly the indications reflect the presence of blood stasis, for example painful abdominal masses, cutting pain below the umbilicus, blood stasis in the uterus etc.

**Ximen P-4**

*Relevant indications*

Chest pain, Heart pain, Heart pain with vomiting, vomiting blood, coughing blood, nosebleed, furuncle and carbuncle, agitated Heart, insomnia, melancholy and fear, fear of strangers, weakness of the shen qi.

**Discussion**

Ximen P-4 is the xi-cleft point of the Pericardium channel (see Diji SP-8 above). Through its dual actions of invigorating blood and moderating acute conditions, Ximen P-4 is strongly indicated for stagnation of blood in the chest and Heart, giving rise to pain. Its important role in the treatment of Heart pain was both emphasised in the classics and is borne out by modern clinical practice and research. By virtue of its ability to clear heat from the blood and stop bleeding, Ximen P-4 is also indicated for hot reckless bleeding in the upper jiao giving rise to nosebleed, and vomiting or coughing of blood.

The second principal group of indications for Ximen P-4 includes a variety of mental and emotional disorders such as agitation of the Heart, insomnia, melancholy and fear, fear of strangers and epilepsy. The relationship between Ximen P-4 and emotional disorders is expressed through its effect on the blood and the Heart qi. The Heart rules the blood and houses the shen, and there is therefore a reciprocal relationship between blood and disturbance of the shen. On the one hand when the blood is stagnant and does not flow freely, essential nourishment will not reach the Heart and the shen may be disrupted. On the other hand, emotional disturbance may lead to stagnation of blood. The Spiritual Pivot in the chapter 'On Original Causes of the 100 Diseases' states: "Internally a person may be injured by worry and anger; when this occurs the qi will rush upwards; when the qi rushes thus the six shu (points) will not move, the warm qi will not circulate and internally the blood will coagulate and not scatter". By resolving stasis of blood Ximen P-4 therefore is able to restore emotional harmony.

Blood stasis in the Heart most commonly occurs as a result of deficiency of Heart qi and yang. These patterns frequently give rise to feelings of fear, melancholy and gloominess, typically seen in patients after a myocardial infarct (the shock of which may further injure the Heart qi). Ximen P-4 is able to regulate the Heart qi, as well as the blood, and is classically indicated for weakness of the shen qi.

Finally there may be symptoms of mental and emotional agitation, as well as haemorrhage, when heat enters the ying or blood levels during febrile disease and rises to disturb the spirit. Thus the Treatise on Warm Febrile Diseases stated: “When the ying system is invaded by heat, the blood is consumed, the shen is disturbed and there is insomnia”. Ximen P-4 is able to calm the shen in such cases by clearing heat from the ying and blood levels.

*Classical combinations*

Heart pain: Ximen P-4, Quze P-3 and Daling P-7.

Heart pain with dry heaves and agitation and fullness: Ximen P-4 and Jiquan HE-1 (Classic of Supplementing Life with Acupuncture and Moxibustion).

Coughing blood: Ximen P-4 and Daling P-7 .

Fear of people, insufficiency of shen qi: Ximen P-4 and Dazhong KID-4.

**Dadun LIV-1**

*Relevant indications*

Irregular menstruation, ceaseless uterine bleeding, menorrhagia, metrorrhagia, bloody urine, nosebleed.

**Discussion**

Dadun LIV-1 is the jing-well point of the Liver channel which encircles the genitals and enters the lower abdomen. Through its action of regulating qi in the lower jiao Dadun LIV-1 is also indicated for a variety of disorders of both urination and menstruation.

As far as menstrual disorders are concerned, the Liver stores the blood, and if Liver qi stagnation transforms to heat and enters the blood, it will give rise to agitation and turbulence manifesting in such disorders as irregular menstruation, ceaseless uterine bleeding, menorrhagia or metrorrhagia.

The Great Compendium of Chinese Acupuncture says “urine red like blood, moxa Dadun LIV-1 and Guanyuan REN-4”. The important action of Dadun LIV-1 on stopping excessive bleeding from the uterus therefore extends to urinary bleeding, and according to Sun Si Miao, even to nosebleed, which is frequently due to upsurging heat of the Liver.

## Ququan LIV-8

*Relevant indications*

Abdominal masses in women due to blood stasis, infertility due to blood stasis, amenorrhoea, lower abdominal swelling, pain of the abdomen and flank, umbilical pain.

### Discussion

The Liver stores the blood and its qi is responsible for the smooth flow of menstruation. When Liver qi stagnates, then menstrual blood may also stagnate. Ququan LIV-8 is indicated in various classical sources for blood stasis in the uterus giving rise to infertility, abdominal masses and amenorrhoea. One specific indication found in a number of sources is the presence of abdominal masses which, when pressed, induce a warm sensation which radiates down the thigh as far as the knee. Ququan LIV-8 is an important point to clear damp-heat from the lower jiao. Clinically the combination of damp-heat and blood stasis is frequently encountered in gynaecological disorders, and the action of Ququan LIV-8 on both these pathogenic factors renders it particularly suited to treating such dual disharmony.

## Dazhui DU-14

*Relevant indications*

Nosebleed.

### Discussion

After ascending to the vertex, the Du Mai descends through the midline of the nose. Dazhui DU-14 is indicated for nosebleed which does not stop, an indication that mirrors the folk practice of placing a key or other piece of cold metal, or a cold sponge, at the back of the neck to stop nosebleed.

*Classical combinations*

Nosebleed: moxa Dazhui DU-14 and Yamen DU-15

### Yinjiao REN-7

*Relevant indications*

Uterine bleeding, irregular menstruation, amenorrhoea, leucorrhoea, infertility, ceaseless flow of lochia after childbirth.

### Discussion

Yinjiao REN-7, literally 'Yin Meeting' is a meeting point of the Ren Mai, Chong Mai and Kidney channels, the three channels that have the strongest relationship with the uterus. The Ren Mai, known as the 'Sea of the Yin Channels' and the Chong Mai, known as the 'Sea of Blood' both originate in the uterus. Their maturation depends on the flourishing of the Kidneys, thus the Plain Questions states: "At the age of fourteen, the Kidney-qi of the female is strong, the reproductive function matures, the Ren Mai flows and the Chong Mai fills, the menses come according to their times, and she can bear offspring". Disorders of menstruation may be shi or xu, due to cold or heat, exterior pathogens or interior disharmony. Due to the close relationship of Yinjiao REN-7 to the uterus, however, it may be selected to treat such disorders as uterine bleeding, irregular menstruation, amenorrhoea, lochiorrhagia and infertility due to any aetiology.

## *Chapter Seven*

# The Concept of Qi

The concept of Qi (sometimes spelled "Chi", pronounced "chee"), or vital energy, is fundamental to traditional Chinese medical thought. There is nothing comparable in allopathic (conventional Western) medicine. While human physiology in allopathic medicine is organized according to specialized function, Chinese medicine is more concerned with dynamics of interrelationships, especially the patterns of vital energy.

Traditional Chinese medicine defines the five main forms of Qi Energy:

**Qi (Matter-Energy):** The vital energy of every living organism and the source of all movement and change in the universe.

**Xue (Blood):** Not only the fluid that circulates in the vascular system, but also the Qi within that fluid that vitalizes its nourishing function as well as its flow. Qi and Xue have mutually interdependent functions.

**Jing (Essence):** The Essential energy of all living organisms which is derived both from the energy we inherit from our parents and from the energy we acquire in our daily lives, principally from air and food.

**Shen (Spirit):** The material/non-material mental-emotional-motivational aspect of consciousness that is stored in the Heart. (Heart is capitalized to remind the reader that the author is referring to the Chinese concept of Heart, not the Western, which views the organ as simply a pump. The Chinese Heart has many other functions including the seat of the Shen. Other organs and organ systems are capitalized to further illustrate this distinction.)

**Jin Ye (Body Fluids):** The functional secretions of the body, including tears, sweat, saliva, milk, mucus, hydrochloric acid and genital secretions. Jin are the lighter, purer and more yang fluids which, via the Lung, moisten and nourish the skin and muscles; ye are the denser, more yin fluids which are processed in the Spleen and Stomach to moisten and nourish the Zang Fu (internal organs), bones, brain and orifices (mucus for sensory orifices and others).

### The Functions of Qi

All five substances are interdependent; however, Qi is central to each of them since it is both the prime activator as well as the recipient of their various functions. The five main functions of Qi are defined as:

Impulsing—the growth and development of the body,

Warming—the maintaining of appropriate body heat,

Defending—against stresses and pathogens,

Controlling—the Blood and Body fluids,

Transforming—metabolizing Qi, Blood and Body fluids.

According to Chinese medicine, the invisible Qi circulates along a system of conduits, the principal ones being the meridians or channels as well as through the Blood (Xue). This Qi is the vital energy which gives life to all living matter. In a way, the Qi conduits resemble those of the vascular or nervous system, since each has a network of main channels and minor capillaries. There are twelve principal bilateral channels of Qi, each intimately connected with one of the viscera of the body, and each manifesting its own characteristic Qi, e.g., Liver Qi, Spleen Qi, etc.

One of the earliest known methods of diagnosis in Chinese medicine was reading the flow of Qi through the meridians and organs. This was done be sensing the energy flow with the hands, fingers, and eyes.

This is still a major technique, and can be accomplished by holding a meridian end point at a given subject's finger or toe, and passing the free hand over the path of the meridian and the corresponding organ. Any changes in the Qi flow indicate an imbalance in relation to the anatomic position where the change occurred, or in the organ. Some practitioners hold the right finger or toe of a female and the left hand or toe of the male. There are also practitioners who treat using methods similar to diagnosis with External Qi Gong.

The following qualities of Qi can be felt by the hands only with a little practice. The "feel" can then be translated into a communicable system which describes the condition of the individual areas.

The following represents some of the information presented in an excellent class on Tui Na taught by Sifu Carl Totten at the Taoist Institute in North Hollywood, California. Many of these qualities of Qi listed below include the associated pathology to which they correspond. Many do not. For those that do not, we'll let you decide what they mean.

**Heat:** From warm to hot, the knowledge of heat measures yang.

**Cold:** From cool to cold, the knowledge of cold measures yin.

**Attracting-Magnetic-Pulling:** When one senses that the energy is being drawn from one's hand into the subject's body, the following possibilities are indicated:

The attracting field is the result of an energy deficiency which is draining energy from its surroundings in order to maintain balance.

The attracting field is overly strong, and it is draining energy from its surroundings.

The examiner's personal energy is not centered or in balance, and, as a result, their energy is being drawn off. The examiner should then center their own energy.

**Repulsing-Pushing Away:** The subject's aura (external yang field) has been emotionally triggered by the presence of the examiner, and is pushing away. This could be indicative of a psychological disturbance, so as to suggest that the patient's body or mind does not want the examiner's hand or person close by.

Internal energy from internal disturbance is affecting the external aura.

**Recoiling:** Injured, or alarmed, sensitive. The energy withdraws and tightens, then relaxes and approaches.

**Tingling, electric:** This indicates the intensity of both yin and yang.

**Hot:** With widely dispersed tingles indicates irritation.

With tingles close together indicates pain. This energy should be approached carefully from a distance in that it could prove painful for the examiner to feel it in the hands. If the energy should flare into the hands, the examiner should relax their muscles and breath the energy into the ground. They should make no resistance to the passage of the energy. This is the energy of excess.

**Cold:** This indicates what is lacking, and its pain is the sharpest.

**Smooth:** Its flow is smooth on the surface, and on the interior.

**Rough:** Its flow is rough, irregular. It is rough on the surface and on the interior. Rough is insufficient, breaking up, diminishing.

**Steady:** Without variation.

**Thick:** Having density.

**Thin:** Having little substance or reserve.

**Solid:** No variation in density.

**Hollow:** Having the external appearance without the internal substance.

**Slow:** A diminished energy unless it is normal for the subject.

**Fast:** Usually indicating that which is excited, unstable, or out of control. To be fast is to burn up quickly.

**Weak:** Almost empty.

**Strong:** Enduring solidity.

**Loose:** Unattached, unstable.

**Tight:** Restricted, taut, as in strangled.

**Sluggish:** A normal energy which is slow. The beginning of disharmony.

**The Qualities of Qi in Meridians**

There are 6 basic functions of Qi. It transforms, transports, holds, raises, protects, and warms. Let's look a each of these in a little more detail. I'll put astericks in front of the ones which are going to be central to understanding the diffence between a diagnosis of Qi Deficiency and Yang Deficiency.

**Transforming:** This refers to things like "Spleen_Qi trnsforms food into Food-Qi, Kidney-Qi transforms fluids, BL_Qi transforms urine, Heart_Qi transforms Food-Qi into Blood."

To clear things up a little for those brand new to TCM, the Stomach "rots" and "ripens" the food one eats, the Spleen extracts the Food Qi from this rotted and ripened food and ....

**Transportation:** The Spleen transports the Food Qi that has been extracted from the "rotted and ripened" food to the Lungs where it mixes with Air Qi which the Lungs have extracted from the air breathed in. "Spleen-Qi transports Food-Qi, Lung-Qi transports fluids to the skin, Kidney-Qi transports Qi upwards, Liver-Qi transports Qi in all directions, Lung-Qi transports Qi downward."

**Holding:** "Spleen-Qi holds the Blood in the blood vessels and fluids, Kidney-Qi and Bladder-Qi hold urine, Lung-Qi holds sweat." There is a TCM syndrome called Spleen Not Controlling Blood. This is a special form of Spleen Qi Deficiency in which the emphasis is on the Qi function of holding. In addition to the usual symptoms of Spleen Qi Deficiency, there will be abnormal bleeding. There may be blood spots in the skin, blood in the stools or urine, abnormal bleeding from the uterus, etc. Please not that Spleen Not Controlling Blood is not the only possible Root of abnormal bleeding. Hot Blood (another TCM syndrome) can be a Root of abnormal bleeding as can be Blood Stasis. Hot Blood and Blood Stasis are Excess problems (problems caused by there being too much of something); Spleen Not Controlling Blood is a Deficiency state (problems caused by there not being enough of something, in this case Spleen Qi). Abnormal bleeding can result from either Deficiency or Excess causes.

One of the possible symptoms of Kidney Qi Deficiency or Bladder Qi Deficiency is urinary incontinence. The person can't make it to the bathroom in time and/or dribbles urine throughout the day. One of the possible manifestations of Spleen Qi Deficiency is diarrhea. In both cases the body isn't holding onto something when it should be. Note the part about "Lung-Qi holds sweat". One of the main diagnostic criteria for Qi Deficiency in general and Lung Qi Deficiency in particular is the person sweats a lot - independently of temperature or activity. Again, something is not being held onto when it should be held onto.

**Raising:** "Spleen-Qi raises the organs, Kidney-Qi rises upward." There is a TCM syndrome called Spleen Qi Sinking. This is another special case of Spleen Qi Deficiency. In this one the Qi function of raising is messed up. The symptoms are those of Spleen Qi Deficiency plus prolapse of Organs. Hemorrhoids and varicose veins may be due in part to Spleen Qi Sinking. Spleen Qi Sinking is classified as a Deficiency syndrome; cases of rebellious Qi (Qi rising when it should be descending) are classified as Excess problems.

**Protecting:** "Lung-Qi protects the body from exterior pathogenic factors." We're talking a special form of Qi here called Protective (Wei) Qi. When a person catches infections easily and/or is weather sensitive, this can be a case of just Protective Qi Deficiency and Lung Qi Deficiency (in the case of infections). Or, it can be a case of longstanding Yang Deficiency.

**Warming:** "This is a function of Yang-Qi. Both Spleen-Yang and Kidney-Yang, especially the latter, have the function of warming the body."

## The Stagnant Qi

Once you've recognized that Qi is Stagnant, the next question is why is the Qi Stagnant? Qi Stagnation (Qi blocked or not flowing very smoothly) can arise from a number of causes.

One of the main ones is emotional problems. What is meant by this is that the person either is repressing emotions or giving in to them too much. Emotions - like energy - only cause problems when they're blocked or inappropriately channeled. Blocking emotions includes things like refusing to acknowledge them, being in denial about them, etc. Inappropriately channeling them includes things like a person who substitutes one emotion for another. Like a person who substitutes feeling anger in order keep from having face a more threatening emotion like fear or feeling helpless and vulnerable. This often is a person who throws temper tantrums, is always angry, and is abusive towards others. The giving in to anger and over- and inappropriately expressing anger is a way to keep from having to face and deal with emotions which are more threatening to the person than anger is. Scapegoating is another form of inappropriately channeling emotions. Instead of confronting the person who is responsible for the original pain and rage, the person will take it out on others. Needless to say, this never works for very long, and the abuser who engages in this starts to require more frequent and more severe "fixes" of taking the anger out on others. The only cure is for the person to eventually confront the true source of the pain and rage.

TCM looks at the effects that various emotions have on energy flow in the body. Each meridian (pathway of energy) has a proper direction of flow, and each emotion will affect energy flow in a different way. Energy in the Stomach meridian is supposed to descend. If it "Rebels" and flows upward instead, a person can experience problems like nausea (not the only possible cause of nausea but one of the possible causes), vomiting, and burping. The flow of energy in the Spleen meridian is supposed to ascend. When it "Sinks" instead of rising, the person can experienced problems like a prolapsed stomach, prolapsed uterus, prolapsed anus, etc.

Each of the emotions have an effect on energy flow. Anger and frustration will cause it to rise inappropriately or to Stagnate. Stagnation can trigger another TCM imbalance. Energy that stays in one place for too long and can't move freely produces Heat, and if this goes on too long, this Heat can change into destructive Fire, and the person has some major health problems. Think of the analogy of an electric wire carrying more electricity than its diameter can safely carry. The thinner wire - unlike a thicker one - will overheat. If it gets too hot this can cause a fire. Another analogy is a pressure cooker. All pressure cookers have a vent for releasing excess pressure. If it didn't and the pressure rose too much, the entire pressure cooker would cxplode. Something similar to this can happen in the body when Qi Stagnates.

Note for those new to TCM: The Liver and the Gall Bladder are the two Organ systems most vulnerable to anger and frustration.

Something else which can cause Qi to Stagnate is Cold. If a person suffers long enough from Exterior Excess Cold (cold weather) and it invades to the Interior, or, if the person is Yang Deficient (not enough Yang energy to warm the body properly), Qi Stagnation can result. Cold slows things down and congeals. Think of a stream or river frozen in the winter. Even if the stream or river doesn't freeze entirely, the water isn't flowing like it usually does. And even the water at the bottom of the stream or river which is still flowing is flowing much slower than it usually does.

An excess of foods that are too Cold or foods that are too Hot also can trigger Qi Stagnation problems.

Mechanical injury can produce Qi Stagnation problems.

Accidents or surgery: In these cases, Blood Stasis (Blood not flowing properly) developing because of the accident (bruises) or after the surgery usually is the more immediate problem, but Qi Stagnation also can result. Blood Stasis if not treated can trigger Qi Stagnation problems just like Qi Stagnation (in particular Liver Qi Stagnation) can trigger Blood Stasis problems if left untreated long enough.

Spinal misalignment also can trigger Qi Stagnation problems. Massage may be able to take care of some of these problems. In other cases the person may need to see a chiropractor or a D.O. (Doctor of Osteopathy). Spinal misalignment can arise due to different causes. Sometimes a person is born with one leg longer than the other. Sometimes an accident will cause the problem. Sometimes cold can cause the problem. In addition to cold being able to trigger Qi Stagnation by causing the muscles to contract excessively, these muscles staying contracted too long because of cold can throw the alignment of the spine off in some susceptible individuals, thus creating further triggers for Qi Stagnation.

There are other possible causes of Qi Stagnation. These are some of the main ones.

I want to make some additional comments here. Once there has been damage to the Liver and/or Gall Bladder whatever the initial cause - emotional, poisoning, virus or bacterial infection, mechanical trauma such as accident or surgery, parasites - the person is going to be more prone to experiencing anger and frustration than before. This is a snowballing situation. Once the Liver is damaged from whatever initial trigger, the person will be more prone to feeling anger, the increased anger will further damage the Liver which results in more anger which then further damages the Liver, and so on. It snowballs - just like a snowball rolled in snow will keep getting bigger and bigger and bigger.

When someone appears very angry suspect and rule in or rule out Liver imbalance and/or pain. People in chronic pain very often will appear and be angry. Even low level chronic pain that a person has learned to ignore consciously can produce this effect. This correlation between pain and anger is not surprising to someone in TCM. One of the possible manifestations of Qi Stagnation is pain. Be it headaches due to Liver Yang Rising or Liver Fire Blazing or pain in the sides due to Liver Qi Stagnation or pains in the lover abdomen that move around a lot. Not all pain is due to Qi Stagnation (there are other possible Roots) but in cases of pain due to Qi Stagnation, that pain can be relieved by the appropriate herbs, acupoints, or massage techniques that get Qi flowing properly again. Sometimes the appropriate herbs may be a combination of different classes of herbs. For example, in cases of pain due to Qi Stagnation due to Cold, herbs to move Qi by themselves won't be enough. You also will need to include warming herbs to correct the Cold which was and is the trigger for the Qi Stagnation. In the case of pain due also to Blood Stasis as well as to Qi Stagnation, both herbs to move Blood and to move Qi will need to be used.

Knowing the basics of TCM and how things work will enable you to analyze more thoroughly than you otherwise would be able to. For example, someone comes in who complains of having felt cold and having trouble warming up for a very, very long time. In this particular case, Yang Deficiency stands out as the major analysis. The Yang Deficiency is so severe that it dwarfs everything else and may even mask some other problems. In cases like this, you can just about bet that there are going to be some Qi Stagnation problems. Yang tonic herbs and herbs to warm the Interior may or may not be enough in one of these particular cases. You may also need to include an herb to get Qi moving properly. When problems go untreated for a very long time and trigger other problems, the other problems can assume lives of their own. In other words, they gain such a foothold that they will continue even if the original imbalance which gave rise to them There is a relation between Qi Stagnation and Phlegm. Qi Stagnation can cause Phlegm, and Phlegm can block the flow of Qi. This is a snowballing relationship.

There are several things which can trigger the formation of Phlegm. If the Spleen is weak, dampness can accumulate. If evil heat and/or dryness are present, these can cause dampness (even normal dampness) to congeal into phlegm. Cold can turn dampness into phlegm - just as cold can freeze water. Wind can trigger the formation of phlegm.etc.

Chinese Herbal Medicine Formulas & Strategies, compiled and translated by Dan Bensky & Randall Barolet, has the following to say about Phlegm in the chapter on "Formulas that Treat Phlegm":

"Although there may be other contributing factor, the basis of all phlegm is the disruption of the transformative and transportive function of the Spleen, and of the Kidney yang which supports them. For this reason, herbs that strengthen the Spleen are included in almost all of these formulas. Similarly, impediment to the flow of qi is both a cause and an effect of phlegm; the smooth flow of qi dissipates phlegm. These principles were concisely summarized by the Ming-dynasty author, Wang Ken-Tang, in Standards of Patterns and Treatments: 'Those who are best at treating phlegm treat the qi instead of (directly treating) phlegm. When the qi flows smoothly, all the body's fluids will then flow smoothly.' Accordingly, herbs that regulate the qi are also included in these formulas."

Remember that one of the functions of Qi is to "transform and transport". This includes fluids as well as food. If the Qi and/or the Spleen (which is the main Organ connected with the production of Qi) are weak, fluids don't get properly transformed and transported, and Dampness accumulates. The Dampness congeals into Phlegm when it sticks around too long.

Spleen Deficiency is the number one Root of Phlegm. However, Lung and Kidney Deficiency also can trigger Phlegm. "If the Lungs fail to disperse and lower fluids and if the Kidneys fail to transform and excrete fluids, these may accumulate into Phlegm. However, the Spleen is always the primary factor in the formation of Spleen."

According to C.S. Cheung, MD. L.Ac., in Comprehensive Management Phlegm Fluid (Tan Yin), the Liver, Heart, and Triple Heater also can participate in the production of Phlegm. (p. 3) "Triple Warmer is responsible for maintaining the patency of Water Channels." "Abnormal Qi activation (Qi Hua) of Triple Warmer or blockage of Qi vessels may interfere with normal circulation and transformation of Fluid: producing Phlegm."

Some authorities believe that any Organ can produce Phlegm, but the Spleen is the main culprit.

The Organ which Phlegm has the most affinity for are the Lungs. However, Phlegm can collect anywhere in the body. It can cause problems in any Organ - like stones in the Gall Bladder or Kidneys. It can block the Heart orifices, and in doing so, "mist the mind", giving rise to some mental illnesses . It can appear in and under the skin in the form of lumps. (Not all lumps and tumors are due to Phlegm.) It can be the cause of swelling of the thyroid as well as some fibroids and lipomas. It can block channels. causing numbness. (Not the only possible cause of numbness.) It can deform joints (like in chronic rheumatoid arthritis. Phlegm can show up about anywhere in the body, but it's especially prone to show up in the Lungs. "Phlegm can the cause of hundred diseases. Evil Spirit of hundred ailments is the Phlegm."

In other words, Phlegm is very versatile in the problems it can cause.

Suspect Phlegm in conditions which are "bizarre" and hard to treat. Phlegm can figure into some very complex clinical pictures. It can take a long time to resolve Phlegm problems once they get established, and especially after they've been around for a while.

The main points to remember is that Qi Stagnation is one of the things which can produce Phlegm, and Phlegm can cause Qi Stagnation. The Spleen is the main culprit involved in the production of Phlegm, but the Lungs and Kidneys also frequently are culprits. Phlegm has a particular affinity for collecting in the Lungs, but it can show up anywhere in the body, including channels. Phlegm can create a lot of different problems throughout the body. Suspect Phlegm if the condition is bizarre, unusually complex, and/or doesn't respond very well to treatment.is corrected.

## General Principles of Syndrome Differentiation

In accordance with the principles of the eight principle syndromes, the status of viscera and qi and blood, the syndrome differentiation of gynecological diseases is based on the clinical characteristics of menstruation, leukorrhea, pregnancy and puerperium as well as their general manifestations.

*A. Syndrome differentiation of menopathy*

The menstrual cycle, the quantity, color, quality and odor of the menses and symptoms such as lower abdominal distension and pain should be particularly emphasized in the diagnosis of menopathy.

a. The menstrual cycle: A short cycle is attributed to blood-heat or qi deficiency, a delayed cycle to blood deficiency or blood-heat, while a shortened period is attributed to blood deficiency or blood cold.

b. The amount of menses: Menorrhagia usually occurs in cases with blood-heat or qi deficiency, and oligomenorrhea in those with blood deficiency or cold blood.

c. The color of menses: A bright red or purplish red color is attributed to heat, a dull red color to cold, a pink color to asthenia, and a dull pale color to asthenia-cold.

d. The quality of menses: A thick, viscous menses indicates a sthenia-syndrome, a thin clear menses denotes an asthenia-syndrome, and a menstrual flow containing blood clots shows a blood-stasis syndrome.

e. The odor of menses: A foul odor is attributed to heat, an odorless menses to cold, and a stinking odor to a serious condition resulting from the putrefaction of stagnant blood.

f. The accompanying abdominal pain: Dysmenorrhea relievable by pressure is attributed to asthenia-syndrome, that aggravated by pressure to sthenia-syndrome, that relievable by warmth to cold-syndrome, while that occurring after the menstrual period signifies an asthenia-syndrome. A preexisting lower abdominal pain which is aggravated during the menstrual period indicates the retention of dampness-heat and the stagnation of qi and blood. Lower abdominal distension during the menstrual period denotes the stagnation of qi.

However, the syndrome differentiation should be based on a comprehensive analysis of the above conditions. Taking the preceding menstrual cycle as an example, it should be differentiated as a syndrome of blood-heat and qi stagnation when it is associated with a prolonged menstrual period, a profuse discharge of bright red or purplish, foul and viscous menses and lower abdominal distension; as a qi deficiency syndrome when the menses is profuse, pale and thin and a bearing-down sensation is experienced in the lower abdomen; and as a syndrome of yin deficiency and blood-heat when the amount of menstrual flow is normal or scanty, the menses is bright red and viscous and abdominal pain is absent.

*B. Syndrome differentiation of leucorrhagia*

The color, character and odor of vaginal discharge may be observed for this purpose. Generally speaking, a yellow and viscous discharge indicates a sthenia or a heat syndrome, while a white and thin discharge indicates an asthenia or a cold syndrome. A foul odor is a sign of sthenia-heat syndrome, while a rank-smelling odor, asthenia-cold syndrome. A yellowish or greenish viscous and foul discharge is attributed to retention of dampness-heat; a whitish, thin discharge accompanied by fatigue or anorexia to spleen deficiency and downward attack of dampness; a continuous dripping of bleedy discharge to yin deficiency and interior-heat with dampness; a profuse thin discharge accompanied by lumbago and weakness to deficiency of kidney-yang; and a grayish, turbid and foul discharge to blood stasis.

*C. Syndrome differentiation of disorders during pregnancy*

Amenorrhea occurring in an adult woman accompanied by symptoms such as nausea, vomiting, desire for sour taste or special food, fatigue, poor appetite, somnolence, smooth pulse, etc., and whose previous menstruation has been normal, is usually a sign of early pregnancy.

Various disorders may occur during pregnancy. Those with excessive movement of fetus, vaginal discharge of pink and thin blood, spiritlessness, shortness of breath and weak pulse are attributed to deficiency of qi and blood; those accompanied by lumbago, fatigue, a bearing-down sensation of the lower abdomen, to kidney deficiency; those with discharge of dark red color, restlessness, dryness of mouth, red tongue and smooth and rapid pulse, to blood-heat.

Cases with morning sickness, anorexia and slow, smooth, weak pulse are attributed to deficiency of spleen-qi and stomach-qi; those with vomiting of bitter or sour fluid and smooth pulse, to adverse flowing of liver-qi and stomach-qi; those with vomiting of mucus, salivation, distention over the stomach, soft-floating and smooth pulse, to retention of phlegm-dampness in the middle-jiao.

Cases with edema, fatigue, epigastric distention and deep and smooth weak pulse are attributed to spleen deficiency; those with edema, fatigue, epigastric distention, lumbago, aversion to cold and deep and slow pulse, to insufficiency of kidney-yang. Those with dizziness, headache, chest upset and nausea appearing in the late stage of pregnancy are attributed to pre-eclampsia.

*D. Syndrome differentiation of puerperal disorder*

There are three criteria for the identification of puerperal disorders in ancient theory. First, the presence or absence of lower abdominal pain is a criterion to determine whether lochiostasis is present or not. Second, the frequency of bowel movement is used to identify whether body fluids are exhausted or not. Third, the amount of milk secretion and appetite are signs indicating the condition of stomach-qi. Besides, the quantity, color, quality and odor of lochia and body temperature must also be observed.

a. Damage of the uterus and Chong and Ren meridians by heat-toxic evil: Profuse and foul lochia, lower abdominal pain and tenderness, fever, headache, thirst and desire for cold drink, red tongue with yellow coating and full and rapid pulse.

b. Retention of blood stasis: Prolonged discharge of lochia which is small in amount, dark purplish in color and contains blood clots and lower abdominal pain and tenderness.

c. Insufficiency of blood and qi: Discharge of light-colored and thin lochia.

d. Stagnation of liver-qi: Lack of lactation, distending pain and induration of breasts, distention of the chest and hypochondrium and poor appetite.

e. Deficiency of qi and blood: Soft breasts without distending pain and lack of lactation with thin and clear milk.

In sum, the principles mentioned above are based on the common manifestations of menstruation and leukorrhea and during pregnancy and puerperium. In clinical applications the physique, qi, blood, pulse and general condition of the patient should all be considered, and the data should be analyzed comprehensively by means of the basic theories concerning the eight principle syndromes, the visceral phenomena, the qi and blood and the meridians.

## An Outline of Therapeutic Principles

Among the therapeutic principles applied in clinical practice, four of them are more commonly used in the treatment of gynecological diseases, namely, tonifying and nourishing the kidneys, dispersing liver-qi and nourishing the liver, invigorating the spleen and regulating the stomach and regulating qi and blood circulation.

*A. Tonifying and nourishing the kidneys*

The kidneys are considered "the basis of innateness" and are where essence-qi is stored. It is essential for the growth, development and reproduction of the human body and plays an important role in the maturation of Tiankui and the activities of the Chong and Ren meridians. In addition, the kidneys are composed of kidney-yin and kidney-yang, which are the essential substances and motive forces for bodily development and reproduction, and both of them must be sufficient and kept in balance in order to maintain the normal condition of the human body. Any forms of disequilibrium, such as insufficiency of kidney-yang, deficiency of kidney-yin, yin-deficiency leading to the hyperactivity of yang or deficiency of both yin and yang, may cause the dysfunction of Tiankui and the Chong and Ren meridians and various gynecological diseases may ensue. Therefore, the principle of tonifying and nourishing the kidneys is commonly applied in gynaecology.

For cases with insufficiency or consumption of kidney-yin, the principles of tonifying the kidneys, nourishing yin and promoting the production of kidney essence and marrow should be applied. The commonly used drugs are Radix Rehmanniae Praeparata, Radix Polygoni Multiflori Praeparata, Fructus Ligustri Lucidi, Herba Ecliptae, Fructus Corni, Colla Plastri Testudinis, Colla Corii Asini, Fructus Lycii and Fructus Mori. The recommended prescription is Zuogui Bolus.

For cases with yin-deficiency leading to hyperactivity of yang, the principle of nourishing yin and suppressing yang should be employed. Decoction of Six Drugs Containing Rehmanniae Praeparata is usually employed, and Os Draconis, Concha Ostreae or Carapax Trionycis Praeparata are added.

Physiologically, the liver and the kidney are the organs that control lower-jiao. The liver stores blood and the kidneys keep essence, and since the essence and blood can be mutually produced, it is considered that the liver and kidneys have a common source. Moreover, the liver and kidneys are the root of the Chong and Ren meridians, and the disorder of liver and kidneys and the impairment of the Chong and Ren meridians may influence each other. Therefore, the principle of nourishing the liver and kidneys may be employed for gynecological disorders with insufficiency of liver and kidneys or impairment of Chong and Ren meridians.

For cases with declination of life-gate fire, the principle of warming and invigorating kidney-yang should be applied. The following drugs are recommended: Cortex Cinnamomi, Radix Aconiti Lateralis Praeparata, Radix Morindae Officinalis, Herba Cistanchis, Colla Cornus Cervi, Fructus Psoraleae, Semen Cuscutae, Cortex Eucommiae, Herba Epimedii, Rhizoma Curculiginis, etc. The representative prescription is Yougui Bolus.

For cases with deficiency of both kidney-yin and kidney-yang, the principle of invigorating both yin and yang should be employed, and the drugs mentioned above may be used in combination.

In sum, tonifying and warming the kidneys are important therapeutic principles in gynecology. But it should be emphasized that yin and yang are a unity of opposites and interconvertible and interdependent, so in dealing with one, the other should be handled simultaneously.

*B. Dispersing liver-qi and nourishing the liver*

Physiologically, the liver serves to regulate the activity of qi and blood, so the nourishment of sinews, vessels and joints and the storage and regulation of blood depend on the liver. Moreover, the Chong meridian is the "blood sea" and relates to the liver. Whenever the liver is impaired by emotional upsets, the Chong meridian may dysfunction and diseases may ensue. Hence, dispersing liver-qi and nourishing the liver are also principles commonly applied in gynaecology.

For cases with stagnation of liver-qi, the principle of dispersing liver-qi to relieve stagnation is recommended. The commonly used drugs are Radix Bupleuri, Rhizoma Cyperi, Pericarpium Citri Reticulatae Viride, Fructus Toosendan, Folium Citri Reticulatae, Rhizoma Corydalis, Radix Linderae, Radix Aucklandiae and Fructus Aurantii. Xiaoyao Powder is considered the representative prescription.

For cases with stagnated liver-qi complicated by fire formation, the principle is to disperse liver-qi and clear away heat. Drugs recommended are: Fructus Toosendan, Herba Artemisiae Annuae, Cortex Moutan Radicis, Fructus Gardeniae, Radix Scutellariae, etc. The representative prescription is Xiaoyao Powder with Moutan Radicis and Gardeniae.

In case of retention of heat in the liver meridian with excessive fire in the liver and gallbladder, the principle of purging liver-fire to remove heat should be employed. The recommended prescription is the Decoction of Gentianae for Purging Liver-Fire.

In case of insufficiency of ying-blood with failure of nourishing the liver, the principles of tonifying yin and nourishing the liver are applied. The common drugs for this purpose are Radix Angelicae Sinensis, Radix Paeoniae Alba, Colla Corii Asini, Radix Rehmanniae Praeparata, Fructus Mori, Fructus Lycii. Fructus Ligustri Lucidi, Fructus Corni, Plastrum Testudinis, etc. The representative prescriptions are the Modified Decoction of Four Drugs and Yiguan Decoction. However, drugs of acrid-warm and fragrant-dry in nature should be used cautiously, otherwise the body fluids and yin may be consumed, the liver-blood be more deficient and complications occur more readily.

In case of insufficiency of liver-blood with upward attack of liver-yang, the principles of nourishing blood, softening the liver, supporting yin and suppressing yang are available. The drugs commonly used are Radix Rehmanniae, Radix Paeoniae Alba, Radix Scrophulariae, Fructus Ligustri Lucidi, Concha Haliotidis, Flos Chrysanthemi, Concha Margaritifera Usta, Concha Ostreae, etc.

In case of yin deficiency and fire hyperactivity with liver-wind stirring inside the body, the principles of tonifying yin, suppressing yang and calming liver-wind are recommended. The drugs commonly used are Radix Rehmanniae, Colla Corii Asini, Plastrum Testudinis, Radix Paeoniae Alba, Concha Haliotidis, Haematitum, Rhizoma Gastrodiae, Ramulus Uncariae cum Uncis, Cornu Saigae Tataricae, etc. The representative prescription is the Decoction of Cornu Saigae Tataricae and Uncariae cum Uncis.

*C. Invigorating spleen and regulating stomach*

Physiologically, the spleen and stomach are considered as the basis of postnatal life and the source of qi and blood production. The spleen serves to govern the transportation and transformation of digested food and to control blood flow. The stomach serves as a receptor for food and is a fu-organ with plenty of qi and blood. The Chong meridian is attached to the yangming stomach meridian. When the spleen and stomach fail to transport and transform the food, to produce enough blood and qi, to keep the blood in the vessels or to eliminate dampness and water, the Chong and Ren meridians will be impaired, resulting in various gynecological diseases such as irregular menstruation, metrorrhagia, amenorrhea, leucorrhagia, vomiting during pregnancy, edema during pregnancy, prolapse of uterus, etc.

In case of hypofunction of spleen and stomach with insufficient production of qi and blood, the principle of regulating spleen and stomach is available. The drugs commonly used are Radix Codonopsis Pilosulae, Rhizoma Atractylodis Macrocephalae, Poria, Rhizoma Dioscoreae, Semen Dolichoris, Pericarpium Citri

Reticulatae, Semen Nelumbinis, Fructus Amomi, Fructus Jujubae, etc. The representative prescription is the Powder of Ginseng, Poria and Atractylodis Macrocephalae.

In case of deficiency of middle-jiao with stagnation of food, the principles of invigorating the stomach and relieving dyspepsia are applicable. The herbs which strengthen the stomach such as Fructus Crataegi, Fructus Oryzae Germinatus, Fructus Hordei Germinatus, Massa Fermentata Medicinalis, Endothelium Corneum Gigeriae Galli, etc., may be supplemented.

For cases with collapse of middle-jiao qi, the principles of invigorating middle-jiao, benefiting qi and lifting up yang-qi are recommended. The drugs commonly used are Radix Astragali, Radix Angelicae Sinensis, Rhizoma Atractylodis Macrocephalae, Radix Glycyrrhizae Praeparata, Radix Bupleuri, Rhizoma Cimicifugae, etc. The Decoction for Strengthening Middle-Jiao and Benefiting Qi or Juyuan Decoction are the typical prescriptions.

In case of qi deficiency with failure of controlling blood, the principles of tonifying qi and controlling blood are employed and supplemented with hemostatics, such as Herba Agrimoniae, Vagina Trachycarpi Carbonisatus, Radix Rubiae Carbonisatus, Os Sepiellae seu Sepiae, Galla Chinensis, Halloysitum Rubrum, Limonitum, Nodus Nelumbinis Rhizomatis Carbonisatus, etc.

In case of incoordination between spleen and stomach with adverse rising of stomach-qi, disease due to stomach-heat is treated with the principles of clearing away heat and keeping the adverse stomach-qi downwards and drugs like Caulis Bambusae in Taeniam, Radix Scutellariae, Rhizoma Coptidis, Haematitum, etc., and the representative prescription is the Decoction of Perillae and Coptidis; disease accompanied by insufficiency of stomach-yin may be treated with drugs for benefiting stomach and producing body fluids, such as Radix Adenophorae Strictae, Herba Dendrobii, Radix Ophiopogonis, Rhizoma Polygonati Odorati, Rhizoma Phragmitis (raw), etc.; disease due to stomach-cold should be treated with the principles of warming middle-jiao and keeping the adverse stomach-qi downwards and drugs like Fructus Amomi, Fructus Myristicae, Rhizoma Zingiberis, Rhizoma Zingiberis Recens, Fructus Evodiae, Flos Caryophylli,

Herba Agastachis, Rhizoma Pinelliae, etc., and the representative prescription is the Decoction of Pinelliae and Poria. However, even if there is no damage of the spleen and stomach, their normal functions should be maintained in the treatment and the potent and greasy drugs are contraindicated.

*D. Tonifying blood and benefiting qi*

Physiologically, woman is specially related to blood and blood is closely connected with qi, so that dysfunction of qi and blood occurs frequently in gynecological diseases. Hence, tonifying blood and benefiting qi is one of the chief therapeutic principles in gynecology. Furthermore, because the heart is the governor and the source of qi and blood, tonifying heart and spleen is a supplemental principle for gynecological diseases in order to promote the coordination of qi and blood and normalize the functions of Chong, Ren, Du and Dai meridians.

For cases with deficiency and collapse of qi and weakening of Chong and Ren meridians manifested as menorrhagia, tonifying qi, lifting up yang-qi and stopping bleeding are the recommended principles. The commonly used drugs are Radix Ginseng, Radix Astragali, Radix Glycyrrhizae Praeparata, Rhizoma Atractylodis Macrocephalae, Rhizoma Cimicifugae, etc., and the Jiuyuan Decoction is considered the representative prescription.

For cases with insufficiency of middle-jiao qi and deficiency and collapse of qi manifested with prolapse of uterus, tonifying and lifting up of qi is the available principle. Radix Astragali, Rhizoma Cimicifugae, Radix Ginseng, Rhizoma Atractylodis Macrocephalae, Radix Glycyrrhizae Praeparata and Radix Bupleuri are the drugs applied, and the Decoction for Strengthening Middle-Jiao and Benefiting Qi is the prescription employed.

For cases with deficiency of spleen and stomach, insufficiency of middle-jiao qi and failure of controlling blood manifested by prolonged menorrhagia, the principles of benefiting qi, invigorating spleen, warming meridians and stopping bleeding should be employed. The commonly used drugs are Radix Ginseng, Radix Codonopsis Pilosulae, Radix Astragali, Rhizoma Atractylodis Macrocephalae, Poria, Radix Angelicae Sinensis (fried), Rhizoma Dioscoreae, Semen Nelumbinis, Receptaculum Nelumbinis Carbonisatus, Radix Glycyrrhizae Praeparata, Fructus Jujubae and Rhizoma Zingiberis Carbonisatus. The Decoction for Invigorating the Spleen and Nourishing the Heart is considered the representative prescription.

For cases with blood deficiency, yin-blood consumption and emptiness of the blood sea manifested by amenorrhea or oligomenorrhea, nourishing blood, tonifying liver and regulating menstruation are the applicable principles. The drugs recommended are Radix Angelicae Sinensis, Radix Rehmanniae Praeparata, Radix Paeoniae Alba, Rhizoma Chuanxiong, Fructus Lycii, Radix Polygoni Multiflori Praeparata and Arillus Longan, and the decoction of four drugs should be employed.

For cases with deficiency of both qi and blood manifested by amenorrhea or delayed menstrual cycle, benefiting qi, invigorating spleen, nourishing blood and regulating menstruation are the principles available. The commonly used drugs are Rhizoma Chuanxiong, Poira, Radix Paeoniae Alba, Rhizoma Atractylodis Macrocephalae, Radix Glycyrrhizae Praeparata, Radix Codonopsis Pilosulae, Radix Angelicae Sinensis, Radix Rehmanniae Praeparata, Radix Astragali, etc. The representative prescription is Eight-Ingredient Decoction for Tonifying Qi and Blood.

For cases with deficiency of both qi and blood but manifested as menorrhagia, benefiting qi and promoting blood production are the principles selected. The Angelicae Sinensis Decoction for Enriching Blood is the typical prescription.

*E. Activating blood circulation and dissipating blood stasis*

This principle is applicable to gynecological diseases caused by the stagnation of blood such as amenorrhea, oligomenorrhea, dysmenorrhea, metrorrhagia, abdominal mass, etc.

For cases with retention of blood stasis and obstruction of meridians manifested with oligomenorrhea, activating blood circulation and eliminating blood stasis are the applicable principles. Semen Persicae, Flos Carthami, Radix Angelicae Sinensis, Radix Salviae Miltiorrhizae, Rhizoma Chuanxiong, Radix Paeoniae Rubra, Herba Leonuri and Herba Lycopi are the drugs commonly employed, and the Decoction of Four Drugs with Persicae and Carthami is the representative prescription.

For cases with stagnation of qi and blood manifested as dysmenorrhea or amenorrhea, the principles of activating blood circulation, regulating qi and dissipating blood stasis are available. The drugs commonly applied are Radix Angelicae Sinensis, Radix Paeoniae Rubra, Rhizoma Chuanxiong, Semen Persicae, Flos Carthami, Fructus Aurantii, Rhizoma Corydalis, Faeces Trogopterori, Radix Salviae Miltiorrhizae, Radix Linderae, Rhizoma Cyperi, Fructus Toosendan, etc. The typical prescription is the Decoction for Removing Blood Stasis Under the Diaphragm.

For cases with impairment of spleen-yang by stagnation of cold and blood with involvement of the Chong, Ren and Dai meridians manifested as dysmenorrhea or amenorrhea, expelling cold, activating blood circulation and promoting menstruation are the recommended principles. The commonly-used drugs are Radix Aconiti Lateralis Praeparata, Ramulus Cinnamomi, Fructus Evodiae, Fructus Foeniculi, Rhizoma Zingiberis Praeparata, Pericarpium Zanthoxyli, etc. The representative prescription is the Decoction for Warming Meridians.

*F. Regulating qi and blood*

Before using this therapy, it is necessary to determine whether qi or blood is predominantly involved. In cases where qi is chiefly affected, the therapy for regulating qi should be employed and supplemented by that for regulating blood. In general, the deficient qi should be tonified, the collapsed qi lifted up, the stagnated qi dispersed and the adverserising qi lowered. For cases with stagnation and sluggish movement of qi, the principles of activating qi circulation and dispersing stagnation are employed. The commonly-used drugs are Rhizoma Cyperi, Fructus Aurantii, Cortex Magnoliae Officinalis, Radix Aucklandiae, Radix Linderae, Pericarpium Citri Reticulatae Viride, Pericarpium Arecae, Semen Citri Reticulatae, Semen Litchi, etc. The representative prescription is the Modified Decoction of Linderae. As for cases with both deficiency and adverse rising of qi, the applicable principles and drugs have been introduced in the section dealing with tonifying the spleen and stomach.

In case where blood is predominantly involved, the therapy for activating blood is the chief measure used and that for regulating blood is applied as a supplemental measure. In general, a tonifying therapy is used for blood deficiency, a dissipating therapy for blood stagnation, a warming therapy for blood-cold and a heat-clearing therapy for blood-heat.

For cases with consumption of ying-blood, tonifying and nourishing blood are the principles recommended. The commonly-used drugs are Radix Angelicae Sinensis, Radix Paeoniae Alba, Radix Rehmanniae Praeparata, Colla Corii Asini, Fructus Lycii, Radix Polygoni Multiflori Praeparata, Arillus Longan, etc. The typical prescriptions are the Decoction of Four Drugs and the Decoction for Invigorating the Spleen and Nourishing the Heart.

For cases with retention of blood stasis, activating blood circulation and dissipating blood stasis are the applicable principles. The commonly-used drugs are Radix Angelicae Sinensis, Rhizoma Chuanxiong, Herba Leonuri, Pollen Typhae, Faeces Trogopterori, Radix Salviae Miltiorrhizae, Herba Lycopi, Herba Selaginellae, Radix Notoginseng, Flos Carthami, etc. The representative prescriptions are the Decoction of Four Drugs with Persicae and Carthami and the Decoction for Removing Blood Stasis in the Lower Abdomen.

For cases with abdominal mass resulting from accumulation of blood stasis, removing blood stasis, dissipating and softening the mass and dispersing stagnation are the available principles. The drugs commonly applied are Semen Persicae, Rhizoma Sparganii, Rhizoma Zedoariae, Radix Achyranthis Bidentatae, Olibanum, Herba Artemisiae Anomalae, Myrrha, Lignum Sappan, Semen Vaccariae, Carapax Trionycis, Concha Ostreae, etc., and the representative prescription is the Pill of Rhei and Eupolyphaga seu Steleophaga.

For cases with accumulation of heat in xuefen and extravasation of blood, clearing away heat, cooling blood and stopping bleeding are the principles employed. The commonly used drugs are Radix Rehmanniae, Radix Paeoniae Alba, Radix Ophiopogonis, Radix Scrophulariae, Cortex Moutan Radicis, Fructus Gardeniae Carbonisatus, Radix Scutellariae, Radix

Sanguisorbae Carbonisatus, Cacumen Biotae Carbonisatus, etc. The recommended prescriptions are the Powder for Clearing Away Heat in the Meridians and the Liangdi Decoction.

For cases with blood-cold syndrome, warming meridians and expelling cold are the recommended principles. However, in the therapy of regulating qi and blood, drugs of a greasy nature and consuming action should not be overused, otherwise qi and blood may be stagnated and damaged.

*G. Clearing away heat and cooling blood*

This principle is indicated for the cases with bleeding due to retention of heat in xuefen.

For cases with preceded menstrual cycle and menorrhagia due to blood-heat, clearing away heat and cooling blood are the available principles. The commonly used drugs are Cortex Moutan Radicis, Cortex Lycii Radicis, Radix Paeoniae Alba, Radix Rehmanniae, Herba Artemisiae Annuae, Cortex Phellodendri, etc. The Powder for Clearing Away Heat in the Meridians is the typical prescription.

For cases with metrorrhagia due to blood-heat, clearing away heat, cooling blood and stopping bleeding are the principles employed. The drugs commonly applied are Radix Rehmanniae, Cortex Lycii Radicis, Plastrum Testudinis Praeparata, Concha Ostreae Usta, Colla Corii Asini, Radix Scutellariae, Nodus Nelumbinis Rhizomatis, Fructus Gardeniae (fried), Radix Sanguisorbae, Vagina Trachycarpi Carbonisatus, Radix Glycyrrhizae, etc. The representative prescription is the Decoction for Clearing Away Heat and Checking Uterine Bleeding.

*H. Warming meridians and expelling cold*

Cold is a yin-type pathogenic agent of an astringent and stagnant nature, which is liable to impair yang-qi and impede the circulation of blood and qi. When cold is retained in the uterus, the Chong and Ren meridians may be obstructed and menopathy may result.

A cold-syndrome may be classified as asthenia-cold or sthenia-cold. For sthenia-cold syndrome, the recommended principles are those of warming meridians and removing stagnation; and for asthenia-cold syndrome, those of nourishing blood and warming meridians. The drugs commonly used for this purpose are Cortex Cinnamomi, Radix Aconiti Lateralis Praeparata, Ramulus Cinnamomi, Herba Asari, Folium Artemisiae Argyi, Fructus Foeniculi, Fructus Evodiae, Rhizoma Zingiberis Praeparata, Fructus Psoraleae, etc. The prescription recommended is the Decoction of Warming Meridians, which may be modified according to whether the asthenia or the sthenia syndrome is predominant.

*I. Clearing away heat and toxic materials*

This principle is mainly applicable to cases due to an attack of exogenous heat resulting in the formation of toxic materials. The drugs commonly used are Flos Lonicerae, Herba Taraxaci, Herba Violae, Herba Patriniae, Rhizoma Paridis, Herba Houttuyniae, Caulis Sargentodoxae, Radix Sophorae Flavescentis, Rhizoma Coptidis, Cortex Phellodendri, Rhizoma Smilacis Glabrae, Flos Chrysanthemi Indici, etc. The recommended prescriptions are the Antiphlogistic Decoction of Five Ingredients and the Antiphlogistic Decoction with Lonicerae, Forsythiae and Sargentodoxae.

Since yin is readily impaired by heat, it is advisable to add some drugs with yin-nourishing and heat-clearing actions such as Radix Rehmanniae, Radix Scrophulariae, etc., to protect yin. Moreover, for the cases with retention of heat-toxin resulting in consumption of qi and blood with mass formation, drugs to activate blood circulation, eliminate blood stasis, soften masses and disperse stagnation should be added, such as Radix Angelicae Sinensis, Radix Paeoniae Rubra, Rhizoma Chuanxiong, Cortex Moutan Radicis, Semen Persicae, Olibanum, Myrrha, Carapax Trionycis, Thallus Eckloniae, Sargassum, etc.

*J. Dispelling dampness and promoting diuresis*

Clinically, disorders caused by dampness usually involve the spleen and kidneys. For cases with retention of fluid and dampness due to spleen deficiency, tonifying spleen, lifting up yang-qi, dispelling dampness and promoting diuresis are the principles available. The commonly used drugs are Rhizoma Atractylodis.

From the yin and yang perspective, the world is transitioning from winter, the most yin season of the year to spring, the most yang season of the year. Nature explodes with the coming of spring. Dormant bulbs once buried under inches of snow erupt and push aggressively up towards the nurturing source of the sun. Tree sap, long stored in the roots, reverses its flow and begins running up to ignite the growth cycle once again. The animal kingdom wakes up and starts the mating cycle so that the young can be raised during the gentler, warmer months.

All of nature is affected by the yang cycle of spring. What effect does it have on us? We are all familiar with the term "spring fever" and what they felt like when we were young and could appreciate the bounties of spring. Often times the burden of responsibilities blinds us to the joy that nature gladly offers in the spring as we hurry into our office buildings to take on the tasks of the day.

According to traditional Chinese medicine, spring is the time of the liver and gall bladder. The emotion most closely tied to the liver and the quality of spring is the explosive nature of anger. You may find yourself becoming easily angered over trivial matters. Anger is the most yang of the emotions and therefore is congruent with the spring. By comparison, the emotion of fear is associated with winter and has a constrictive quality. Just as the sap of a tree reverses its directional flow upwards, our emotions also find their way to the surface and may explode forth more easily in the spring than at any other time of year. Other emotional difficulties related to anger that may bubble up are impatience, frustration, resentment, rudeness, edginess, arrogance and aggression.

Rather than beating up yourself and everyone else with whom you come in contact, you may want to consider eating foods that will help relieve the liver. Chinese medicine teaches that the liver is the organ that is most susceptible to congestion and when congested throws the body into disharmony. This disharmony may be the root cause of the pent up emotions that may be bursting forth.

The first bit of advice to relieve the liver is to eat less. Limit your intake of highly processed foods and increase your intake of lightly steamed vegetables and whole grains. The taste of spring is sweet so emphasize those grains, vegetables and legumes that have a sweet flavor. Honey is an excellent detoxifier if used sparingly. Honey mixed with apple cider vinegar has a particularly beneficial effect on the liver. Mix one teaspoon of each in a cup a water to detoxify and activate the liver.

The reason vinegar is beneficial is that it has a bitter and sour taste which has a detoxifying effect on the liver. If heat signs are prevalent such as having a red face, thirst, and constipation, then substitute lemon, lime or grapefruit juice for the vinegar. Other bitter foods that can be used for detoxification purposes include rye, romaine lettuce, asparagus, amaranth, and quinoa.

To help build the liver, concentrate on an intake of chlorophyll rich foods provided by cereal grass sprouts that are so readily available in grocery stores. Other green foods that are beneficial are kale, parsley, and collard greens.

# *Chapter Eight*

# Management & Research on Some Disorders

## Acupuncture in Infertility

Acupuncture as a therapeutic intervention has been extensively studied and is increasingly practiced in the United States. A recent survey of acupuncture released by an NIH Consensus Development panel indicated that although there are inherent problems of design, sample size, and appropriate controls in the acupuncture literature, promising data exist for the use of acupuncture in treating nausea and vomiting , postoperative pain, addiction , and general pain syndromes . As a medical technique, acupuncture has also been reported as an adjunct in the treatment of various gynecologic problems.

Although conventional treatment options for female infertility have been well established, there have been few systematic reviews of complementary or alternative approaches to the treatment of infertility. In light of an increasing trend in the use of complementary and alternative medicine (16) and common inquiry and utilization of such approaches by patients suffering from infertility, we intend to review the existing scientific rationale and clinical data based on which acupuncture may exert an influence on the outcome of female fertility.

In examining the potential usefulness of acupuncture in enhancing female fertility, it is appropriate first to give some theoretical background for acupuncture. Although the theory of acupuncture stems from underlying traditional Chinese medicine premises that would define etiologies for infertility in terms of energy disturbance of imbalances, or organ deficiencies and excesses, we intend to review the existing literature by examining modern medical aspects of the central and peripheral modes of action of acupuncture as they impact on the hypothalamic-pituitary-ovarian axis and the pelvic organs, respectively. Moreover, the effect of acupuncture on anxiety and stress and ensuing potential indirect effects on female fertility will also be discussed.

*Background:* Acupuncture is the manipulation of thin metallic needles inserted into anatomically defined locations on the body to affect bodily function. The US Food and Drug Administration has recently removed acupuncture needles from the category of experimental medical devices and now regulates them just like it does other devices, such as surgical scalpels and hypodermic needles, under good manufacturing practices and single-use standard of sterility .

The general theory of acupuncture is based on the premise that there are patterns of energy flow (Qi) through the body, which are essential for health. Disruption of this flow is believed to be responsible for disease. Acupuncture can correct imbalances of flow at identifiable points close to the skin.

According to the proposed international acupuncture nomenclature by The World Health Organization in 1991 ,the meridian system consists of 20 meridians interconnecting about 400 acupoints. These acupoints correspond to specific areas on the surface of the body, which demonstrate higher electrical conductance because of the presence of higher density of gap junctions along cell borders. They act as converging points (or sinks) for electromagnetic fields. A higher metabolic rate, temperature, and calcium ion concentration, are also observed at these points. In principle, positive (anode) pulse stimulation of a point inhibits the organ function, whereas negative (cathode) pulse stimulation enhances that function. This forms the basis of electroacupuncture, which applies small electrical needles inserted in specific acupoints.

Effects of acupuncture on the hypothalamic-pituitary-ovarian axis and menstrual cycle:

Although traditional Chinese medicine understanding of acupuncture is based on ancient medical theory, a modern and scientific neuroendocrine perspective has begun to evolve in the past two decades. Mayer et al. first reported that acupuncture analgesia was induced through endorphin production and antagonized by the narcotic antagonist naloxone. Other studies similarly suggested that certain effects of acupuncture are mediated through the nervous system, within which ß-endorphin and other neuropeptides have been implicated.

Acupuncture was shown by Petti et al. (20) to cause a significant increase in ß-endorphin levels during treatment, which lasted for up to 24 hours. ß-endorphin is derived from its precursor protein pro-opiomelanocortin, which is present in abundant amounts in neuronal cells of the arcuate nucleus of the hypothalamus, pituitary, medulla, and in peripheral tissues including intestines and ovaries (23-25). Pro-opiomelanocortin cleaves to form adrenocorticotropic hormone and ß-lipoprotein. Further cleavage of ß-lipoprotein yields neuropeptides including ß-endorphin. Aleem et al. (26, 27) demonstrated the presence of immunoreactive ß-endorphin in follicular fluids of both normal and polycystic ovaries.

The influence on gonadotropin secretion and the menstrual cycle by endogenous opioid peptides is believed to be mediated by their action on GnRH secretion (28). The hypothalamic ß-endorphin center and the GnRH pulse generator, in fact, are both situated within the arcuate nucleus. Quigley et al. (29) first reported an increased opioid inhibition of LH secretion in hyperprolactinemic patients with pituitary microadenomas. Ching (30) and Orstead and Spics (31), respectively, showed that opioid peptides suppress GnRH release in rats and rabbits.

The role of these neuropeptides, including ß-endorphin, in the regulation of GnRH secretion in humans has recently been reviewed by Kalra et al. (32) and Pau and Spies (33). Rossmanith et al. (34) demonstrated the role of opioid peptides in the initiation of the mid-cycle LH surge in normal cycling women. Meanwhile, measurement of ß-endorphin in ovarian follicular fluid of healthy ovulatory women revealed much higher levels than that in circulating plasma (35). The highest level of ß-endorphin was noted to be in the preovulatory follicle.

Because acupuncture treatment impacts on ß-endorphin levels, which in turn affect GnRH secretion and the menstrual cycle, it is logical to hypothesize that acupuncture may influence ovulation and fertility. Animal studies have revealed that acupuncture treatment normalized GnRH secretion and affected peripheral gonadotropin levels (36, 37). Various investigators have shown that in normally ovulatory or anovulatory women, acupuncture also influenced plasma levels of FSH, LH, E2, and P (38-40). Acupuncture as a surrogate for hCG in ovulation induction was successfully used by Cai (41). Chen and Yu (42) showed that electroacupuncture normalized they hypothalamic-pituitary-ovarian axis, and in another study Chen reported that 6 of 13 anovulatory cycles responded to acupuncture treatment.

A series published from the University of Heidelberg in Germany used auricular acupuncture on 45 infertile women suffering from ovulatory dysfunction such as oligomenorrhea and luteal phase defect. The control group received medical treatment including bromocriptine, dexamethasone, levothyroxine, clomiphene citrate (CC), and gonadotropin. Although the investigators concluded that resumption of ovulatory cycles occurred significantly more often in the acupuncture group compared to the control group, pregnancy rates were not different between the two groups. However, interpretation of study data was very difficult due to the heterogeneity of the patient population and treatment modalities. Moreover, seven pregnancies in the acupuncture group were actually achieved with hormone treatment 6 months after acupuncture was stopped.

Another study by Stenver-Victorin et al. evaluated the use of electroacupuncture for ovulation induction on 24 oligo/amenorrheic women with polycycstic ovarian syndrome (PCOS). The percentage of ovulatory cycles in all subjects was shown to improve from 15% (in a total of 3 months before treatment) to 66% up to 3 months after treatment. Responsive patients were noted to have significantly lower body mass index (BMI), waist-to-hip circumference ratio, serum T concentration, serum T/sex hormone-binding globulin ratio, and serum basal insulin level. They suggested that, in these selected patients with PCOS, acupuncture could be considered as an alternative or adjunct to pharmacological ovulation induction.

A recent prospective randomized controlled study by Paulus et al. compared pregnancy rates in a total of 160 patients undergoing IVG. Acupuncture was performed in 80 patients 25 minutes before and after ET. After controlling confounding variables, clinical pregnancy rate for the acupuncture group (42.5%) was significantly higher than the control group (26.3%).

Peripheral effects of acupuncture:In addition to the central modulation of the hypothalamic-pituitary-ovarian axis, the effects of acupuncture on the autonomic nervous system have been well documented. In the early 1980s, Yao et al. reported long-lasting cardiovascular depression induced by acupuncture stimulation of the sciatic nerve in unanesthetized hypertensive rats. In the human, acupuncture was also shown to be sympathoinhibitory. After acupuncture, sympathetic nerve activity as measured by norepinephrine level, skin temperature, blood pressure, and pain tolerance threshold was shown to be decreased.

Endometrial thickness, morphology, and uterine artery blood flow have been implicated as important parameters for success of implantation of human embryos .Despite conflicting results in the utilization of these parameters during various stages of treatment to predict outcome in IVF, it is generally believed that adequate endometrial thickness is required to optimize pregnancy rate. Because endometrial thickness is a function of uterine artery blood flow, Sher and Fisch reported a novel method of using vaginal sildenafil in an attempt to improve uterine artery blood flow and endometrial development in patients undergoing IVF.

With its central sympathoinhibitory effect, acupuncture may contribute to reduce uterine artery impedance and therefore, increase blood flow to the uterus. In fact, Sterner-Victorin et al. demonstrated this when they performed acupuncture in 10 infertile women who were down-regulated by GnRH analog to avoid the effect of endogenous hormone on the uterine artery blood flow.

Pulsatility index in the uterine artery and skin temperature (on the forehead and lumbosacral area) were evaluated in three time periods-before, right after, and 2 weeks after acupuncture treatment (twice a week for 4 weeks). Pulsatility index and skin temperatures were found to be significantly decreased and increased, respectively, both right after and 14 days after acupuncture treatment. This effect was hypothesized to be caused by central inhibition of sympathetic activity.

### Acupuncture and Stress Reduction

It has been well documented that infertility causes stress and stress reduction may, in turn, improve fertility. However, the relationship between stress and infertility is that of a vicious cycle. Social stigmatization, decreased self-esteem, unmet reproductive potential of sexual relationship, physical and mental burden of treatment, and the lack of control on treatment outcome are just some of the factors that can lead to psychological stress in any couple pursuing infertility treatment. In turn, stress may lead to the release of stress hormones and influence mechanisms responsible for a normal ovulatory menstrual cycle through its impact on the hypothalamic-pituitary-ovarian axis.

The use of acupuncture for reducing anxiety and stress possibly through its sympathoinhibitory property and impact on ß-endorphin levels has been reviewed, and the efficacy of acupuncture in depression has also been studied. Because the pharmacological side effects of anxiolytic and antidepressant drugs on infertility treatment outcome are largely unknown, acupuncture may provide an excellent alternative for stress reduction in women undergoing infertility treatment. Hence, the practice of acupuncture to treat identifiable patho-physiological conditions has been a subject of intense research. The underlying physiologic mechanisms of acupuncture such as the release of opioids and other peptides in the central peripheral nervous system, and its inhibition of the sympathetic nervous system have been increasingly established. Promising results from credible trials have emerged for the use of acupuncture in treating various pain syndromes, substance abuse, and chemotherapy-induced nausea and vomiting.

Although the definitive role of acupuncture in the treatment of female infertility is yet to be established, its neuroendocrine effect on the hypothalamic-pituitary-ovarian axis and the preliminary clinical data reviewed here justifies further clinical trials to systematically examine the efficacy of acupuncture in treating various conditions related to female infertility such as ovulatory dysfunction associated with PCOS. The peripheral impact of acupuncture in improving uterine artery blood flow and hence endometrial thickness also provides encouraging data regarding its potential positive effect on implantation.

Whether these potential beneficial effects of acupuncture on the reproductive system can be translated into improving infertility treatment outcomes will eventually mandate randomized controlled studies of adequate design. Because acupuncture is nontoxic and relatively affordable, its indications as an adjunct in assisted reproduction or as an alternative for women who are intolerant, ineligible, or contraindicated for conventional hormone induction of ovulation deserves serious research and exploration.

Appropriate training, credentialing, and certification of acupuncture practitioners by state agencies can facilitate the integration of acupuncture into the treatment of female infertility, and healthcare in general. The NIH Consensus Conference agreed that this is necessary to allow the public and other health practitioners to identify qualified acupuncture practitioners. With the help of the US Department of Education, issues of training and licensure of non-physician and physician practitioners have been addressed. There is sufficient evidence to acupuncture's value to expand its use into conventional medicine and treatment of female infertility, and to encourage further studies of its underlying mechanisms as well as to establish its clinical value. We have described in details the etiology and suggested treatment lines in chapter fifteen.

Dry mouth (also known as xerostomia) is a painful condition caused by a decrease in the amount of saliva in the mouth when salivary glands do not work properly. Saliva is a natural defense for teeth and plays a major role in preventing tooth decay by rinsing away food particles and neutralizing harmful acids.

A decrease in saliva puts patients at risk for cavities, gum disease and discomfort since foods that are consumed adhere to the teeth longer. Dry mouth can be caused by medications like antihistamines, decongestants, antidepressants and diuretics and can often be treated by the dentist.

The quality of life of patients suffering from dry mouth is often profoundly impaired. Symptoms include extensive dental decay, infections of the tissues of the mouth, difficulty in speaking, eating and swallowing, ulceration or soreness of the mouth, an altered sense of taste and difficulty in wearing dentures.

However, "typical treatment options for dry mouth have been short-term at best," according to Warren M. Morganstein, DDS, MPH, and associate dean at the Baltimore College of Dental Surgery, University of Maryland Dental School. "Studies have found that acupuncture was a viable option to successfully treat dry mouth pain in patients and provide long-term relief."

After undergoing head and neck radiation therapy, seven patients with dry mouth were treated using acupuncture. Patients were seen once a week for four to five weeks, followed by two or three biweekly sessions. Dr. Morganstein found that eight months after treatment, all patients reported a reduction in dry mouth symptoms, as well as an increase in saliva flow and the ability to eat and speak, and improved sleep.

In the United States, acupuncture is performed primarily by licensed, non-physician acupuncturists. Additionally, physicians and a small number of dentists have been trained in medical acupuncture.

Acupuncture is effective in increasing the amount of saliva and, by doing so, alleviating or decreasing the symptoms of dry mouth.

To Ease Dry Mouth Pain:

Brush and floss twice a day

Chew sugarless gum

Avoid alcohol and caffeine

Avoid smoking

Avoid overly salty foods

Drink plenty of water

Avoid citrus juices (tomato, orange, grapefruit)

Avoid dry foods, such as toast or crackers

Use over-the-counter moisture replacement therapies

Visit the dentist regularly

While Western medicine tends to view menopausal disorders as a problem with hormone levels, Oriental medicine sees them as a deficiency of Qi (energy flow) and an imbalance between the Yin and Yang in the body. In order to correct this imbalance, many women are now turning to meridian therapy in the form of acupuncture.

In meridian therapy the acupuncturist stimulates certain meridians in the body to encourage the flow of Qi and balance the Yin and Yang. In menopause, the most likely imbalance is between the upper (Yang) half of the body and lower (Yin).

In a healthy body, the Yang Qi produced by the upper warmer descends and the Yin Qi generated by the lower warmer ascends. The Qi above and below interact and maintain health. However, when this interaction is obstructed, the Qi stagnates and causes a variety of symptoms.

When the Qi stagnates, Yang Qi becomes heat unable to descend. This can cause stiffness in the shoulders, headache, ringing in the ears, nose and throat problems and the infamous hot flashes as the heat in the upper body tries to dissipate.

When the Yin Qi is obstructed and does not go up it can cause such problems as backache, stomachache, menstrual irregularities and cold feet.

Many menopausal disorders are associated with emotional and psychological factors. Anxiety, quarreling and stress can overwork the kidneys and weaken them. If the kidneys are weak and are not able to stabilize the Qi, it moves upward and causes palpitations, headaches and insomnia that can lead to even more anxiety. If the liver is weakened symptoms may include irritability and emotional instability.

There are various treatments for menopause disorders, but meridian therapy is considered one of the most effective. In addition, a happy marriage and a healthy sex life help to activate the lower warmer and prevent blood stagnation.

The most common complaints acupuncturists treat are stress-related conditions such as anxiety and insomnia. Stress induces the fight or flight reaction, controlled by the autonomic nervous system.

The nervous system is divided into the voluntary and the autonomic. The voluntary nervous system is how we are able to control our muscles and movements. The autonomic nervous system works to maintain a state of balance in relation to external and internal conditions through the involuntary regulation of the internal organs, blood vessels and glands.

The sympathetic and parasympathetic nervous systems make up the two opposites of the autonomic nervous system. Ideally, there should be a balance between these two systems. A long-term imbalance prevents healing and leads to disease.

The sympathetic nervous system controls functions that include those associated with action, fight or flight. The parasympathetic system is passive, controlling the functions of rest and repair.

Stress is the most common cause of sympathetic system activation. Therefore, most patients are sympathetic dominant. That is, their sympathetic nervous system is activated most of the time, interfering with the functions of the parasympathetic. This is a result of our modern lifestyles.

If a person has sympathetic nervous system dominance, they will experience tight muscles (especially neck), rapid pulse, shortness of breath, reduced digestion and elimination, dizziness, cold extremities, headaches, sleep disturbances, bacterial infections, heart palpitations, low back pain, joint pain, etc. After long-term sympathetic dominance, the adrenals become depleted.

Since chronic stress activates the autonomic nervous system, it is outside of our control (involuntary).

This is why it is very difficult for a person to reset his or her own sympathetic nervous system dominance.

When the parasympathetic nervous system dominates, the exact opposite occurs.

The immune system is activated. The pupils dilate, heart rate decreases, digestive functions increase, appetite increases, blood vessels open, blood pressure is reduced, and muscles relax.

Acupuncture balances the autonomic nervous system, gradually adjusting the condition of the body. After acupuncture, people are usually relaxed or sleepy, indicating the parasympathetic system has been stimulated. Rest and repair has begun.

The prescription for wellness is the same as the prescription for combating chronic illness: reduce the impact of stress.

**Obesity**

People often puzzled over the "weight" topic and the many factors that affect it. Every day you can see new articles, ads, or other information on how to lose weight. I've wondered what acupuncture can add to the discussion.

The prevailing East Asian medical prescription for health is acupuncture, Chi Gung, and diet. Acupuncture addresses blockages and imbalances. Chi Gung also moves chi (life energy) to maintain and support the balance. Good diet increases chi. In Western terms, you do these three things to optimize your metabolism.

Americans spend over $40 billion per year to lose weight, but the percentage of overweight Americans continues to increase. Something must be wrong with the approach. Perhaps there is more in the equation than calories, fat content, gender, age, heredity, and cardiovascular exercise.

Studies show that Americans are the most anxious eaters in the world, obsessing about calories, fats, and the latest scientific fad of what is or isn't healthy. The experts conclude that worrying about food is not good for your health, and a more relaxed and social approach toward eating could break our unhealthy habit of binges and fad-diets. We could eat less and actually enjoy it more.

Why were people in the 1950's so much smaller than we are today? It certainly was a time of abundance. Moms who stayed home and cooked may be part of the answer. They prohibited snacks and insisted on everyone eating dinner together. This along with smaller portions and a more labor intense lifestyle are a part of the answer. There was less fast food and no super sizing.

You won't see Europeans and Asians jogging or spending hours at the gym, but they don't have the weight issues we Americans have. They don't eat in their cars, or obsess about carbs and fats either. They are less stressed, take more vacation time, and in general are less ambitious.

Maybe it isn't just the red wine or the olive oil that the French eat, but how they eat that keeps them in better health. While they eat unhealthy foods, they have very strict and stable rules: they eat small portions, don't go back for seconds, don't snack, and seldom eat alone. Communal meals are long leisurely affairs.

We all accept that exercise gets muscles and blood moving. What if you could get things moving in all of your organs as well as in the muscles? Then, the Kidneys could remove the water and help decrease bloating and water weight. Pancreas/Stomach brought into balance would decrease cravings. The Liver tuned up would affect hormones and emotional balance. Lung can move our chi so that we feel more resilient. All of these organ systems in balance and not fighting each other let us crave less, eat less, and have more energy.

In many Asian countries, the population does some sort of daily stretching and breathing routine. They move all of the joints and loosen muscle tightness, which increases chi flow, gradually working through the stuck places in the body. This is not cardiovascular exercise but medical Chi Gung, Tai Chi, or SoTai. Maybe we westerners have it wrong in our extreme workouts, with our notion that no pain is no gain. Can billions of Chinese be wrong?

If your hips are tight and you take up running, you will still have tight hips and a block in your circulation. In contrast, doing a daily chi exercise will gradually remove the tightness. In the beginning you may want to do an intensive program with acupuncture, but in the end you only need a maintenance program. You are never too old, too sick or too big to start moving your chi.

**Facial Rejuvenation**

Facial Rejuvenation Acupuncture is a non-surgical method of reducing the signs of the aging process. It is a rejuvenation and revitalization process designed to help the whole body look and feel younger. The treatment is based on the principles of Oriental Medicine and involves the insertion of hair-thin needles into particular areas of the face, ears, neck, hands, trunk, and legs along channels or meridians of energy called Qi (pronounced chee). As your practitioner, I will choose specific points to move energy in your body according to your individual needs. As well as focusing on particular areas of your face, the treatment will improve your overall appearance and bring out your inner radiance. Facial Rejuvenation Acupuncture specifically affects the face while simultaneously treating the underlying factors that contribute to the aging process.

Facial Rejuvenation Acupuncture may erase as many as five to fifteen years from the face, with results apparent after just a few treatments. Fine lines may be entirely eliminated and deeper wrinkles diminished. Bags under the eyes can be reduced, jowls firmed, puffiness eliminated, droopy eyelids lifted and double chins minimized. Other likely results include: moisturizing of the skin with increased local circulation of blood and lymph to the face; increased collagen production, muscle tone, and dermal contraction; tightening of the pores; brightening of the eyes; improving of hormonal balance to help acne; and reduction of stress evident in the face. It allows your own beauty to come from within.

If one is concerned with looking and feeling younger and slowing down the aging process, this treatment is for you. Facial Rejuvenation Acupuncture is suitable for people with deep wrinkles, fine lines, bags under the eyes, sagging, puffiness, drooping eyelids, double chin, large pores, dry skin or acne and more. Different methods are emphasized and specific points chosen according to how the aging process is working within you. A person with excess puffiness, for example, would require a different treatment than someone with dry skin. Unlike surgical or chemical treatments - such as Botox, Dermabrasion or a Facelift – acupuncture can treat you as a whole person. It works not only on a body level, but on a mental/emotional level as well. Thus if you are struggling with self-esteem concerns around your appearance, Facial Rejuvenation Acupuncture can help you to address those issues as well.

Generally, a Facial Rejuvenation series consists of 12 treatments. While effects are evident after the first or second treatment, they become more noticeable and lasting on or about the seventh session. Depending upon your condition and lifestyle prior to treatment, you may respond faster or slower to treatment. After the initial series, maintenance sessions can prolong your results for five to ten years. Adding appropriate herbs, diet, exercise and rest will also help to supplement the treatment.

Acupuncture has proven itself over the course of several thousand years, treating a wide range of conditions in billions of people. The use of Acupuncture in Cosmetology–especially in preventing and reducing wrinkles–has already attracted great attention in Japan, Hong Kong, and Sweden. Acupuncture's effectiveness is due to its direct manipulation of the body's energy system by balancing flow, removing blockages or adding energy when necessary. A 1996 report in the International Journal of Clinical Acupuncture reported that among 300 cases treated with Facial Acupuncture, 90% had marked effects with one course of treatment. The effects included: the skin becoming delicate and fair, improvement of the elasticity of facial muscles and leveling of wrinkles, a ruddier complexion, and overall rejuvenation–not confined to the face.

As early as the Sung Dynasty (960AD-1270AD) Acupuncture Rejuvenation practices were employed for the Empress and the Emperor's concubines. Acupuncturists discovered and utilized ways to change the energy flow within the body to initiate the healing process for rejuvenation. Even for those unfamiliar with the principles of Chinese Medicine, it is known that increased circulation helps the body to look and feel better.

While not a replacement for surgery, Acupuncture Facial Rejuvenation is an excellent alternative. It is far less costly than cosmetic surgery and is safe, virtually painless, has no side effects or risk of disfigurement. Unlike surgery that may have an extended recovery period with swelling and discoloration, there is no trauma from Facial Rejuvenation Acupuncture. While Facial Rejuvenation Acupuncture cannot reshape one's nose or chin, it is a more subtle rejuvenation that takes years off one's face–safely and naturally while improving overall health. Facial Rejuvenation Acupuncture treats the underlying cause of why someone is aging instead of masking the outward symptoms and allowing further decline and dysfunction to continue within the body. It allows your own beauty to come from within.

Facial Rejuvenation Acupuncture is contraindicated for some pituitary disorders, heart disorders, diabetes mellitus, high blood pressure, individuals who have a pacemaker or who have a problem with bleeding or bruising, or who currently suffer from migraine headaches. Facial Rejuvenation Acupuncture should not be done during pregnancy, during a bout with a cold or flu, during an allergic attack or during an acute herpes outbreak.

## Acupuncture for Labour

A recent research suggests that acupuncture may help control pain during childbirth.

Previous studies have found that acupuncture may be helpful in treating low back pain, acute dental pain and recurrent headaches. Acupuncture has also been used to treat morning sickness and to induce labour (labor).

To evaluate, researchers from the Universities of Exeter and Plymouth, UK conducted a computerised literature search of several databases. They identified three trials that fitted their quality standards. In the first trial, 106 women who received acupuncture along with conventional medication were compared with 92 women who were given only conventional care. It was found that the acupuncture group was less likely to request for pain medications than those who did not receive acupuncture. Almost all women treated with acupuncture said they would use the complementary treatment again for labour (labor) pain.

The second trial involved 90 women who were randomly assigned to a group that received acupuncture or a group that received conventional care. Both groups were also given the requested pain medication or non-pharmacologic pain management techniques such as a bath or shower. It was found that women in the acupuncture group requested less of one pain medication, but similar levels of other pain medications than those in the comparison group. The acupuncture group also reported a higher level of relaxation than their peers and was less likely to request non-pharmacologic pain treatment.

In the third trial, 106 women received acupuncture and 102 women received placebo acupuncture, in which superficial needles were applied to non-acupuncture points. None of the women knew whether they received acupuncture or the sham treatment. The acupuncture group reported less pain up to two hours after acupuncture and two hours after giving birth than those who received the sham treatment. The women who received acupuncture requested less pain medication than their counterparts.

Overall, the data suggest that acupuncture can be another option for pregnant women for labour (labor) pain management if future trials support acupuncture's effect.

## Hypertension

High blood pressure, or hypertension, is a major risk factor for heart attack and stroke. Middle-aged Americans face a staggering 90 percent chance of developing the condition, according to a new report in the Journal of the American Medical Association.

But the drugs used to treat it must be taken daily, usually for a lifetime. And they may have side effects, such as fatigue, depression and dizziness.

So Zusman is looking for alternatives for relieving hypertension. He thinks he may have found one in the ancient Chinese technique of acupuncture.

"There is an extensive literature from Asian and Russian communities that acupuncture does indeed lower blood pressure," he says.

American researchers have already shown that special acupuncture needles, when gently inserted into specific points on the skin, can stimulate nerves that reach up into the brain and to cells in the brain that control blood pressure.

"There's evidence from our laboratory and many other laboratories to suggest that the cells quiet down after acupuncture," says Dr. John Longhurst professor of medicine at the University of California, Irvine.

When those cells "quiet down," or become less active, blood vessels relax.

"A substantial number of our patients have responded with significant reductions in blood pressure," he opins.

Perhaps most amazing, acupuncture's benefit can be long lasting. Some patients who received the acupuncture treatment nine months ago still have normal blood pressure.

"The implication," says Zusman, "is that 12 acupuncture treatments over a six-week period will produce a cure."

In this case, the doctors defined "cure" as maintaining normal blood pressure for one year without medication. And that, for some patients, may now be within their reach.

Have you ever known someone with cold hands or feet? I met someone so cold that it was a shock to shake his hand. In 75 degree weather, how could someone's hand feel like 30 degrees? In East Asia it's called cold invasion.

Cold invasion is not the same as having a cold. This internal cold condition interferes with the body's health maintenance system known as defensive chi. I've heard doctors say that being cold will compromise the immune system, making a person more susceptible to illness. This sounds like another way of describing the loss of defensive chi, due to cold invasion.

In the Western hemisphere, the concept of cold invasion seems odd. Perhaps it seems odd because we are just not familiar with the expression. What about the expressions "catching cold," or "catching a chill?" Why do we call a rhinovirus a "Cold" virus?

The western medical advice given to a patient with a cold includes "stay warm and dry." So, there is western acceptance that exposure to cold has a negative impact on our health. There is obviously a relationship between cold and a cold virus.

In the West we think of being invaded by an organism. In the East, the idea is that physical cold impacts the body. This is also how the cold invasion symptoms show up. There can be cold acupoints on the abdomen, internal cold, or cold at the extremities. Poor circulation is frequently identified as the cause.

Circulation can create problems including being cold, but it is not the root cause. What causes poor circulation? The causes are varied and sometimes indirect: trauma, surgery, exposure to cold, inflammation, medication, prolonged illness, etc.

Since medications can induce an internal cold condition, you can get worse (or at least not get any better) by medicating when you are already cold internally. This inhibits healing.

The presence of cold is a sign or symptom. Until cold is gone, the body will have a harder time healing and have a harder time fighting off potential illnesses.

In general, it can be difficult to sort out which causative event occurred first. With acupuncture, it doesn't matter. We have several diagnostic tools to determine where the circulation is a problem, and have techniques to correct it.

## *Chapter Nine*

# How Acupuncture Works

Several theories have been advanced to explain acupuncture's effectiveness in this regard. There is speculation that the needle insertions stimulate the body's production of such natural opiates (painkilling chemicals) as endorphins or enkephalins. Others have posited that the minor stimulation of acupuncture selectively acts on impulse transmission to the central nervous system, thus closing certain neurological "gates" and blocking the transmission of pain impulses from other parts of the body. Some Western observers studying the method have suggested that acupuncture analgesia is plainly a placebo analgesia—which does not, however, detract from its effectiveness. Chinese assertions that acupuncture can actually cure disease defy rational clinical practice and have yet to be substantiated by Western medical researchers.

In trying to find ways to unite or just bring closer the mysterious transformational techniques of the East to the reductionism theories of the West, our Western medical science has tried to organize a logical explanation of how the insertion of tiny acupuncture needles can reduce and even dissolve pain in the human form.

This research takes a look at the different approaches the Biosciences have attempted in explaining the way holistic acupuncture works in healing. This research will take a look at the biochemical, biomechanical, as well as bio-electromagnetic theories that have been developed in trying to explain the healing aspects of the Ancient Art of Acupuncture.

The Ancient Art of Acupuncture is the needling of specific points along "meridians" or channels that run throughout our body. Acupuncture can be traced back as far as the Stone Age in China, when stone knives and pointed rocks were used to relieve pain and diseases. "These instruments were known by the ancients as "bian".

In the Han Dynasty (206 BC to 220 AD) an Analytical Dictionary of Characters "Shuo Wen Jie Zi" describes the character "bian" as meaning a stone to treat disease." Later these stones were replaced by needles made of bamboo and slivers of animal bone, then finally in the Shang Dynasty bronze casting techniques made metal needles possible, which conducted electricity and Qi. This led to the mapping of the meridian system or channels of energy within the body.

Acupuncture remained relatively unheard of until 1974 when James Reston, a reporter for the New York Times accompanied President Nixon on a trip to China where they witnessed an appendectomy and several demonstrations of serious surgeries being performed with acupuncture as the only anesthetic using Acupuncture Anesthesia. Despite many efforts to prove it's efficiency, Western science has never been able to reconcile how Acupuncture works. They can prove "that" it works, but not "how" it works?

## Biochemical Theories

Most of the scientific studies of acupuncture have been centered on the analgesic aspects of pain relief. Acupuncture is definitely effective in treating pain; it works 70% to 80% of the time, far greater than the placebo, which only has about 30% efficiency.

The problem with attributing all of acupuncture's effects to the placebo effect, which is based on a "suggestive way" or the fact that one just wants to believe that it works, was the fact that veterinarians in China have used acupuncture successfully to treat animals.

Dr. Bruce Promeranz, working at the University of Toronto, was very involved in research done on acupuncture analgesia. By activating small myelinated nerve fibers, acupuncture applications send impulses to the spinal chord, midbrain and pituitary-hypothalamus in the diencephelon. Neurological research done in the late 70's discovered the naturally occurring chemicals in the body known as endorphins. By binding to the opiate receptors that are found throughout the nervous system, endorphins are able to stop pain.

The hypothalamus-pituitary releases Beta-endorphins into the blood and cerebral spinal fluid to create an analgesic effect by causing incoming pain signals from reaching the brain. Pomeranz discovered that pre-treating rats with a drug called Naloxone, a drug known to block the healing endorphins, could not achieve acupuncture pain relief. This finding suggested that endorphin release caused by acupuncture stimulus was an important mechanism behind acupuncture's pain relieving effects.

Pomeranz was then interested in the effects of electrical stimulation and manipulation of acupuncture needles. What he also discovered was the difference between high frequency, low intensity vs. low frequency, high intensity application.

The low frequency, high intensity produced an analgesic effect which was slower at the onset but longer in duration and also having cumulative effects. Therefore, repeated treatments produce more and more benefits for the patient.

The high frequency, low intensity produced a very rapid analgesic effect, which is great for acute pain but shorter in duration with no cumulative effects.

There are presently 100 different neurotransmitters and neuroendocrine substances in the body, of which the endorphins constitute only one class. Hence, there is much work to be done in testing and researching these chemicals and their possible effects with acupuncture.

### Biomechanical Theories

The biomechanical questions had to do with the presents of meridians in the body. These are the channels in the body, which are filled with our life force, energy – Qi. The meridians are said to circulate Qi throughout the system of the body. In an attempt to locate the meridians anatomically, two French Drs. Claude Darras and Pierre De Vernejoul injected human studies with radioactive isotopes into acupuncture points.

A solution of an ionic salt of technetium was injected and followed over a period of time with a gamma ray camera. The radioactive technetium followed the exact same pathways of the meridian channels described and illustrated in several hundred-year-old acupuncture charts of the human body! To ensure that the Drs. were measuring meridians and not blood vessels or lymphatic channels, some patients received technetium injections adjacent to non-acupoint skin regions as well as in nearby blood and lymphatic channels. The radioactive tracers tended to diffuse outward from the injection site into a typical small circular pattern.

In 1975, Dr. Liu YK researched the location of acupoints present at sites of motor nerves.

His work realized that acupoints correspond to regions where motor nerves enter skeletal muscle and where there is a great density of motor nerve terminal elements at the surface.

As well, there was found to be dense clusters of encapsulated autonomic nerve mechanoreceptor sites at these points.

Further research was done on Dr. Liu's work. Dr. Watari published a report in Beijing, China in November 1987, based on his work. He found that histologically, volume density of corresponding acupoints to blood vessels are elevated fourfold and that of nerves 1.4 times over that of surrounding tissues. These vessels and fibers mingle to form glomerular structures.

This was exciting new biomechanical evidence in both identifying the meridian channels in the human body and the fact that the acupuncture points on the body have corresponding volume densities that increase with stimulation.

### Bio-electromagnetic Theories

Science has long been aware of an electrical phenomenon called the "Current of Injury".

This happens when tissue in the body undergoes trauma or microscopic damage to an area of skin. When skin cells are pierced, as with an acupuncture needle, they start leaking electrically charged ions into the surrounding areas of tissue. A weak electrical battery-like charge is created. This electric current is called the current of injury, which is know to stimulate a healing response from the nearby cells.

This does not explain how stimulating acupoints with low level, non-invasive lasers could achieve the same therapeutic effects.

The electrical conductivity of acupoints has been known for several decades thanks to the work of Nakatani in the 1950s and by Dr. Robert Becker in the 1970s. Becker's work on the Large Intestine and the Pericardium meridians found that the points along these channels showed significantly more electrical conductivity than areas of skin with non-acupoints.

In 1986 German scientist Fritz-Albert Popp and Chinese biologist, Chang-Lin Zhang developed a model they called the "Standing Wave Superposition Hypothesis". This research attempts to accommodate the holographic nature of acupuncture such as the homunculus or miniature representation of the whole body represented in the ears and the feet. The theory also strives to explain the anomalous skin resistance properties of acupuncture points as well as the apparent interconnectivity between them.

In the Zhang-Popp model, it is shown that the body is composed of sodium, potassium and other electrically charged inorganic ions such as proteins and DNA which when accelerated will emit EM radiation in accordance with conventional physical theory.

With these many types of charges oscillating in the body, an interference pattern is produced formed by the various waves of various wavelengths.

The highest combination of wave amplitudes forms the acupuncture points and meridians by means of constructive interference. At these points the skin is at the highest in electrical conductivity. This conductivity depends on the internal electrical field, which is determined by the interference pattern from the superposition of the numerous waves. Hence, the standing wave pattern of a sick person would have a varied pattern from that of a healthier person.

The treatment of acupuncture with needles in the acupoints would cause a disturbance in the standard wave pattern caused by new boundaries formed by the needle. The needle activates the current of injury response resulting in a change in the EM field, producing changes in the biological response, which may promote healing. It is this theory, which implicates the EM fields of the entire body.

The principle of the Connective Tissue Continuum is another approach at viewing the correlation of acupuncture to the bio-electromagnetic theory. From a cellular level through to the bodies' connective tissue, these living organisms are considered a continuum. Not only is the entire cell now known to be mechanically and electrically interconnected in a "solid state", but, all the cells in the body are in turn interconnected to one another via the connective tissues.

The function of connective tissues is to keep the body organized, acting as a lace work between the major organs and tissues, to strengthen the wall of arteries, veins, intestines and pathways and to provide fascia and the skeletal structure attachment to the muscles. It is believed that connective tissues may be largely responsible for the rapid intercommunication that enables our body to function effectively as a coherent whole, and is therefore central to our health and well-being. Recent studies with Nuclear Magnetic Resonance has shown that the muscles in living human subjects provide evidence of a "liquid-crystalline-like" structure.

Liquid crystals usually undergo rapid changes in phases or transitions when exposed to electromagnetic fields. Liquid crystals will also respond to changes in temperature, hydration, pressure and shear forces. Biological liquid crystals carry static electric charges and are influenced by pH, salt concentration and dielectric constant of the solvent.

There are many types of liquid crystals, from those which are most liquid, to those which are most solid. Those that are most liquid can flow as water does, and even though all molecules tend to be aligned in one direction, individual molecules can move very freely and change places with each other while maintaining their common orientation. The ones that resemble solid crystal will have order and will remain flexible and responsive. It is already widely recognized that all the major constituents of living organisms may be liquid crystal such as lipids of cellular membranes, DNA, possibly all proteins, especially cytoskeletal proteins, muscle proteins, and proteins in the connective tissues such as collagens and proteoglycans. It is through this "liquid network" that scientist believe an acupuncture response is solicited.

By looking at the Bioscience attempts in explaining the way holistic acupuncture works in healing, we are introduced to some very notable concepts. Observing the biochemical view, we see, by Pomeranz research, that the hypothalamus-pituitary releases Beta-endorphins into the blood and cerebral spinal fluid to create an analgesic effect by causing incoming pain signals from reaching the brain. The low frequency, high intensity produced an analgesic effect which was slower at the onset but longer in duration and also having cumulative effects. Therefore, repeated treatments produce more and more benefits for the patient. The high frequency, low intensity produced a very rapid analgesic effect, great for acute pain but, shorter in duration with no cumulative effects.

Biomechanically, Drs. Claude Darras and Pierre De Vernejoul injected human studies with radioactive isotopes into acupuncture points. A solution of an ionic salt of technetium was injected and followed over a period of time with a gamma ray camera. The radioactive technetium followed the exact same pathways of the meridian channels described and charted in several hundred-year-old acupuncture charts of the human body!

Dr. Liu YK researched the location of acupoints present at sites of motor nerves.

His work realized that acupoints correspond to regions where motor nerves enter skeletal muscle and where there is a great density of motor nerve terminal elements at the surface.

Bio-electromagnetic theories are based on the current of Injury, which is know to stimulate a healing response from the nearby cells.

The electrical conductivity of acupoints researched by Nakatani in the 1950s and by Dr. Robert Becker in the 1970s found that the points along the channels showed significantly more electrical conductivity than areas of skin with non-acupoints.

The Zhang-Popp model, shows us that the body is composed of sodium, potassium and other electrically charged inorganic ions such as proteins and DNA which when accelerated will emit EM radiation in accordance with conventional physical theory.

The acupuncture needle activates the current of injury response resulting in a change in the EM field, producing changes in the biological response.

The Connective Tissue Continuum embraces the concept that the cytoskeletal structure of each individual cell in the body is a homunculus of the connective tissue in which it creates. Magnetic Resonance has shown that the muscles in living human subjects provide evidence of a "liquid-crystalline-like" structure. Liquid crystals usually undergo rapid changes in phases or transitions when exposed to electromagnetic fields. It is through this "liquid network" that scientist believe an electromagnetic response from acupuncture is solicited. This research represents much of the current biological views on how acupuncture heals and tries to explain the Biomedical Basis of Holistic Acupuncture.

Acupuncture is one of the key components of the system of traditional Chinese medicine (TCM). In the TCM system of medicine, the body is seen as a delicate balance of two opposing and inseparable forces: yin and yang. Yin represents the cold, slow, or passive principle, while yang represents the hot, excited, or active principle. Among the major assumptions in TCM are that health is achieved by maintaining the body in a "balanced state" and that disease is due to an internal imbalance of yin and yang. This imbalance leads to blockage in the flow of qi (vital energy) along pathways known as meridians. It is believed that there are 12 main meridians and 8 secondary meridians and that there are more than 2,000 acupuncture points on the human body that connect with them.

Preclinical studies have documented acupuncture's effects, but they have not been able to fully explain how acupuncture works within the framework of the Western system of medicine that is commonly practiced in the United States.9-14 It is proposed that acupuncture produces its effects through regulating the nervous system, thus aiding the activity of pain-killing biochemicals such as endorphins and immune system cells at specific sites in the body. In addition, studies have shown that acupuncture may alter brain chemistry by changing the release of neurotransmitters and neurohormones and, thus, affecting the parts of the central nervous system related to sensation and involuntary body functions, such as immune reactions and processes that regulate a person's blood pressure, blood flow, and body temperature.

With a cultural history that includes thousands of years of acupuncture, Asians implicitly accept the nature of it. Westerners are warming up to it. Researchers, doctors, & lawmakers continue to examine or conduct trials of many modalities (drugs, surgeries, etc.) that include acupuncture, all with the goal of improving care of patients. Even without the recent bad press of many popular medications, the data supporting acupuncture continues to grow.

Acupuncture isn't just showing up in news items in the Wall Street Journal, USA Today, and the New York Times. Medical organizations are conducting research, and medical journals are reporting on the notable benefits of acupuncture, or showing how it works. These include The Journal of the American Medical Association (JAMA), The Annals of Internal Medicine, Human Brain Mapping Journal, Medicine and Science in Sports and Exercise, The Anatomical Record, The World Health Organization, and The National Institute of Health. With support from reputable medical journals and establishments, it is clear that people know it works and they want to know more.

What are they saying that acupuncture does or what it can help? No one is claiming acupuncture is a panacea. It is a set of protocols based on a different medical model. The experts are reporting on acupuncture's specific effects or specific conditions that improved with acupuncture:

Corrects breach orientation pregnancies;

Reduces nausea and vomiting;

Osteoarthritis pain relief and improved function;

Increases fertility;

Reduces cortisol, increases IgA antibodies, releases serotonin;

Affects the visual cortex and auditory cortex of the brain;

Increases beta endorphins; and

The World Health Organization lists dozens of other known conditions acupuncture treats.

Acupuncture is one aspect of Traditional Chinese Medicine that has flourished in China for over 2,500 years. Presently, it is practiced widely throughout Asia and Europe. The United States has followed suit, and Acupuncture is now accepted as one of the newest forms of health care in this country. Some insurance plans pay for acupuncture treatments.

Acupuncture treats diseases and its syndromes, strengthens the immune systems and the physical body, prevents diseases and achieves longevity. A lot of research has confirmed that acupuncture can regulate and balance the endocrine system and hormone levels. So, it is useful to treat reproductive disorders. Acupuncture is not however a cure all and does not take the place of surgery.

Acupuncture is based on the knowledge of vital energy flow to the whole body. This energy travels through pathways called meridian, etc. Once this energy is deficient or blocked, then the body stops functioning normally and will eventually become sick. An Acupuncturist is trained to find these deficiencies or blocks. Through complex diagnostic techniques, he or she determines if the energy supply is ample, if it is flowing the correct direction and speed. Then, with the application of needles and needling techniques, he or she is able to restore the flow of energy back to normal. The body returns to its normal function, pain is relieved, other symptoms disappear, vital energy and health is restored.

As a side effect of the restoration of ample and correct energy flow in the body, studies have shown that Acupuncture could influence the central and peripheral nervous systems. Evidence indicates that it releases endorphins from the brain making it particularly effective in pain control. Among a host of factors, acupuncture also affects the metabolism and production of sugar levels in the blood, as well as affects the endocrine system, and digestive system.

In the Chinese medical paradigm, all the major organs in the human body have corresponding energetic pathways along the surface of the body which are called channels or meridians, and these meridians have points which have certain energetic functions. In Chinese medicine this disease is considered to be a disturbance of prenatal qi (energy), what we in the West would call our genetic makeup. Prenatal qi governs a person's organization, creation, and continuing re-creation. This qi originates in the kidneys, therefore the kidney channel or meridian must be considered in treatment. There is also the factor of stagnation of dampness and coldness in the body, which Chinese medicine considers to be an excessive yin or deficient yang condition. Put in simpler terms, the qi is too cold and not moving well, therefore the qi must be warmed to help it move. A technique called moxibustion is used to alleviate the dampness and cold, and bring warmth (yang energy) into the body. Moxibustion is the burning of a wool-like herb called mugwort near the skin's surface on preselected points along meridians.

In 1998 a study published in the Archives of Internal Medicine showed that Medical doctors refer their patients to acupuncturists more than any other alternative care provider. the study also revealed that 51% of medical doctors believe that acupuncture is efficacious and of value!

There are numerous theories as to the mechanism of how acupuncture works. Acupuncture is used to treat various ailments in animals. The restoration of function in animals has often been used as a way of demonstrating acupuncture's effectiveness and explaining away the placebo affect which some attribute to it.

A study performed at the University of Medicine and Dentistry of New Jersey has finally provided the scientific proof of how acupuncture works.

The study monitored twelve patients using functional magnetic resonance imaging (MRI). This instrument allows researchers to see what parts of the brain are receiving increased blood flow. Increased blood flow to a certain area of the brain indicates that that part of the brain is being stimulated. Pain was induced in the patients by using a tiny filament to prick the inside or outside of the upper lip. It was found that activity subsided in 60 to 70 percent of the entire brain.

Wen-Ching Liu, an assistance professor of radiology at the University of Medicine and Dentistry of New Jersey and co-author of the study stated, "It is important for Western Medicine to recognize that these acupoints really mean something I regard to pain relief." Dr. Lee concluded, "So many people with pain, whether from cancer, headache, or a chronic, unexplained condition, rely on medications such as morphine, which can become addicting. Acupuncture has no side effects, and other studies have shown the pain relief it provides can last up for months."

## How Acupuncture Works

### *Kundu-Led Sin Theory*

Eminent authors and researchers Dr.Debasish Kundu and Dr.Choo Led Sin opined that , so far we know from the philosophy of classical chinese acupuncture that ailments take place from the abnormality or increase or decrease of the life energy in various parts or organs of the body , the type of needling and depth of insertion are also measured according to this increase(shi) or decrease(xu) of the life energy.

In the various body parts or organs life energy flows through the yin and yang poles of the meridians, simultaneously, yin and yang are inter-connected through the capillary and neuro-fibrous network in a meridian and when needles are inserted into the specific points of a meridian, while stimulating the specific region or organ concerned the stimulation (deqi) also affects the central nervous system and the feedback or 'immune response' acts as a catalyst to optimize the energy levels of the yin and yang poles of the meridian resulting the desired therapeutic effect.

With painless acupuncture techniques becoming popular day by day the deqi or stimulation is now a days produced by adding electronic stimulator to needles.

## *Chapter Ten*

# Acupuncture Anesthesia

Greek word algesis means sensation of pain. Acupuncture can effectively reduce pain thus it can also be used to reduce sensation of pain of a specific part or organ which may then subjected to surgical treatment.

Researchers have established that internal secration of a morphine like substance called endorphine and the immune response of the neuro transmitters to the segmental stimulation are the parts of this pain relieving mechanism.

Anesthesia, absence of physical sensation in part or all of the body. The term more commonly refers to a reversible condition that is induced using anesthetic drugs. These drugs may be injected, inhaled, or applied directly to the surface of the body. Each year about 40 million patients in the United States receive anesthetic drugs for surgery, obstetrics, dentistry, or other medical procedures. Induced anesthesia may be local, involving only part of the body, or general, involving lack of sensation in the entire body as well as a loss of consciousness. Localized anesthesia can also be a result of natural causes, such as nerve injury, leprosy, or diabetes. The lack of sensation caused by these conditions is not easily reversible, and patients' unawareness of pain and other sensations can put them at risk of serious harm. This article focuses on induced anesthesia used in medical procedures.

Anesthesia is distinct from analgesia. An analgesic, or pain-relieving drug such as aspirin, may relieve a headache, but a person who takes an aspirin still feels other physical sensations, such as pressure, heat, cold, and vibration. In contrast, anesthetic drugs block all physical sensations, though for medical purposes their ability to block pain is among their most important effects. Pain is a crucial warning system that tells us when our bodies are in danger, but without anesthesia, pain would make surgery and various other medical procedures much more difficult—or even impossible.

The sensation of pain results from communication between nerve cells in the brain, spinal cord, and elsewhere in the body (see Nervous System). The process begins when certain nerve cell endings, known as pain receptors or nociceptors, are stimulated. Pain receptors are located in the skin, joints, muscles, the linings of the body cavities, and elsewhere in the body. Nerve impulses travel from pain receptors along nerve fibers to the spinal cord and then to the brain. Pain impulses are relayed through a brain structure known as the thalamus and then to the cerebral cortex, the area of the brain that interprets messages and generates the conscious sensation of pain. At several points along their journey from pain receptor to cerebral cortex, pain impulses can be modified. For example, chemicals known as endorphins, the body's natural painkillers, interact with nerve cells in the brain and spinal cord to dampen the sensation of pain.

The various drugs used in anesthesia work by several different mechanisms to block the transmission or perception of pain and other sensations. Some sleep-producing drugs used as part of general anesthesia are injected into a patient's veins. These drugs are taken up by organs, muscles, and brain tissue and interfere with the complex and poorly understood biochemical mechanisms of consciousness. Anesthetic drugs that are inhaled dissolve in the blood and circulate to the brain. There they interact with brain cells, especially cells in the cerebral cortex that are involved in sensory perceptions. Opiates, a family of opium-derived pain relievers that includes morphine, codeine, and fentanyl, act like the body's own natural endorphins to dampen the sensation of pain. Drugs used as local anesthetics block pain impulses in a specific part of the body, preventing these nerve impulses from reaching the brain. These drugs interfere with the chemicals inside nerve fibers that are involved in transmission of nerve impulses.

Anesthetic also spelled Anaesthetic, agent which produces a local or general loss of sensation, including pain. General anesthesia involves loss of consciousness, usually for the purpose of relieving the pain of surgery. Local anesthesia involves loss of sensation in one area of the body by the blockage of conduction in nerves.

Drugs of various kinds have been used for many centuries to reduce the distress of surgical operations. Homer wrote of nepenthe, which was probably cannabis or opium. Arabian physicians used opium and henbane. More recently powerful rum was administered freely to British sailors before emergency amputations were carried out on board ship in the aftermath of battle.

In 1799 Sir Humphry Davy, British chemist and inventor, tried inhaling nitrous oxide (laughing gas) and discovered its anesthetic properties, but the implications of his findings for surgery were ignored. By the early 1840s parties had become fashionable in Britain and the United States at which nitrous oxide, contained in bladders, was passed around and inhaled for its soporific effect. Itwas soon found that ether, which could be carried much more conveniently in small bottles, was equally potent. In the United States several young dentists and doctors experimented independently with the use of nitrous oxide or ether to dull the pain of tooth extractions and other minor operations. In 1845, Horace Wells, an American dentist, attempted to publicly demonstrate the use of nitrous oxide anesthesia for dental extractions. Unfortunately, the demonstration was unsuccessful.

Historians argue about who should be credited with the first use of true surgical anesthesia, but it fell to William Morton, an American dentist, to convince the medical world that general anesthesia was a practical proposition. He administered ether to a patient having a neck tumour removed at the Massachusetts General Hospital, Boston, in October 1846. Crawford Long, an American surgeon, had used ether in his practice since 1842 but did not make his findings public until 1849.

A few weeks after Morton's demonstration, ether was used during a leg amputation performed by Robert Liston at University College Hospital, London. In Britain, official royal sanction was given to anesthetics by Queen Victoria, who accepted chloroform from her physician, John Snow, when giving birth to her eighth child, Prince Leopold, in 1853.

Early anesthetics had unpleasant side effects (often causing vomiting on recovery) and were somewhat hazardous, since the dose needed to produce unconsciousness and full muscle relaxation (so that the surgeon could work unimpeded) was not far short of that which would paralyze the breathing centre of the brain. In addition, the early anesthetics were administered by simple devices consisting of glass or metal containers for sponges soaked in ether or chloroform (which was introduced as an anesthetic in 1847) and allowed no control of dosage.

Modern inhalation anesthetics such as trichlorethylene and halothane have a much widersafety margin and are administered, mixed with oxygen and nitrous oxide, from an anesthetic machine. The anesthetist can control the flow and composition of the gas mixture precisely and, using a tube placed down the trachea (windpipe) after the patient is unconscious, can, if necessary, maintain respiration by mechanical means. Delivering the gas mixture to the lungs through a close-fitting endotracheal tube also prevents accidental inhalation of mucus, saliva, and vomit.

With respiration artificially maintained it is possible to paralyze the muscles with drugs like curare, a neuromuscular blocking agent, so that proceduresrequiring full muscle relaxation, such as chest and abdominal surgery, can be carried out under light anesthesia.

Many short operations can be carried out under anesthesia produced by injecting an agent such asthe barbiturate sodium thiopental (Pentothal) into a vein, either as a single dose or intermittently through a saline drip. Patients are also commonly put to sleep by this method before the administration of an inhalation anesthetic is begun, since it is a distress-free procedure, and unconsciousness occurs smoothly within 10 or 15 seconds of starting the injection.

Local anesthetics work by blocking the passage of impulses along nerves. Cocaine was thus used for eye operations in 1884 by a Viennese surgeon, Carl Koller, acting on the suggestion of Sigmund Freud. A solution of the drug was applied directly to the part to be operated on. Soon it was being injected under the skin to facilitate small, local operations, and it was later successfully used for larger procedures by injecting it into the trunks of nerves supplying a part. Now, synthetic cocaine substitutes are widely used.

Major operations on the lower half of the body can be carried out after injecting a suitable local anesthetic into the fluid-filled space between the spinal cord and its outer membrane coverings (spinal anesthesia). Painless childbirth can be achieved by an epidural block, which involves injecting the anesthetic agent through a fine tube threaded into the space surrounding the tough membrane covering the lower end of the spinal cord, thus dulling the emerging nerves that supplythe pelvic organs.

In recent years much interest has been shown in acupuncture anesthesia, whereby apparently painless major operations are carried out after the insertion of acupuncture needles into specified points on the skin. Often an electric current is passed through the needle used. The results of some research into the efficacy of acupuncture have suggested that the stimulation of the peripheral nerves by the needles triggers the release of endorphins, a group of neurochemicals that have pain-killing effects.

## Theories of Pain

There have always been two theories of the sensation of pain, a quantitative or intensity theory and a stimulus-specific theory. According to the former, pain results from excessive stimulation of every kind: e.g., excessive heat or cold, excessive damage to the tissues. This theory in its simplest form entails the belief that the same afferent nerve fibres are activated by all of these various stimuli; pain is felt merely when they are conducting far more impulses than usual. But knowledge acquired in the 20th century has shown that the quantitative theory—at least in its classic form—is wrong. Peripheral nerve fibres have been found to bestimulus-specific, each one excited by certain forms of energy. The stimulus-specific theory proposes that pain results from interactions between various impulses arriving atthe spinal cord and brain, that these impulses are brought to the spinal cord in certain non-myelinated and small myelinated fibres, and that the specific stimuli that excite these nerve fibres are noxious, or harmful.

In the somatic tissues there are certain kinds of nerve fibre that do not give rise to pain, no matter how many there are orhow frequently they are stimulated. Included in this category are mechanoreceptors that report only deformation of the skin and the larger afferent nerve fibres from muscles and tendons that form part of the organization of posture and movement. No matter how they are excited, these receptors never give rise to pain. But the smaller fibres from these tissues do cause pain when they are excited mechanically or chemically.

Warmth and cold fibres are specific. Warmth fibres are excited by rising temperature and quieted by falling temperature, and cold fibres respond similarly with cold stimuli. Although pain arises from very hot and very cold stimulation and with intense forms of mechanical stimulation,this occurs only with the activation of afferent nerve fibres that specifically report noxious events. When no noxious events are occurring, these nerve fibres are silent.

In contrast, the quantitative theory seems to apply to the viscera, where afferent nerve fibres used in reflex organizationalso report events giving rise to pain. In the heart, for example, the same nerve fibres are excited by mechanical stimulation as are excited by chemical substances formed in the body that cause pain. Also, in the bladder, rectum, and colon, nerve fibres activated by substances that cause pain are the same as those activated by distension and contraction of the viscera. This means that the same nerve fibres are reporting the state that underlies the desire to urinate or defecate and the sensation underlying the pain feltwhen these organs are strongly contracting in an attempt to evacuate their contents. In the heart, rectum, and bladder, therefore, pain appears to be due to a summation of impulses in sensory nerve fibres and is not mediated by a special groupof fibres reserved for reporting noxious events. It must be pointed out, however, that not all researchers accept the argument.

## Lower-level Pain Pathways

### *Tissues*

Not all the tissues making up the body give rise to pain; furthermore, each tissue must be stimulated in an appropriate way to invoke its particular sensation of pain. Skin, being the outer covering of the body, easily raises the warning of pain, but other tissues that do not come in direct contact with the outer environment are just the opposite. Thebrain, for example, can be pierced, cut, and burned in neurosurgery, while the patient would require only local anesthesia of the pain-sensitive scalp. The lung, liver, and spleen also do not give rise to pain, no matter how they are stimulated. Pain arises from hollow viscera when the passage of their contents is obstructed and the musculature must undergo strong contraction and stretching. Pain cannot be induced by cutting or burning the wall of the intestine, but pulling on the mesenteric tissue that fixes the intestines to the posterior wall of the abdomen causes pain. The reason for these differences is clear. Tissues are sensitive to the kinds of damage they are likely to meet during life and not to those that they probably will never meet.

Although the warning function of pain is obvious, it is not equivalent to nociception, the perception of forces likely to damage the tissues of the body. First, nociception can occur without pain and pain without nociception; also, the sensation of pain is only a part of the total act of nociception. There are reflex effects as well, such as a local reflex withdrawal from a sudden noxious stimulation of the skin. There are autonomic effects, such as a rise in blood pressure, quickening of the heart rate and respiration, and other excitatory sympathetic nervous effects. There may even be shrieking or howling, warning other animals that something dangerous and painful is occurring.

*Pathological conditions*

Acute and chronic pain differ in many ways. Acute pain occurs with sudden damage, such as stepping on a nail or biting the tongue. Chronic pain is the pain of pathological conditions—the pain that accompanies gout, arthritis, inflammation, or cancer. Each type of pain has effects on the nervous system.

The effect of acute inflammation of the joints on nerves reporting the state of the joint and on the central nervous system has been studied by inducing arthritis in animals. In this condition, locally formed chemical substances excite the small myelinated and nonmyelinated afferent fibres that report noxious events.

Most of these nerves, sensitized by the inflammatory exudate, begin to fire impulses continuously. This flow of impulses to the dorsal-horn neurons of the spinal cord increases their excitability so that many of them also begin to fire continuously. Neurons that are normally excited only by noxious stimulation now respond to light touch as well. Meanwhile, motor neurons in related areas also fire spontaneously, and stimuli that would not normally cause withdrawal reflexes now cause a prolonged reflex response. There is no change in the motor neurons themselves; the change is in the firing threshold of peripheral neurons comingfrom the inflamed area and in the interneurons between the afferent nerve fibres and the motor neurons. These interneurons are ultimately connected to the brain, so that the state of increased sensitivity is passed on to related cerebral neurons. Eventually, neurons in the cerebral hemispheres continuously and spontaneously generate impulses. Other neurons of the brain start responding to movements of the affected joints that normally would not do so.

In some people with chronic painful conditions, the constant pain impulses change the character of neurons of the thalamus and cortex. For example, one patient who had had atoothache 10 days before he had an operation on the thalamus for parkinsonism suddenly got the pain of toothache again when the thalamus was stimulated electrically. Normally, no pain can be induced by stimulating that part of the thalamus.

*Peripheral nerves*

Most of the afferent nerves making up the dorsal roots are nonmyelinated fibres. These fibres are activated by warmth within a physiological range (and by higher temperatures likely to damage the body), by chemical substances (including those made in the body), and by strong mechanical stimulation such as pricking and crushing. The smaller myelinated fibres report mechanical stimulation of the skin, noxious stimulation, and cold.

As stated above, pain is not the inevitable result of the firing of nonmyelinated fibres reporting noxious events. These fibres may fire at a slow rate without causing pain; they may even continue to fire for an hour or so without pain. Furthermore, the pain threshold does not correspond with the onset of activity in the nonmyelinated fibres, for pain can increase while the discharge of nerve impulses decreases.

*Spinal cord*

The stimulus-specific organization of the peripheral nerve fibres is not continued within the spinal cord, as the various afferent nerve fibres do not transmit their impulses exclusively to neurons of only one kind of sensibility. In the dorsal horns (the spinal region that receives afferent impulses) a few neurons are purely nociceptive, but most neurons reporting noxious events receive both noxious and mechanoreceptive input. These latter are called convergent neurons. The size of the peripheral field (the area of the body from which it receives stimuli) of a dorsal-horn neuron continually varies, depending on the state of excitability of the neuron. Furthermore, events in the peripheral field affect future responses. For example, repeated input along a group of afferent nerve fibres produces a gradually decreasing response in the central nervous system. This is called habituation. Also, the region of decreased response spreads from local neurons that received the input to neighbouring neurons.

The state of excitability of a dorsal-horn neuron depends on many variables. If it is very excitable, it will respond to impulses from many afferent peripheral nerve fibres; if it is relatively inexcitable, it will be affected only by those peripheral fibres that are habitually connected to it and located near it. A neuron excited by many afferent fibres receives input from a larger area than a neuron receiving onlyfrom the fibres most nearly related to it. For this reason the area of skin or deep tissue connected to neurons of the dorsal horn varies and changes. In experiments using damaged skin, it has been found that a barrage of nerve impulses from the damaged region increases the excitability of the dorsal-horn neurons. Once this hyperexcitable state has been set up, it continues for a time without further input from peripheral nerves. In this state of local excitability, some dorsal-horn neurons receive an input from the area of damaged skin that they would not receive were the skin in a normal state.

The convergent neurons mentioned above can have their activity inhibited by tactile stimulation of a region near their peripheral fields or of a homologous region on the opposite side of the body. Also, their responsiveness to stimuli can be increased by damage to the skin in their peripheral fields.

From these convergent neurons and from other neurons of the dorsal horns, there arise tracts of long fibres that cross the midline and lead to the thalamus and other nuclei of the brain. These constitute the spinothalamic tracts. The other main pathway of pain impulses ends in the reticular formation of the medulla oblongata and pons and is known as the spinoreticular tract. It is believed that spinoreticular inputto the brain serves the autonomic responses and emotional components associated with pain, whereas the spinothalamicserves conscious sensation, with its exact temporal and spatial aspects. Neurons around the central spinal canal that receive input from the bladder and colon and their overlying somatic tissues may be connected to an ascending tract that stays within the gray matter in the neighbourhood of the central canal.

## Higher-level Pain Pathways

*Brain*

Many regions of the brain can influence the input arriving at the lower levels of the nervous system. This so-called descending inhibition can be selective, with different regions of the brain inhibiting certain inputs to the spinal cord. Some regions reduce mechanoreceptive input, and others reduce noxious and warmth inputs. Descending inhibition can also reduce input from the skin while increasing that related to movement.

Prominent regions of influence are those that themselves receive noxious input. For instance, the lateral reticular nucleiof the medulla oblongata cause a constant inhibition of input brought to the spinal cord by the nonmyelinated fibres. In the rat (in which the discovery was first made), descending inhibition can be so effective that a noxious input does not enter the spinal cord. In other words, normally painful stimuli cause no reaction or concern, and there is no change in bloodpressure, respiration, and other reflex activities. In these circumstances it seems that pain simply is not felt.

Electrical stimulation of the nucleus ceruleus, a small nucleuswith widely ranging axons, and the nucleus raphe magnus, a nucleus in the central reticular formation of the medulla, inhibits input from noxious stimulation of the skin, and it also inhibits activities of dorsal-horn neurons receiving mechanoreceptive input. Since it was discovered that pain could be obliterated in this manner, attempts have been made to stop the chronic pain of cancer and other conditions by implanting electrodes in the brain. These can be placed in relevant parts of the brain so that constant stimulation can inhibit the input coming from the region of the pain.

This built-in system for obliterating or reducing pain can normally be brought into play by stress. Furthermore, it has always been known that one pain can mask another. A volley of nerve impulses reaching the brain via the spinothalamic and spinoreticular tracts and causing a moderate degree of pain is stopped when the cells of origin of this tract are inhibited. Experiments have shown that this suppression can be brought about by a more severe pain or by a pain in a larger area of the body, which causes descending inhibition of neurons of the spinal tract. This descending inhibition is the main mechanism of acupuncture analgesia.

The reticular formation consists of a vast number of small interconnected neurons occupying the central area of the brain stem. Parts of the reticular formation, hypothalamus, and thalamus excite the cerebral hemispheres and keep the cerebral cortex active and alert—partly in response to noxiousinput. In fact, it may be said that pain reaches consciousness in the thalamus. The thalamus receives noxious input from the spinal cord in two regions, a lateral part called the ventrobasal complex and a medial part consisting of several nuclei. The ventrobasal complex is concerned with the accurate temporal and spatial localization of conscious sensation, while the medial nuclei are concerned with the emotional, affective, and autonomic components of pain and other sensations. The ventrobasal nuclei relay impulses to thesensory areas of the postcentral gyrus. Noxious stimuli also cause responses in many areas of the cortex and the deeper islands of gray matter. This is to be expected, for, of all sensations, pain is the least pure sensation:

it startles, it excites, and it has unpleasant qualities. All these aspects of pain are added by different parts of the brain.

*Central pain*

Pain arising within the central nervous system when there is no damage to the body is known as central pain. The most common central pain is due to lesions in or near the thalamusand is called the thalamic syndrome. This condition is characterized by diminution in sensibility as well as severe pain when any stimulus exceeds a certain threshold.

With central pain there is both spontaneous pain and excessive pain on stimulation of all kinds. The pain may occur in the entire half of the body, affecting even visual and auditory inputs, or it may occur in a restricted region, such as the upper limb and side of the face or the lower limb.

*Referred pain*

The term referred pain is used to describe pain felt in a region where it does not originate but to which it is "referred." It is usually used to mean pain arising in hollow viscera and felt in somatic tissues, such as the body wall. Referred pain is alwaysreferred in one direction—from deep to superficial tissues. It ispain referred from an unknown or unfamiliar part of the body to a known or familiar part.

Certain regions of the dorsal horns of the spinal cord receive both nerve fibres from the viscera and nerve fibres reporting noxious events in the skin and musculature. For example, afferent nerve fibres from the heart come to the same regionsas those from the muscles and skin of the chest wall and upper limbs. From these two body tissues, visceral and somatic, there is an intermingling of inputs, and there is similar convergence in the thalamus. This anatomical arrangement is likely to form the basis of referred pain, although the mere convergence of impulses from viscera and soma onto the same neurons does not alone account for the false localization of visceral pain. It is probable that in sensory areas of the brain, the skin is served by a large number of neurons, the muscles with fewer, and the viscera with least, the visceral representation in the cortex being very small compared to that of the somatic tissues. It is supposed that, as the input to these sensory regions of the cortex usually comes from the skin and body wall, localization of the visceral input will be to these tissues and not to the viscera, the cortical region of which is small and relatively unused.

*Changes in the cerebral cortex*

Normally, electrical stimulation of the sensory region of the postcentral gyrus does not cause pain. But in many patients who have a painful state on the opposite side of the body, such as a painful amputation stump or damage to the mediannerve of the hand, stimulation of this region reproduces the pain. Pain also arises from stimulation of the white matter deep in this area.

In these cases the character of the sensory region of the cortex changes in such a manner that neurons that normally never cause pain when stimulated now invariably produce the pain from which the patient is suffering. Also, the cortical area subserving the limb enlarges. For instance, the sensory area receiving impulses from the opposite lower limb is normally at the upper end of the postcentral gyrus. If there is a painful amputation of the limb, then the area of cortex in which electrical stimulation induces the pain spreads downward from the normal area to include the trunk area andsometimes the upper limb area.

Anesthesia induces unconsciousness and loss of sensation prior to surgery. During surgery, the anesthesiologist monitors the patient's condition and increases or decreases the dosage of anesthesia as needed. General anesthesia, which is usually used for major surgery, produces an absence of pain and sensation in the entire body, loss of consciousness, muscle relaxation, and amnesia. These effects make complicated surgical procedures easier to perform. For instance, muscle relaxation and loss of consciousness prevent movement by the patient, helping doctors perform more accurate surgery. Surgery under general anesthesia is less traumatic for the patient because he or she remembers nothing about the procedure.

*General Anesthesia in Surgery*

Anesthetic drugs must be administered throughout the length of an operation in order to maintain the proper depth of general anesthesia. Most commonly, general anesthesia is produced with a combination of several different drugs, each used for a specific effect, such as producing sleep, pain control, or muscle relaxation. General anesthesia often begins with the injection of a sedative medication, such as midazolam. A patient may also receive medications to reduce the production of saliva, which could cause choking, and of stomach acid, which could damage the lungs if inhaled. Propofol and sodium pentothal are common sleep-inducing drugs that are administered intravenously. These drugs act rapidly but their effect does not last long, so they are often used for the early stages of anesthesia. Anesthesia is then maintained for the length of the surgical procedure with longer acting drugs. Isoforane and desflurane are sleep-inducing drugs that are inhaled. They are mixed with oxygen in an anesthesia machine, then inhaled by the patient through a facemask. Nitrous oxide, a gas that produces light anesthesia when inhaled alone, is often used in combination with other anesthetic drugs to increase their effect. Commonly used muscle relaxants include curare and vecuronium, which work by blocking impulses from nerves to muscles. These drugs paralyze muscles throughout the body, including those involved in breathing. For this reason, doctors place patients who are under general anesthesia on a breathing machine. A pain-blocking drug such as fentanyl is also injected as part of general anesthesia.

Anesthetic drugs can have various side effects, including nausea and vomiting or changes in blood pressure, breathing, and heart rate. In addition, many surgical patients already have other illnesses, such as problems with the heart, blood pressure, lungs, kidney, liver, or nervous system. These problems can make anesthetic drugs more dangerous. To detect and correct any complications that may develop, an anesthetized patient's blood pressure, heart rate and rhythm, blood oxygen concentration, breathing rate, exhaled carbon dioxide, and temperature are monitored throughout surgery. The patient is also observed for signs such as tearing, sweating, and wrinkling of facial muscles that can indicate anesthesia depth may be lightening.

Using a combination of anesthetic drugs enables doctors to use lower doses of each drug and maintain the proper depth of anesthesia while minimizing the risk of side effects. This strategy, along with better monitoring of anesthetized patients and the development of improved anesthetic drugs, has greatly improved the safety of anesthesia in recent years. In the last decade alone, the number of deaths attributed to anesthetic drugs has dropped 25-fold, to about 1 in every 250,000 general anesthesias.

Anesthesia is reversed simply by halting the administration of anesthetic drugs. Any remaining anesthetic gases in the body are gradually exhaled, and as their concentration in the body falls, consciousness returns. The muscle relaxant circulating through the body is removed by the liver and kidneys, and its effects can also be reversed with other drugs. Medications to control pain continue to be given after the operation.

Local anesthesia is commonly used for a variety of relatively minor procedures, such as dentistry, sewing up wounds in the emergency room, and operations on the toes and fingers and other superficial areas of the body. Local anesthesia is less complicated and often safer than general anesthesia because it involves fewer drugs and has less effect on blood pressure, heart rate, and breathing because there is no loss of consciousness. In dental procedures, local anesthesia is advantageous because protective reflexes such as the gag reflex, which helps prevent choking, remain intact.

Local anesthetics are most commonly administered by injecting them into the part of the body that needs to be anesthetized. They can be injected directly into the tissue being operated on, a technique known as local infiltration. Or, they can be injected near the nerves that carry pain impulses from a particular part of the body, a technique known as nerve block. Topical anesthesia is the application of a local anesthetic directly onto the surface of a mucous membrane, such as the eye or the lining of the throat or nose.

Regional anesthesia is produced by injecting a local anesthetic around the spinal area, thus anesthetizing a larger area of the body than in local anesthesia. Spinal anesthesia is a type of regional anesthesia in which the anesthetic is injected into the fluid around the spinal cord. Epidural anesthesia is a similar technique, but the anesthetic is injected into the spinal canal between the membranes that surround the spinal cord. Spinal and epidural anesthesia block sensation everywhere in the body that is lower than the site of injection. These techniques are frequently used in childbirth and in surgery on the lower half of the body, such as prostate gland removal and surgery on the hips or knees.

The earliest known local anesthetic was cocaine, but it is rarely used today because it can cause convulsions and nervousness, and it is addictive. The most commonly used local anesthetic today is lidocaine. Procaine, more commonly known by its brand name Novocain, is sometimes used as a local anesthetic, particularly in dental procedures. However, it does not last as long as lidocaine, and it is more toxic. Bupivacaine is a very long acting local anesthetic that is useful for long operations and provides a greater duration of pain relief after surgery. To help allay patients' anxiety, a sedative is often given as a part of local anesthesia.

All local anesthetics can be toxic if injected in too high a dose. Particularly when used as part of spinal or epidural anesthesia, local anesthetics may cause a dangerous fall in blood pressure. Many people experience nervousness and discomfort when local anesthetics are injected with epinephrine, a drug that constricts blood vessels to help keep the anesthetic in the area where it is needed. However, true allergic reactions to local anesthetics are very rare.

An anesthesiologist is a medical doctor specially trained to administer anesthesia (see Medicine). In the United States, an anesthesiologist must complete two or three years of residency training in an anesthesiology hospital program after finishing medical school and the required internships. An anesthetist is any person who administers an anesthetic, regardless of qualification. Nurses trained to give anesthesia under the direction of a physician or to assist an anesthesiologist are called nurse anesthetists.

In the operating room, an anesthesiologist is in charge of administering anesthetic drugs and is responsible for recognizing and treating complications that may develop during surgery, such as a heart attack or a sudden change of blood pressure. The anesthesiologist is trained to understand how anesthetics work and how they may interact with each patient's health problems and other medications they may be taking. Before surgery, the anesthesiologist makes sure patients are healthy enough to undergo surgery and answers questions from patients and their families. After surgery, the anesthesiologist monitors the patient as he or she gains consciousness and decides when the patient may be moved out of the recovery room or, in the case of outpatient surgery, sent home. Trained to deal with emergencies in the operating room, anesthesiologists are often called on to help with resuscitation in the emergency room and with care and stabilization of patients in the intensive care unit.

Acupuncture is a traditional Chinese medicine that stimulates specific points in the body in order to restore a proper balance of various chemicals. This practice is used to treat a range of conditions, including chronic pain, drug addiction, arthritis, and mental illness.Although today's anesthetic drugs are usually effective and safe, the risk of side effects and, in very rare cases, permanent organ damage or death, causes some patients concern. While scientists continue to search for better and safer anesthetic drugs, some doctors and patients have begun to investigate alternative means of inducing anesthesia.

Acupuncture, an ancient Chinese technique that involves inserting special needles at specific points on the body, is sometimes used for surgical anesthesia. The needles are rotated manually or, more often, connected to a device that sends electrical current along the needles and into the body. Acupuncture is thought to block pain by causing the release of pain-blocking endorphins and preventing pain impulses from being transmitted along the spinal cord to the brain. It can be used alone or in combination with sedatives or painkillers. Acupuncture is used as part of surgical anesthesia in most Chinese hospitals today. Scientific studies have been unable to establish how effectively acupuncture can block pain during surgery. However, the technique has been shown to reduce the nausea and vomiting that sometimes occur as a side effect of general anesthesia.

Another alternative means of inducing anesthesia is hypnosis, which can be useful for patients who cannot tolerate anesthetic drugs. However, it requires a great deal of preparation by the patient. Before surgery, a patient must go through several training sessions with a hypnotist. Only about 10 percent of people are capable of reaching a state of hypnosis deep enough for surgery to be performed. Hypnosis is also useful as an addition to anesthetic drugs. It can help allay patients' anxiety before surgery and help diminish complications such as nausea, vomiting, and pain afterwards. Hypnosis is helpful in easing the pain of childbirth and promoting healing in severely burned patients.

Early Operation with Ether American dentist William Morton pioneered the use of ether as an anesthetic in 1846. He used it first to extract a tooth and then, to remove a tumor from a patient's neck. The discovery of anesthesia removed one of the major obstacles to the progression of surgery.

Minor surgery has been performed for thousands of years, often with opium, alcohol, or Cannabis used to stupefy the patient. However, these drugs were unable to block the pain and shock of surgery to enable lengthy operations or operations involving the interior of the body.

## The Greatest Medical Discoveries of the Millennium

The medical discoveries of the past 1,000 years have saved countless lives and have doubled the life expectancy of people in many parts of the world. In this October 1999 Encarta Yearbook article, physicians Meyer Friedman and Gerald W. Friedland explore ten discoveries that fundamentally changed the way scientists and physicians were able to improve human health.

Modern anesthesia—the ability to produce a controlled, reversible state of unconsciousness, amnesia, and muscle relaxation—began in the mid-19th century. Nitrous oxide was first used as an anesthetic in 1844 by the American dentist Horace Wells. In 1846 American dentist William Morton used ether to produce general anesthesia for surgery. Crawford Long, an American surgeon, had been using ether since 1842, but he did not publish his results until 1849. British physician Sir James Simpson first discovered the anesthetic properties of chloroform in 1847. Chloroform anesthesia became more popular after another British physician, John Snow, administered it to Queen Victoria of England for childbirth in 1853.

Anesthesiology became an established branch of medicine in the United States during the early 20th century. The American Society of Anesthesiologists, which sets standards of safety and ethics for anesthesiologists, was founded in 1905. The Board of Anesthesiology, which maintains educational standards, was established in 1938. Anesthetic drugs were also improved throughout the 20th century. The first intravenous anesthetic, sodium pentothal, was introduced in 1932 by American physician John Lundy. The muscle relaxant curare, originally used in hunting by Native American tribes in South America, was first used in surgery in 1942. Better inhalation anesthetics were also developed to replace ether, which is flammable, and chloroform, which is toxic.

The history, mechanisms, and clinical applications of acupuncture in the anesthesia setting are addressed herein. Special emphasis is placed on the role of acupuncture in pre-operative preparation of certain types of patients, intra-operative application of acupuncture-assisted anesthesia, and post-operative management of surgical and anesthesia complications. Advantages of acupuncture analgesia and other symptomatic control, functional maintenance and restoration, reduced mortality, and acceleration of discharge are further explored.

The clinical efficacy of acupuncture has been reviewed elsewhere. The scientific merits and physiological phenomena achieved through acupuncture have been demonstrated through the use of various types of advanced technologies,1-5 including myoneural electrophysiology studies, radioactive tracer survey and imaging, and single-photon emission computed tomography. Other research, including thermographic studies and studies of kinesiology phenomena, have demonstrated clinical and physiological responses to acupuncture, although the findings remain controversial.

The growing acceptance of acupuncture is undeniable as seemingly greater numbers of physicians begin to take interest. The National Institutes of Health currently endorses the application of medical acupuncture in many areas. Since February 1996, the Food and Drug Administration has classified acupuncture devices as general medical, rather than investigational, devices.

The primary goal of using acupuncture pre-operatively is to complement and enhance the medical preparation rather than to replace it. Acupuncture preparation of a patient for surgery does not replace a sound medical evaluation and diagnostic testing whenever indicated. Assessments should be made of the potential surgical structures, co-existing anatomical and physiological abnormalities, general physical condition, and the patient's psychological and socioeconomic status. Energetic and meridian conditions must also be addressed. Normalization or optimization allows the patient to safely undergo surgery and recover uneventfully.

During this phase of acupuncture application, the principles used are primarily meridian regulations, optimization of physiological function, and enhancement of endogenous opioid activities for the immediate pre-operative period.

Korean Hand Acupuncture, Auricular Acupuncture, and a short form of either Traditional Chinese Medicine (TCM) or French Energetic Acupuncture are the most applicable techniques during the pre-operative period. Two of the most commonly applied examples are:

*Cardiac Patients*

**Korean Hand Therapy (KHT):** 12 Shu Mu, Pericardium, KA 18, and KI 11 Shu Mu, Heart, KA 16, and KI 12

**Auricular Acupuncture:** Heart and Kidney points3,29

**Distinct Meridian:** BL 1, SI 10, and HT 1 (K, HT points could be an alternative approach)1,12

TCM pattern diagnosis and prescriptions2,3*

**French Energetics:** Shao Yin and Tai Yang regulation, or Distinct Meridians1*

Japanese Meridian Therapy30*

*Constitutional balance

*Pulmonary Patients*

KHT12

**Auricular Acupuncture:** Lung1, 2, Asthma1, 23,29

**Distinct Meridian:** LI 15, LU 1, LI 18, KHT corresponding points. KD 11, KC 1, KD 19

TCM 2,3*

French Energetics1*

Japanese Meridian Therapy30*

***Note:** Items with an asterisk should be applied only by physicians well-trained in those areas.

Recommendations for the pre-operative acupuncture preparation of patients are primarily safety, simplicity, short-term improvement oriented, and minimal duration. Acupuncture is to be used particularly for cardiac and pulmonary patients who are receiving maximally-tolerated medical treatments and still remain dyspneic, having chest pain, etc. For other symptoms associated with the surgical target, i.e., pain and nausea/emesis, acupuncture should be used only if necessary.

Other co-existing diseases (diabetes mellitus, for instance) appear to be minimally indicated in acupuncture pre-operative preparation. The patient's blood glucose level usually can be controlled satisfactorily within hours with a computerized insulin pump. Use of acupuncture in this type of case appears redundant and unnecessary.

In other medical conditions including seizure disorder, coagulation disorder, or blood loss, acupuncture should not be used to replace medical treatment; there appears to be little value in the enhanced medical effect of acupuncture within the short pre-operative period in these areas.

## Intra-Operataive Preparation with Acupuncture

*Principles of Acupuncture Surgical Analgesics*

Acupuncture does not produce a true anesthesia in any form; it does, however, have a profound analgesic effect and produces sedation.2,8,13-18

## Enhancement of Endogenous Opioid Activities

Numerous studies have demonstrated acupuncture stimulation and induced enhancement of various types of neurotransmitter activities in the central nervous system.2,3,5,8,13,19,20 b-Endorphin activity in the peri-aqueduct increases by 2 to 21/2 times the baseline level; the duration can be up to several hours at times. Other neurotransmitter activities, including serotonin and norepinephrine, have also been demonstrated. Findings indicate that norepinephrine may play some role in the management of acute pain, while serotonin appears to be more important in the control of chronic pain.

To initiate the endogenous opioid activation effect, points LI 4 for surgical procedures above the clavicle, LI 11 for surgical procedures below the clavicle and above the diaphragm, and LR 3 for procedures on the lower extremities must be selected. These points can sometimes be used in combination to produce an enhanced effect.

Studies reporting a failure to produce this endogenous opioid activation effect have been shown. However, in reviewing those studies, it appears that the endorphin-related points as described above were not used. In other cases, the points have been stimulated at too high a frequency. According to Stux and Pomeranz,2 the opioid-related stimulation was mediated through the low-frequency stimulation of A-beta fibers. Therefore, the actual needling and the application of electro stimulation should not produce a sharp pain. This stimulation should be applied approximately 20 to 30 minutes immediately prior to surgery to produce the desired level of effectiveness. It has also been suggested that a similar acupuncture application within 24 hours prior to surgery, and then again within 20 minutes prior to surgery, may produce an enhanced effect.

## The Nervous System

The application of acupuncture in the proper combinations can induce a series of changes along the ascending pain pathway and the descending inhibitory system.1,2,9,14-16,21 In this manner, the most significant areas affected seem to involve spinal cord interneuron activation. The activation of these neurons prevents the "wind up" mechanism of intensified pain. Also, the acupuncture activation of Raphe Magnum Nucleus and stimulation of the hypothalamus seem to attenuate acute pain perception.

Interruption of peripheral nerve (a-delta conduction) is perhaps not a true acupuncture effect. There are several devices available that are able to completely block out the pain from incision. They involve the use of electrical stimulation at a high frequency (200-300 Hz) at the incision site or along the major nerve trunk innervating the incision site. Other alternatives include an electrical stimulator connected to needles along the nerve trunk, or 2 long electrodes that are placed either transcutaneously or percutaneously along both sides of the incision. This type of high-frequency stimulation (>400 Hz) can produce analgesia in less than 5 minutes.

## Point Selection

*LI 4*

Contralateral or bilateral, used for surgeries above the clavicle, and sometimes used in chest surgeries (Chinese). Initiates uterine contraction; contraindicated in pregnancy unless the induction of labor is desired.

*Indications:* Relieves pain in the head and otolaryngological conditions, fever, URI, trismus, and urticaria; induces uterine contraction.

*MH 6*

"Luo Point" of Principle Meridian, "Master Point" of Yin Wei Mo, and "coupled point" of Chong Mo.

*Indications:* Mental symptoms of excess Fire, cardiac arrhythmia and angina pectoris, nausea and vomiting, hiccups, and gastrointestinal "fire."

*TH 6*

Zhigon is the "branch ditch," Fire point, and Luo point.

*Indications:* Shoulder and arm pain, chest wall pain, post-thoracotomy, intercostal neuralgia, sore throat, and constipation.

*TH 5*

Waiguan is the "outer gate," Luo Point, Master Point of Yang Wei, and coupled point of Dai Mo.

*Indications:* High fever, chest and neck inflammatory conditions, tinnitus, migraines, enuresis, central nervous system diseases, and upper extremity joint pain.

*LR 3*

Ta Chong is the "great pouring," Shu/Wood point, and source point.

*Indications:* Headaches, vertigo, hypertension, insomnia, hepatitis, mastitis, thrombocytopenia, irregular menstruation, chest wall pain, and urinary retention.

*ST 36*

Zusanli is "three measures on the leg," he/earth point, and special command point for stomach (strengthening).

*Indications:* Gastroenteritis, pancreatitis, digestive disorder, shock, weakness, fatigue, allergies, constipation or diarrhea, lower abdominal distention, breast diseases, and nausea/vomiting.

*SP 6*

Sanyingjiao is "three yin junction."

*Indications:* Abdominal distention, borborygmus, diarrhea, gynecological disorders, urinary retention and incontinence, sexual dysfunction, eczema, and urticaria.

Ear Points (Pain Control-Related)3,29

*Master Point 1*

Shen Men. Divine Gate. Wonder point.

*Master Point 2*

Sympathetic.

*Master Point 3*

Thalamus. Subcortical. Pain control point.

*Master Point 7*

Tranquilizer point. Relaxation point.

Anatomical corresponding points.

Lung Point: Skin incision.

KHT (Hand Points)12

Corresponding points.

Basic prescriptions. Upper Heater/Jiao. Middle Heater/Jiao. Lower Heater/Jiao.

Shu Mu points for internal organ surgeries.

Basic Principles Of Electrical Stimulation To Acupoints (Intra-operative And Immediately Pre-Operative)1,2,6,8,9,14,20,22

*Meridian (Body) Points*

Low frequency direct current 2-4 Hz.

Ipsilateral or bilateral.

LI 4 or 11; contralateral.

Moderate output, starting 20 minutes pre-operatively.

*Auricular Points*

Low frequency 2-4 Hz, may induce electro-coagulation in 15 minutes, and difficulty in removing the needle. Also may attenuate effects with time.

Starting at 5 minutes pre-operatively.

Local Point/Area Stimulation Adjacent To Surgical Site

High frequency 400-1000 Hz.

Graded increase in output intensity according to adaptation.

10-15 minutes immediately pre-incision, and removal immediately prior to incision/scrubbing.

*KHT12*

E-beam stimulation after incision to supplement pain control and symptomatic treatments.

Point Combinations in Surgical Analgesia

Skin Incision

*LI 4, LI 11.*

*Auricular Therapy:* Lung point, Shen Men.

20-30 minutes of electrical stimulation at 2-4 Hz.

Oral, Facial

*LI 4, ST 44, MH 6.*

*Auricular Therapy:* Tranquilizer, Thalamus, and corresponding points.

Chest Wall Procedures

*LI 11, TH 5 or 6, ST 41 or 44.*

*Auricular Therapy:* Tranquilizer, Thalamus, corresponding points.

Intrathoracic Procedures

*LI 11, TH 6, MH 6, CV 17, GV 14.*

*Auricular Therapy:* Sympathetic, Heart, Lung.

Upper Abdominal Procedures

*LI 11, ST 36, SP 6, MH 6.*

*Auricular Therapy:* Sympathetic, Stomach, Heart, corresponding points.

Pelvic Procedures

*LI 11, ST 36, SP 10, MH 6, Dai Mo.*

*Auricular Therapy:* Pelvis, Sympathetic, corresponding points.

Genital-Rectal Procedures

*LU 6, SI 7, SP 6, LR 1, KI 6.*

*Auricular Therapy:* Sympathetic, Heart, Shen Men.

Upper Extremities

*LI 4, TH 5, MH 6, GB 21, and GB 34.*

*Auricular Therapy:* KI, LU, SP, corresponding points.

Lower Extremities

*LI 11, ST 36, GB 34, KI 3, LR 3.*

*Auricular Therapy:* KI, LU, SP

Obstetrical

Hyperemesis gravida26

*MH 6, ST 36, 40, LR 3.*

*Auricular Therapy:* LR, ST Sympathetic (Shen Men).

KHT: KA 8, 12, 16, 18, KK 9, KF 5

Conversion of breech position of fetus

- Moxibustion BL 67

- KHT: KA 1, 3, 5, 6, 8, KI 19, KT 23, KF 5

Induction of labor (or abortion)

- LI 4, SP 6

Labor (not as effective and convenient as epidural anesthesia)27

- BI 23, 26, 30, 33, SP 6, LI 4, MH 6, Chong Mo, Dai

*Other Systems Used Intra-Operatively:*

Nasal, facial, scalp, and "Barefoot Doctor's Anesthesia Points."

In the intra-operative application of acupuncture, body point needles should be removed if they interfere with the surgical site (likewise, auricular points in facial surgeries). Electrical stimulation is to be used only at points accessible to the anesthesiologist. Additional points may be added through microsystems (e.g., hand, scalp, and auricular points). The number of needles should be kept to a minimum. Continuous electrical stimulation (especially at a high frequency and/or long duration) should be avoided.

**Post-Operative Preparation with Acupuncture**

Acupuncture may be used to enhance and supplement symptomatic medical treatments and to restore physiological functions.1,2,6-8,10-12,22,28 It is not necessary to use acupuncture to completely supplant the use of medications. However, the supplementary use of post-operative acupuncture can decrease the amount of opioids and/or other symptomatic control medications needed to relieve post-operative pain, thus facilitating early ambulation, fluid and food intake, and hospital discharge. Moreover, in situations in which medications are not applicable or effective, acupuncture can be helpful.

**Acute Pain Management**

Basic principles are the same as intra-operative point combinations, but points closer to the surgical site can be used with proper aseptic techniques.

*KHT (hand acupuncture) system.*

Curious Meridians (very effective in acute conditions).

Nausea/Vomiting Control29

*MH 6, ST 36, LR 3.*

*Auricular Therapy:* Sympathetic, Stomach.

*KHT: KA 8, 12.*

Post-Extubation Spasm of the Larynx

*MH 6, KI 3.*

*Auricular Therapy:* Lung points.

*KHT: KE 8, KA 20, 24, KM 5.*

Urinary Retention

Deep-drainage K-UB (Distinct Meridian).

*SP 9, LR 8.*

Chong Mo.

*Auricular Therapy:* Sympathetic corresponding points.

Paralytic Ileus

*LI 11, ST 25, 36, SP 4.*

*Auricular Therapy:* LI, SI (constipation points).

*KHT: KI 19, KE 22.*

Hiccups

*MH 6.*

*Auricular Therapy:* Diaphragm. Stomach. Tranquilizer.

*KHT: KK 9, KB 20, KM 10.*

## Conclusion

The use of acupuncture to complement medications has many advantages in pre-operative preparation of patients with co-existing diseases. This is especially evident in patients with chronic cardiopulmonary diseases. Pre-operatively, acupuncture treatments can alleviate chronic symptoms and enhance responses to medications within a short period. This effect frequently carries through the intra-operative and post-operative periods to facilitate recovery and early hospital discharge.

During the immediate pre-operative period, application of acupuncture should be simplified: no more than 1 to 4 body points and/or up to 4 auricular points are used; the duration of stimulation is reduced to 20 minutes.

Intra-operatively, acupuncture-assisted anesthesia is recommended to bypass the disadvantages of incomplete blockage of pain by the use of acupuncture alone. Moreover, acupuncture enhances the results of regional and local anesthesia, and allows for a reduction in the dose of intravenous opioids and sedatives or the total dose of general anesthetics needed. Further titration and definition of the impact of acupuncture to general anesthesia can be assessed with the aid of moderate anesthesia depth-monitoring devices currently available.

Post-operatively, the treatment of symptoms can be achieved effectively with proper use of acupuncture in conjunction with medications. The supplementary use of post-operative acupuncture can decrease the need for opioid and/or other symptomatic control medications and thus facilitate early ambulation, fluid and food intake, and discharge.

Acupuncture anesthesia is successfully used in tonsillectomy, subtotal or total thyroidectomy, hernia treatment, extraction of teeth, scissorian section, surgical treatment of ovary or uterus, ligation of haemorrhoids, repair of stomach wall etc.etc. and even in brain tumour operation.

# *Chapter Eleven*

# Laser Acupuncture

It is also called acu-laser or laser therapy, laser ray is beamed on the acupuncture points, this technique has acclaimed much popularity due to it's easily assecible faster, painless and effective properties.

The theory of laser was first discussed by Prof.Albert Einstein in1917. A laser is a beam of monochromatic, coherent, monophasic, light energy. Laser is the short form of Light Amplification by Stimulated Emission of Radiation. In late 1950's Schawlow and Townes demonstrated an optical laser. In 1963 Theodore Kaiman invented the first laser based on gemstone 'ruby', thereafter, lasers based on liquids and gases are introduced.

Helium-Neon lasers are commonly used in laser therapy.

It may be used on the local, distal and the ah-shi points as well as on the dangerous points as well as tender, hyper-sensitive parts rich in nerve and blood supply such as the eyes, face, neck and ear(auriculotherapy) and even on a cracked skin.

The intensity of the laser beam is very low, hence there is no chance of any mishap. The commonly used apparatus has two functions first to detect location of a point using the phenomenon of higher electrical conductivity of the skin at the acupuncture points and an adjacent acoustical device that give signal when the electrode touches a specific point and generates the laser beam through the same electrode.

Although laser acupuncture has been researched and practiced quite extensively in China, Russia, Spain and Germany for over 30 years, the procedure is almost unheard of in the U.S. Combining the low-level laser biostimulation effects, a well-known photobiological phenomenon, and acupuncture points, the procedure has been proven to be both effective and practical. The procedure is non-invasive, produces no pain, and no heat, and it is environmentally clean, and best suitable in pediatric, geriatric care and needle-phobic adults. Laser acupuncture is not intended to replace needle acupuncture, but rather to add to our acupuncture modalities and broaden the effectiveness of acupuncture.

Since laser was first invented in 1960, it has slowly found acceptance in the Western medical community, particularly in dermatology applications such as removal of dark spots, tattoos, and acne scars. Recent technological advances in laser devices have prompted even wider applications in cosmetic procedures, dental treatments, and eye surgery. While most of these applications require high laser power, lower level laser power was first investigated in the early '70s in the applications of "biostimulation" and later suggested to replace traditional metal acupuncture needle with the "light needle".

Beginning in 1973, extensive clinical laser acupuncture was conducted and results were published in China. In the United States one of the most notable laser acupuncture researchers is Dr. Margaret Naeser, Ph.D., Lic.Ac., Dipl.Ac., a research professor of Neurology, Boston University School of Medicine, and a licensed acupuncturist in Massachusetts, who has been doing research since 1984 and has published a textbook and many papers on the related topics.

Laser should be no stranger to anyone in this modern life. It is in the heart of entertainment devices such as CD players, computer's CD-ROM drives, and the latest DVD players. The laser used in these consumer gadgets has power output no higher than about 100 milliwatts (mW). One milliwatt is one-thousandth of a watt, and one watt is expressed as a unit of work energy, or joule, per second. In general, laser acupuncture uses laser power between 5 to 500 mW (Class IIIb lasers). For comparison, the cutting lasers used in surgery are often greater than 100 Watts.

Another important parameter of laser is wavelength. Like radio waves, light travels in a pattern of waves that has peaks and valleys. The distance between the peaks or valleys is called wavelength and is usually measured in nanometers (nm). One nanometer is one-billionth of a meter and a meter is 39.37 inches.

For example, visible light such as violet, green, and red are between 400 nm and 700 nm. The light spectrum just below 400 nm is ultraviolet and beyond 700 nm, infrared. Unlike room ambient light, which scatters and contains many different wavelengths, laser light is coherent, or concentrated, and emits one single frequency. In other words, coherent (laser) light travels in a repetitive wave pattern that carries one specific wavelength. In order for laser acupuncture to be therapeutic, the useable wavelengths must be in the range of 600 to 1000 nm. Otherwise, the hemoglobin or water may block the laser beam and desirable energy penetration cannot be achieved.

Although laser acupuncture has been investigated since the late 1960s, the cumbersome, bulky and expensive helium neon gas tube laser apparatus in these earlier days had prevented more extensive clinical use. No applications of laser acupuncture procedure would be commercially viable without a novel laser source, e.g., a semiconductor laser diode. In the early 1990s, this author (SL) had worked with 30 mW, 780 nm (infrared) laser diodes, two-tenths of an inch in diameter, with a cost back then of less than $100 (in volume quantities). A variation of this laser diode (5 mW, 670 nm) is now found in inexpensive laser lecture pointers. In her laser acupuncture textbook, Dr. Naeser has listed some treatment protocols for hand and foot laser acupuncture using a laser pointer and a microamp TENS device.

With red-beam laser, there is only a shallow penetration suitable for treating points such as Jing-Well points at the ends of the fingers and toes. Infrared lasers (e.g., 780 or 904 nm, for example), on the other hand, have up to 1 - 1.5 inches of penetration and are best used on arm or leg points, back shu and ahshi points. When a 5 to 20 mW laser beam is shown onto the skin, it produces no feeling - no heat, no cold, and no pain. The only possible risk is that the laser will harm the retina if one stares directly into the source of the laser beam.

Lastly, the treatment time, or light exposure time, is a function of the power and type of ailment. In general, the higher the power, the lower the treatment time; more exposure time is needed on joint pain than for soft tissue pain; and with chronic conditions than for acute. Often this parameter is expressed in terms of energy density (joules/cm2), as dosage. Protocols can be established and repeated to treat a particular disorder, with appropriate modifications on a case by case basis, often per TCM indications for point selection, etc. As stated above, one watt (W) is one joule per second. In order to determine the amount of seconds necessary to emit one joule/cm2 from a given laser, you must know the following laser parameters: the mW output converted to Watts, and aperture size, in cm2, of the laser probe you are going to use to stimulate the acupuncture point. The following formula is used to calculate the necessary time to produce 1 joule/ cm2:

With a 5 mW Laser (0.005 Watts), with a 0.5 cm diameter aperture on the probe tip, the Beam Spot Size is 0.196 cm2. The necessary time to emit 1 Joule per cm2 (Energy Density) is computed as follows:

**Formula:** (Average Output Power in Watts x Seconds) / Beam Area in cm2 = 1 Joule per cm2

(0.005 Watts) x (X Seconds) / 0.196 cm2 = 1 Joule per cm2

0.005 X = 0.196

X = 0.196 / 0.005

X = 39.2 Seconds

Thus, 39.2 Seconds of exposure time is required to emit 1 Joule per cm2 with the 5mW laser, with a 0.5 cm diameter aperture on the probe tip (Beam Spot Size of 0.196 cm2).

Acupuncture points are often treated with 4 to 8 joules per cm2, or about 2.5 to 5 minutes exposure time if using the laser probe in the example given above, especially to obtain an anti-inflammatory effect when treating chronic pain.

**Photo-biostimulation**

The idea of biological changes from the stimulation, or biostimulation, of light is actually nothing new. This so-called photo-biostimulation is how vitamin D is produced in our bodies when ultraviolet rays in the sunlight strike the skin. It has been suggested that the laser biostimulation is also of a photobiological nature. The exact mechanism of the biological and physical effects of low level laser radiation is still unknown. Much like the acupuncture development in ancient China, much of the laser acupuncture research work reported to date is empirical observation. However, two Finnish physiologists, Dr. Reijo Makela and Dr. Anu Makela, in their 1999 paper pointed out that the "trigger" function of laser light of specific wavelengths can cause biochemical, electrochemical, and structural changes at the cellular level which may in turn alter the outcome of diseases.

For example, at wavelengths of 628-652 nm, as Drs. Makela point out, phenyl pyruvate is turned into phenyllalanine, which is a naturally occurring amino acid from which tyrosine is formed. Tyrosine in turn is the precursor of dopa, dopamine, norepinephrine, epinephrine, and thyroid hormones. The increase of dopamine relieves a variety of symptoms of a well known dopamine-deficiency illness- Parkinson's Disease. Together the two Finnish doctors have treated over 12,000 patients with laser based acupuncture over about fourteen years.

In China, laser acupuncture has been applied clinically to help treat over 200 diseases in the last 30 years. In a paper published in 1999, in The Journal of Alternative and Complementary Medicine, Branco & Naeser observed success in treating pain in 33 of 36 hands (91.6%) with carpal tunnel syndrome, including 14 hands where surgery had failed to provide pain relief. While laser acupuncture can help treat many treatable ailments already treated with needle acupuncture, the advantages of laser acupuncture over needle acupuncture are several:

The laser is totally non-invasive; it produces no pain and there is no possibility for infection when used properly. It is also often used successfully in the treatment of chronic wounds that have not healed.

The laser is suitable for children, frail elderly, and needle-phobic adults. For example, the British Journal of Anesthesia recently published a controlled study from he University of Vienna, Austria, where a double-blind, randomized, placebo-controlled study with 40 children, ages 3 - 12 years, undergoing strabismus surgery, found the incidence of post-operative vomiting to be significantly lower (25%), than the placebo group (85%), following red-beam, 670 nm, 10 mW, laser irradiation of P 6, at 15 minutes before induction of anesthesia and 15 minutes after arriving in the recovery room.

In another study with cerebral palsy (CP) children and adults, from Japan, the low-level laser therapy was observed to reduce the spasticity. For example, Asagai et al., (1994), used low-level laser therapy on acupuncture points to treat spasticity in 150 cases of CP (ages 10 months to 20 years). Two semiconductor laser diodes [60mW or 100mW, continuous wave, 810 nm wavelength (near infrared)] were used for 15 to 30 seconds per point. Improvement was reported in the majority of the 150 babies and children; exceptions were those with severe joint contracture. In addition, in 42 cases whose hands were normally involuntarily clenched, 34 cases (81%) were able to open their hands with less effort. The authors quote Kamikawa et al. (1982) who hypothesize that low-level laser therapy (LLLT) may cause vascular dilatation through the sympathetic nervous system, and reduce tonic muscle spasms in muscles which had been in a hypoxemic state. The authors concluded:"..Compared with conventional methodology, laser therapy has proved to be a simple, reliable and noninvasive method which enabled painless suppression of spasm ... The effect of LLLT lasted from one to several hours in patients with severe spasticity ... the authors feel that LLLT is particularly useful as a supplementary or adjunctive therapeutic modality to improve the overall efficacy of physical rehabilitation and functional training in children with cerebral palsy."

The laser is more cost effective in the long run and environmentally friendly since needles must continue to be disposed of and purchased, while the laser apparatus can be reused over and over again.

There are only a few contraindications with low-level lasers:

Do not shine the laser beam directly into the eye, it would harm the retina.

Do not shine the laser on the unclosed fontanelles of babies, it may promote bone growth there, before the skull should be closed.

Just as with needle acupuncture, do not use the laser on standard "forbidden" acupuncture points with pregnant women. It is helpful, however, to use a 5 mW, continuous wave, red-beam laser on acupuncture point UB 67, five minutes per day toward the end of pregnancy, to help revert a fetus that is in the breech position. This was successful, for example, in 85% of 615 cases treated at the Shanghai Medical University (the control group had a 65.7% spontaneous conversion rate). The use of the red-beam laser on UB 67 is easier than moxibustion.

Just as with needle acupuncture, do not use the laser directly on a cancerous tumor. Red-beam laser, however, may be used on P 6 to help stop nausea and vomiting, as mentioned above, in the study with children undergoing surgery.

Because of the ease of use of the laser acupuncture, acupuncturists around the world increasingly add it to their scope of practice. The low-level laser devices are regulated in the U.S., however, regarding their medical application. In the U.S., the Food and Drug Administration (FDA) Center for Devices and Radiological Health (CDRH) has the responsibility for implementing and enforcing the laws and regulations which apply to radiation-producing electronic products and medical devices.

## US Federal Drug Administration and Regulation

In its June, 1999 update of Laser Facts CDRH stated that no biostimulation laser therapy devices have been approved by the FDA for humans. Therefore, it is illegal to make any claims of clinical effectiveness despite positive research data from US and elsewhere in the world. Why? The FDA still considers low-energy lasers (classified as Class IIIb: 5 to 500 mW) to be "Investigational" at the time this article is written. As a reminder, acupuncture needles were only dropped from the "Investigational" list by the FDA about 5 years ago. However, at the time when the FDA made this new ruling, it was estimated that over 12 million Americans had already turned to acupuncture for treatment.

Because of the "Investigational" nature, some FDA guidelines need to be observed if low-level lasers are to be used by a licensed acupuncturist in this country. Among the rather lengthy guidelines, the most important issue is that the acupuncturist must first obtain Institutional Review Board (IRB) approval regarding two areas: 1) The exact type of laser the licensed acupuncturist will be using (e.g., power, wavelength). 2) The exact manner in which the licensed acupuncturist proposes to use this laser to treat which conditions (e.g., energy density or dosage from the laser to be used on specific acupuncture points, disease conditions, etc.).

An independent IRB can be set up to consist of at least five members, who meet at regular intervals to review applications from acupuncturists who wish to obtain approval for the use of low-level laser acupuncture. In addition, an IRB-approved patient Informed Consent Form is required in the private practice acupuncture office. With these guidelines in mind, one can understand why laser acupuncture, which is rather common in countries like China, Spain, Germany, Russia, Austria, Czech Republic, and Hungary, lags in clinical use, and is mostly unknown within the acupuncture profession in the U.S. However, the FDA's stand on the LLLT might be changing.

In dialogue with the FDA over the years, it has recently been "suggested" to some LLLT practitioners that if low-level lasers are permitted within the defined scope of the practice of medicine, as defined by a given State, that it is permissible to use the low-level lasers without an IRB approval and the Consent Form may not be required. At the time this article is written, this verbal understanding has not been put into writing by the FDA. Thus, legally, it would appear that the original "Investigational Use" label for Class IIIb lasers may still be in effect with the requirements of IRB approval and Informed Consent.

A key issue in this possibly new FDA policy, regarding potentially less restrictive use of low-level lasers in the U.S., is the necessary inclusion of low-level laser therapy into the scope of medical practice (e.g., scope of acupuncture practice) as defined by each State. In the 1993 scope of acupuncture practice guidelines in Massachusetts (Dr. Naeser's home State), the State of Massachusetts included laser acupuncture within the scope of acupuncture practice. Other states like Arkansas, Florida, Wisconsin, and New Mexico also have such inclusion. In

California, despite having the majority of the U.S. acupuncturist population, in July, 2000, Governor Davis vetoed a bill in which the laser acupuncture was supposed to be included within our scope of practice. The bill, SB 466, after passing the Assembly and Senate with only one opposing vote, was vetoed by Governor Davis as soon as it reached his desk because of his concerns with low-level lasers. Through this article and future education of acupuncturists regarding the use of low-level laser in the profession, it is the author's wish that when a similar bill is introduced next year, California acupuncturists will have a clearer common goal as to why low-level laser is important to the practice of Traditional Chinese Medicine (TCM) as a whole.

As we are stepping into the new Millennium, to an ever-changing technological world, the area of TCM has amazingly endured and flourished from many previous millennia. Laser acupuncture, instead of being seen as an unfit, high-tech gadget within the realm of an ancient medical system, should be gracefully absorbed into this enduring system as another effective and elegant modality, which is part of other TCM modalities. Laser acupuncture therapy is safe and easy to apply, carries no pain or side-effects, has zero potential for infection, is not invasive, and is environmentally clean. Only through collaborative efforts (and governmental understanding) more comprehensive treatment protocols may be developed.

## *Chapter Twelve*

# Auriculotherapy

Auriculotherapy is a therapeutic intervention in which the auricle of the external ear is utilized to alleviate pain, dysfunction and disease as represented and manifest throughout the body.

The auricle of the ear is a complete Microsystem of the human body. All vertebra, sympathetic/parasympathetic nerves, spinal nerves, visceral organs and the central nervous system, and including all anatomical sites and many functional points are represented on the ear. They total over 200 specific acupuncture points.

Ear acupuncture has been developed largely outside China. It is quite clear that there are some ancient Chinese manuscripts that mention the use of the external ear for acupuncture, but classical Chinese acupuncture applies to the body rather than the ear. The detailed ear map that is now being used by most acupuncturists was developed by Dr. Paul Nogier in France in the early 1950's.

Ear acupuncture was known to the ancient Egyptians. Ear cauteries have been found in the pyramids; these were used for burning or scarring specific ear points for conditions like sciatica. Hippocrates also mentioned that the external ear could be used to treat conditions such as impotence

In 1637 a Portuguese doctor, Zactus Lusitanus, described the use of auricular cautery for sciatica, and in 1717 Valsalva demonstrated the use of ear acupuncture for toothache. These early European and Middle Eastern experiments with ear acupuncture are a completely separate discovery; they have nothing to do with the growth and development of acupuncture in China. Sciatica seems to have been a disease that was particularly amenable to this crude form of acupuncture, and studies in the mid-nineteenth century indicate that 56 per cent of people who were treated with ear cautery for sciatica, obtained relief from their symptoms.

It was this crude form of acupuncture that interested Dr. Nogier in the early 1950's. Some of his patients had received ear cautery and obtained relief from pain, and therefore Dr. Nogier began to develop and investigate this form of treatment. He soon produced an ear map and since the early 1950's he has refined and developed this technique. One of his earliest findings was that if there was pain in the body then the equivalent part of the ear also became painful.

If the hand is painful then the part of the ear representing the hand also becomes painful when slight pressure is applied to the relevant part of the ear. If the painful ear point is punctured with a needle then the hand pain will be relieved. According to folklore the pirates used to wear a gold ear ring through his ear lobe ,the gold ring is supposed to increase the visual ability of the pirate, so that he can see ships to plunder before he is seen by them! Strangely enough, the ear ring usually seems to be placed in the eye point on the ear lobe.

All systems of acupuncture began originally in China with the Yellow Emperors Classic of Internal Medicine compiled in 500 B.C. In this text, the six yang meridians were B.C. connected to the auricle of the ear. Whereas the six yin meridians were indirectly connected to the ear by its corresponding yang meridian. These ancient Chinese ear acupuncture points were scattered over the auricle of the ear. Ancient Egypt, Greece, and Rome between 500 B.C. and 100 A.D.. had recorded clinical uses of earring's and other forms of ear stimulation for various problems particularly in the treatment of sexual and menstrual disorders which Hypocrite's and Galen recorded. After the fall of Rome approximately 200 A.D.. ancient medical records were found in Persia where the medical treatment for sciatic pain was cauterization on the ear.

From 1500-1700 the Dutch East Indian Company, while merchant trading in China brought many Chinese acupuncture procedures back to Europe including the use of ear acupuncture.

It was the Dutch East Indian Company that saw acupuncture being used in the orient where medicine was placed next to the needle site and they then developed the Western hypodermic needle from Chinese acupuncture needles. Sporadic clinical reports in Europe were discussed with the use of ear cauterization to relieve sciatic pain.

Then in 1957, Dr. Paul Nogier, a physician from Lyon, France observed the occurrence of scars on the ears of a patient who were successfully treated for sciatic pain by French lay practitioners. Dr. Nogier then developed a somatatopic map of the ear based upon the inverted fetus concept. His work was first presented in France and then published by a German acupuncture society and then finally translated into Chinese. In 1958, a massive study was initialed by Nanking Army Ear acupuncture research team which verified the clinical accuracy of Dr. Nogier's inverted man concept of the little man on the ear. During the cultural revolution, the "barefoot doctors" were taught the easy techniques of ear acupuncture to bring healthcare to the Chinese masses.

In 1980, a double blind experimentally controlled research study at UCLA Pain Management Center department of anesthesiology UCLA School of Medicine conducted a research study by Richard J. Kroeuning M.D., Ph.D and Terry D. Oleson Ph.D. This study reported in PAIN verified the scientific accuracy of auricular diagnosis. There is a statistically significant level of 75% accuracy achieved in diagnosing musculoskeletal pain problems in 40 pain patients. Specific areas of height and tenderness and increased electrical activity on the ear predicted specific areas of the body where some pain or dysfunction would be identified whereas the body free of pathology corresponded to non-active points on the ear.

Research that followed throughout the United States utilized both the Chinese and the French Auricular acupuncture points for the treatment of chronic pain problems and the withdrawal from narcotic, alcohol and nicotine. International meetings of the World National Organization in 1990 culminated in a standardization of names of auricular anatomy in location of ear reflex points.

## Body And Ear

Both ear and body acupuncture take their origins from China. However body acupuncture has remained essentially unchanged whereas ear acupuncture has been greatly modified by the discoveries of Dr. Paul Nogier and further research is continuing to yield never developments in auricular diagnosis and treatment.

Body acupuncture is based upon a system of 12 meridians, 6 yin and 6 yang meridians. The ear is a self contained microsystem that affects the whole body.

Acupuncture points are anatomically defined in the areas of the skin. They are set at fixed specific locations in body acupuncture and can always be detected. In ear acupuncture , the auricular point can be detected only when there is a problem without he corresponding part of the body in which the ear point represents. The deqi that accompanies stimulation of the body acupuncture point is not observed in stimulation the ear acupuncture point.

In both body and ear acupuncture, the points are localized regions of lowered skin resistance or higher skin conductivity. When there is pathology in an organ represented in the meridian point or the auricular point the epidermal skin conductance of the acupuncture point is high.

Ear acupuncture points are ipsiladeral or same side as the pain or pathology. This representation on the ear is due to two contralateral projections from the ear to the opposite side of the brain and from the opposite side of the brain back to the opposite side of the body. Using traditional Chinese medicine theory, ear points are ipsilateral because Qi flows up the ipsilateral meridian.

Ear acupuncture provides a more scientifically verified means of identifying areas of pain or pathology in the body than traditionally Chinese medicine approaches such as tongue or pulse diagnosis. In auricular diagnosis one can identify specific problems in the body by detecting areas of the ear in which there is discolored, flaky, tender, or have high skin conductivity. This increased conductance is measured by a probe and is repeatable and verifiable. The subtle changes in auricular diagnosis may identify conditions in which the patient and the physician may only be marginally aware of.

Both ear acupuncture (auriculotherapy) and body acupuncture can be chemically utilized to relieve pain pathology. They both can be used together or applied separately. Healing not just pain relief. Both body acupuncture and ear points do not simply reduce the experience of pain but also facilitate natural healing processes within the body. Auricular therapy facilitates the natural self regulating homeostatic mechanisms of the body by diminishing over active body functions and increasing underactive physiological processes. Both body acupuncture and auricular therapy can have deep physiological and psychological affects.

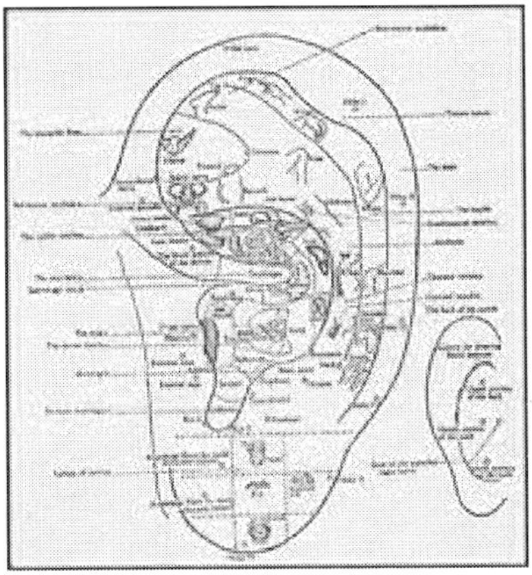

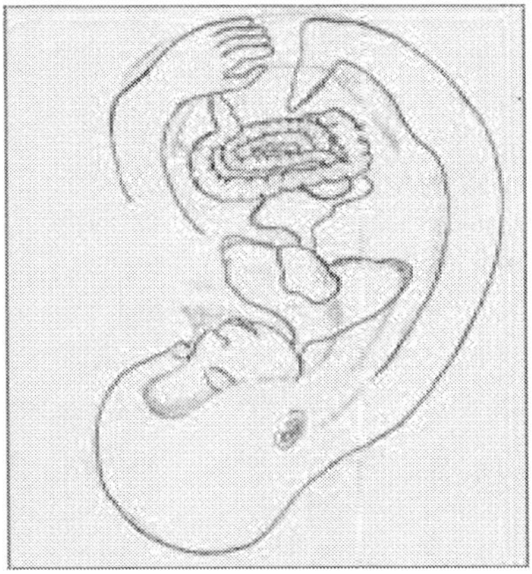

Take a look at the illustrated diagrams. The shape of the auricle (ear) clearly resembles a near-term foetus in the inverted position in the mother's womb. You will need to understand that the classic Chinese Acupuncture points on the ears are in a similar position to the various anatomical areas of the foetus.

For example, all the head acupoints are located on the ear lobe, e.g. tonsils, throat, sinuses etc. All the major organs of the foetus are located in the 'well' or concha of the ear as is their acupoints e.g. lungs, heart, liver, etc. and the lower limbs of the foetus are positioned at the 'top' of the ear as are the acupoints, e.g. knees, toes, ankles etc. This is a very simple explanation of the Chinese Foetus Representation, further study will help you understand it fully.

Direct evidence of endorphinogenic response to auricular therapy has been provided by Abbot et al in 1980, they observed a significant increase in endorphins after acupuncture stimulation was combined with nitric oxide inhalation. Whereas the controlled subjects given nitric oxide without acupuncture showed no elevation of the endorphins.

The primary side-effects of ear acupuncture (auriculotherapy) is that the ear itself can become tender and inflamed. Auricular therapy and acupuncture generally is not recommended for patient with pace-makers and during pregnancy. While auriculotherapy does not require the use of needles, ear points may be sensitive to any applied simulation through auriculotherapy treatment. Infection is almost never heard of in auricular therapy and acupuncture and if a patient is afraid of needles, auricular electrical stimulation is the preferred treatment.

**Embryological Basis**

Dr. Paul Nogier noted that the ear was composed of tissue from each of the three primary types of tissue in the developing embryo. His theory was that each type of embryological tissue on the ear accounts for a different somatotopic functions related to the auricle. Ectodermal tissue, superficial tissue is found in the ear lobe in the helix teal. The ectoderm become the skin, hair, sweat gland, cornea and lens of the eye. Nose, epithelium, teeth, nerves, spinal cord, subcortex of brain, cerebrum and pituitary gland, pineal gland and adrenal medulla.

The mesodermal tissue: the middle tissue is found in the anithelix scaphoid fossa, the triangular fossa. The mesoderm becomes the musculoskeletal system of muscles, joints, bones, cardiac muscles, smooth muscles, connective tissue, blood cells from the bone marrow, lymphatic tissues, genial organs, kidney, and the adrenal cortex.

The third type is the endodermal tissue, the deep tissue which is found in the concha. The endoderm becomes the gastrointestinal digestive tract, the lungs, tonsil and the respiratory system. The internal organs like the liver, pancreas, bladder, urethra.

The neurotein system: natural pain relievers, endorphins, enkephalins, are indigenous morphine chemicals which are found within the pituitary and other parts of the central nervous system and encephalon is subfactor of endorphin. These neurotransmitters occur in the brain at the same site where opiate receptors are found. Both body and ear acupuncture have been found to raise the blood serum and cerebral spinal fluid levels of endorphins and enkephalins. Naloxone is a opiate antagonist which blocks morphine endorphin.

Research report from UCLA by Simons & Oleson 1993, Mayer et al 1977, were the first investigators to provide scientific evidence that there was neurophysiological and neurochemical basis for acupuncture and auriculotherapy in human subjects. They demonstrated that the acupuncture stimulation of the body through Large Intestine 4 points, led to a significant increase in pain threshold. They were then able to yield statistically significant reversal of elevated pain threshold by intravenous administration of 0.8 mg of an opiate naloxone. The acupuncture had raised dental pain threshold by over 27 %. There was no treatment control group which showed a 6.9% in dental pain threshold. A total of 20 of 35 acupuncture subjects showed increased pain threshold greater than 20% contrasted with only 5 out of 40 subjects in the controlled condition exhibiting a 20% elevation of pain threshold. Naloxone given to acupuncture subjects reduced the pain threshold to the same level as the control group.

Direct evidence of endorphinogenic response to auricular therapy has been provided by Abbot et al in 1980, they observed a significant increase in endorphins after acupuncture stimulation was combined with nitric oxide inhalation. Whereas the controlled subjects given nitric oxide without acupuncture showed no elevation of the endorphins.

Both body and ear acupuncture (auriculotherpy) are used for a broad variety of clinical dysfunction and diseases including headaches, chronic backaches, hypertension, asthma, dental disorders, addiction.

The theoretical understanding of auriculotherapy can be perceived from knowledge of standard anatomical and neurophysiological treatises and theories, and additionally to from the use of Chinese energetic theories. The neurological basis for auriculotherapy is based upon a somatotropic map in which a brain map of the body exist in neurons on the cerebral cortex through the thalamus and the brain stem. The brain map is similar to the auricular map exhibiting a inverted fetus orientation.

The ear is intervened by the auricular temporal nerve formed by the mandibular ranus of the trigeminal nerve, cranial nerve V. The major and minor auricular nerves are formed by the nerves of the cervical plexus C2, C3 and finally the auricular Rami of the facial nerve, cranial nerve VII and the glossopharyngeal nerve, cranial nerve IX and the vagus nerve, cranial nerve X. This dense enervation of five different afferent nerves of somatic and visceral nature give abundant intervention of the ear.

The basis of this neural anatomy and embryological and comparative autonomy, auricular reflex therapy was composed and utilized by Rueben Durinjan. The therapy developed by Melzack and Wall 1965, date control theory, the inhibitory interneuron in the spinal cord is differentially effected A fiber C fiber input. Fast conducting A fibers carry information about touch affecting inhibitory interneurons in the spinal cord to suppress the experience of pain. Slow conducting C fibers carry information about pain. Inhibiting these same inhibitory interneurons results in a further increase in neural discharges which are sent towards the brain activating the conscience experience of pain.

TENS (transcutaneous electrical nerve stimulation) suppresses pain by activating A-Fibers which inhibit the input from C fibers. Acupuncture stimulation tends to activate C fibers which activates super spinal gating systems which then send descending input to the spinal inhibitory neurons which suppresses the pain message. Secondary, stimulation produced analgesia is a pain inhibitory system that has been demonstrated by brain stimulation by the periactiductal central gray matter which reduces the responses to pain in rats, cats, monkeys, and humans. This peripheral stimulation and ear acupuncture points may peripherally activate the pain inhibitory system.

Auricular therapy is needle-less stimulation of the auricle, or external ear, using electrical probe for alleviating pain, dysfunction and disease as manifest in other parts of the body.

Auricular therapy uses electricity to diagnose auricular acupoints. It uses electricity, laser or colored filters to treat auricular acupoints. It is performed by a physician, acupuncturist or therapist.

Auricular therapy is the bioenergetic and biomechanical approach to wholistic health care and pain management. It is a form of needle-less acupuncture. It is a diagnostic method and a therapeutic treatment of the microsystem. It is rooted in acupuncture teachings and research and it is the easiest and most "western" approach to acupuncture.

*How does auriculotherapy work?*

Auriculotherapy works by stimulating the central nervous system through the cranial nerves/spinal nerves on the auricle of the ear. This stimulation results in a neurotransmitters being stimulation within the periactal ductal gray and pituitary and spinal cord of the central nervous system. This stimulation of neurotransmitters modulates the pain and modulates nerve function beginning the healing process within the body to that organ or body part.

*Does auriculotherapy hurt?*

Using acupuncture needles on the ear, pain may last one to three seconds with the placing of the needle. Otherwise, acupuncture needles should not hurt on the ear. If electrical stimulation is used or lasers are used on the ears, there should be little to no pain at all perceived by the patient.

*What problems is auriculotherapy good for?*

Auriculotherapy is good for acute painful problems alleviating pain almost immediately or within 24 to 48 hours. Auricle therapy is good for chronic degenerative conditions such as osteoarthritis, rheumatoid arthritis and other chronic painful conditions like spinal stenosis and other chronic central nervous system conditions such as multiple sclerosis. Other conditions include diseases and dysfunctions of the gastrointestinal, genital urinary and cardiovascular systems. Auricular therapy should not take the place of acute orthodox medical care in life threatening situations.

*How frequently should I be treated?*

In most cases, treatment for most chronic conditions may be treated once or twice per weeks. However, in some acute conditions and very serious conditions auriculotherapy may be applied daily for approximately one week to 10 days.

*How does one perform auriculotherapy?*

It is performed by a therapist using electrical means to diagnose auricular acupoints. There are over 200 auricular acupoints on each ear that represent all parts of the body and many functional areas of the human organism. These points represent anatopical and neurological and physiological functions.

The physician therapist uses a hand held wand and a diagnostic probe similar to a pen that measures differences in skin conductivity between the hand and the acupoint on the ear. The positive and negative polarity of that relationship and if it is extremely negative or extremely positive, with the touch of a button, the instrument stimulates the ear with electrical stimulation either positively or negatively as needed. With this the physician auricular therapist will be able to diagnose pain, dysfunction and disease whether it be somatic, visceral or psychological in origin. These diagnostic aids, through research performed at UCLA, prove to be quite accurate for a simple test — on study yielding over 75% accuracy in a double-blind study.

People who do not want ear acupuncture or auricular therapy should, obviously, not have it, but it would be wise for anyone with the following conditions to abstain from ear acupuncture or auricular therapy.

These conditions include:

First trimester pregnancy

First two months of constitutional homeopathic treatment

Patients with pacemaker or spinal cord stimulator

Neonates children less than one days old

Patients with no external ear

Individuals with a known genetic abnormalities of CCK enzyme produced in the central nervous system. (This enzyme, which is produced in the brain, neutralizes the neuroprotients that are released with acupuncture. Only a very small percentage of the population is affected. As of today, there is no simple test to identify these patients other than a trial of acupuncture or auricular therapy.

*Are there side effects?*

The primary side effect of ear acupuncture or auricular therapy is tenderness or inflammation to the ear itself. Auricular therapy and acupuncture generally have almost no side effects, especially if one is using auricular therapy with electrical stimulation. If the therapist is using the Elector-Therapy Association's guidelines for treatment, there are virtually no negative side effects.

Infection is possible when the skin is pierced with the acupuncture needle, but is almost never heard of in auricular therapy. If the patient is afraid of needles, auricular therapy, rather than ear acupuncture should be performed.

Ear acupuncture is only about 50 years old. Paul Nogiers a neurlogist from Lyons, France became involved with this discovery when a woman entered his office one day in the early 1950s. She said she had back pain for years. Dr. Nogiers said perhaps he could help her. She remarked "No. I had back pain for years but is was cured by a woman in the Mid East. She burnt my ear and the pain has been gone since." Dr Nogiers scientific curiosity was aroused as he saw a scar on her ear. From that point he searched for other areas on the ear that might relieve ailments and discovered that the ear has points communicating with the in Germany a lecture on the subject. A Chinese contingency photographed his slides and they pursued the subject by using the Red army as subjects. They developed a map of the ear which we present here in our website. Dr Nogiers published many works on the subject and recently died at the age of 88.

In 1972 a Japanese physician, Dr. Y. Omura began a detoxification program at Lincoln Hospital in New York City to see if acupuncture could remove the cocaine withdrawals. Indeed it worked and Dr. Michael Smith and others followed his work for that treatment. As a side affect, Dr. Omura found that many of his addicted patients had quit smoking and many also lost weight. This lead to the use of acupuncture to help people quit smoking and lose weight.Our second picture in the Atlas shows points that you can use for pain relief or other ailments.

# *Chapter Thirteen*

# Atlas of Acupuncture Points

## Acupuncture Points

*Figure 1: Anterior View of Meridians*

Acupuncture involves the insertion of very fine needles into the body to stimulate acupoints, of which the major ones are shown on this chart These points are located along 14 meridians traversing the head, arms, legs, and trunk. With the exception of the Ren and Du meridians, all meridians are symmetrical, traversing both sides of the body.

(**Note:** Although this chart shows meridians on both sides of the body, only one side is labeled). These meridians are channels through which Qi (vital energy) flows throughout the body. If the flow of Qi is insufficient or interrupted, then the body's yin and yang become unbalanced, and illness may result.

**Note:** The first point of the Ren Meridian (RN 1) cannot be seen in this figure.It is located between the scrotum and the anus in men, and between the posterior commissure of the labia and the anus in women.

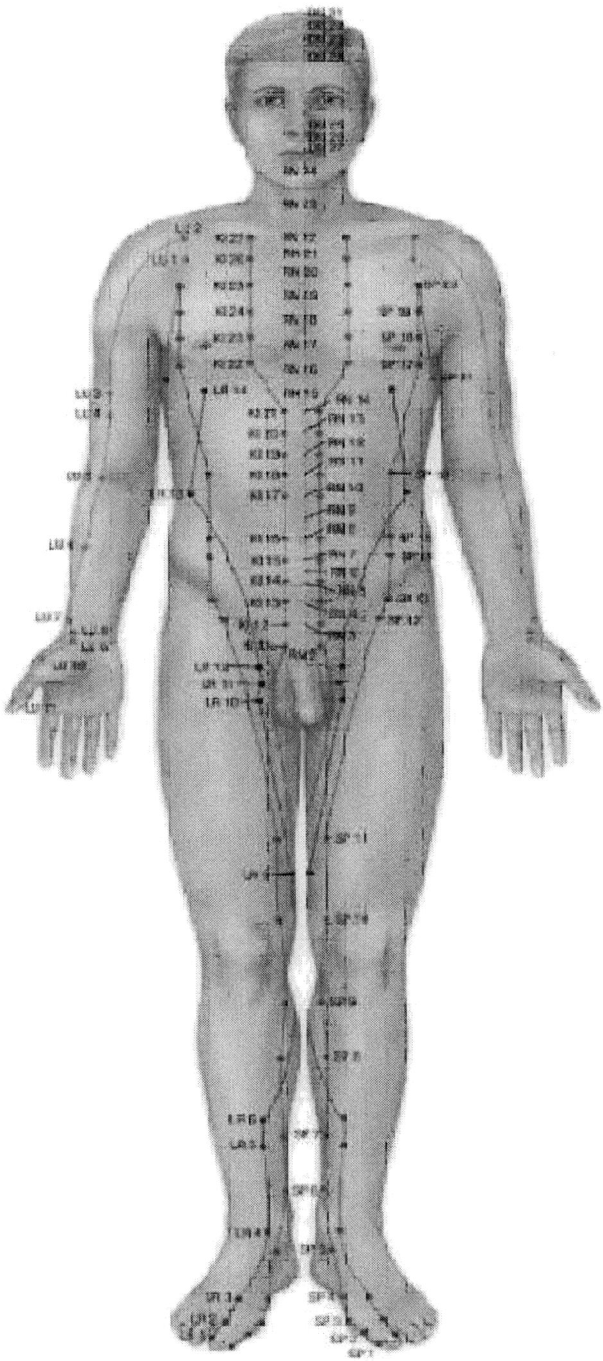

## Acupuncture Points:

*Figure 2: Posterior View of Meridians*

Acupuncture removes blockages in the flow of Qi by diffusing lactic acid and carbon monoxide that accumulate in muscle tissue and cause stiffness and stagnation of blood. This stiffness creates abnormal pressure on nerves, lymph nodes, and blood vessels, which adversely affects the function of the skeletal system and internal organs.

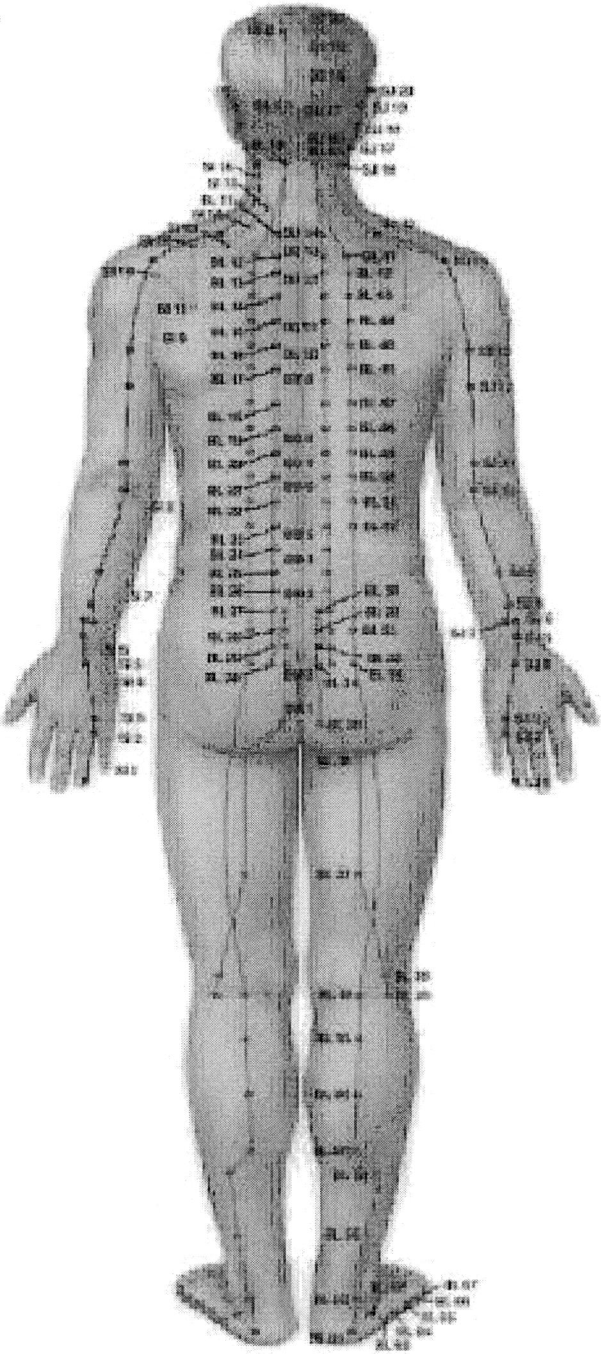

**Acupuncture Points:**

*Figure 3: Lateral View of Meridians*

**Notes:** Points KI 1, DU 28, and HT 1 cannot be seen in this figure. KI 1 is located on the sole of the foot at the depression that appears dring plantar flexion (at the junction of the anterior third and posterior two-thirds of the line connecting the base of the second and third toes and the heel).

DU 28 is located under the upper lip, at the junction of the labial frenulum and upper gum HT 1 is located at the apex of the axillary fossa, just medial to the axillary artery.

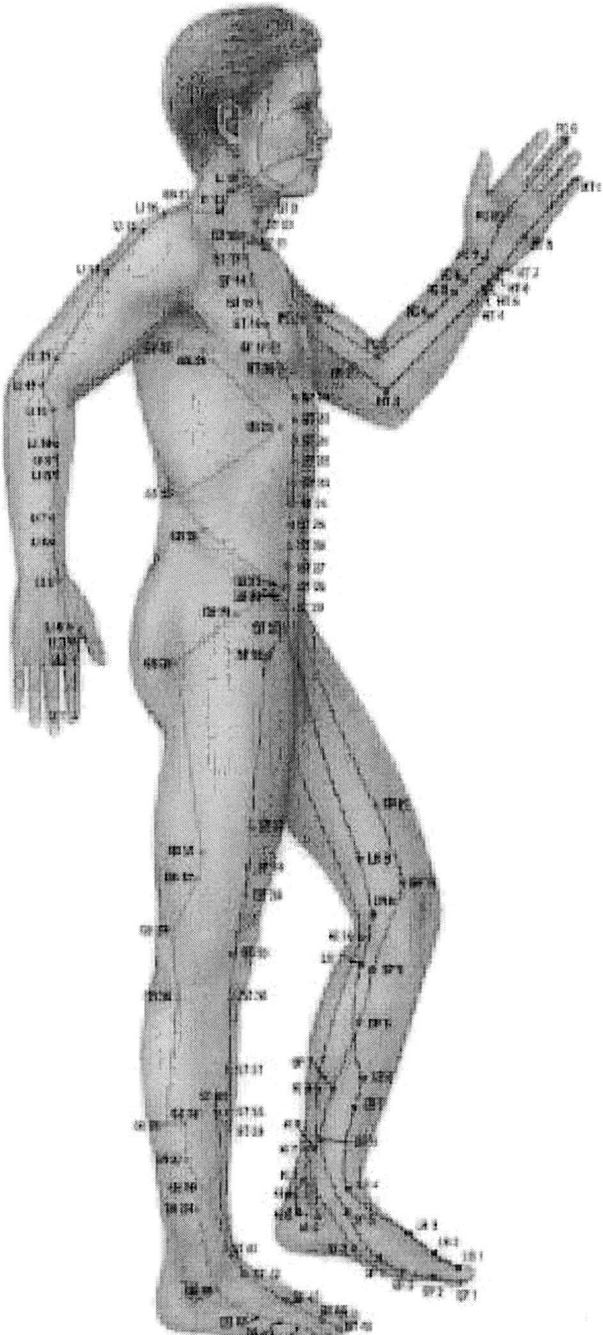

## Acupuncture Points:

*Figure 4: Meridians of the Head (lateral View)*

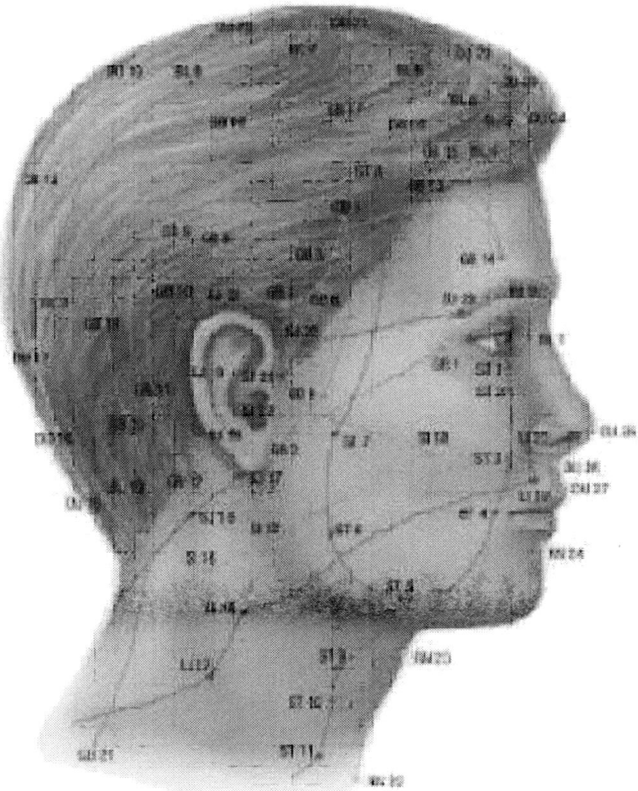
GB 14
ST 3
ST 4
ST 9
ST 10
ST 11

## The Chong Meridian

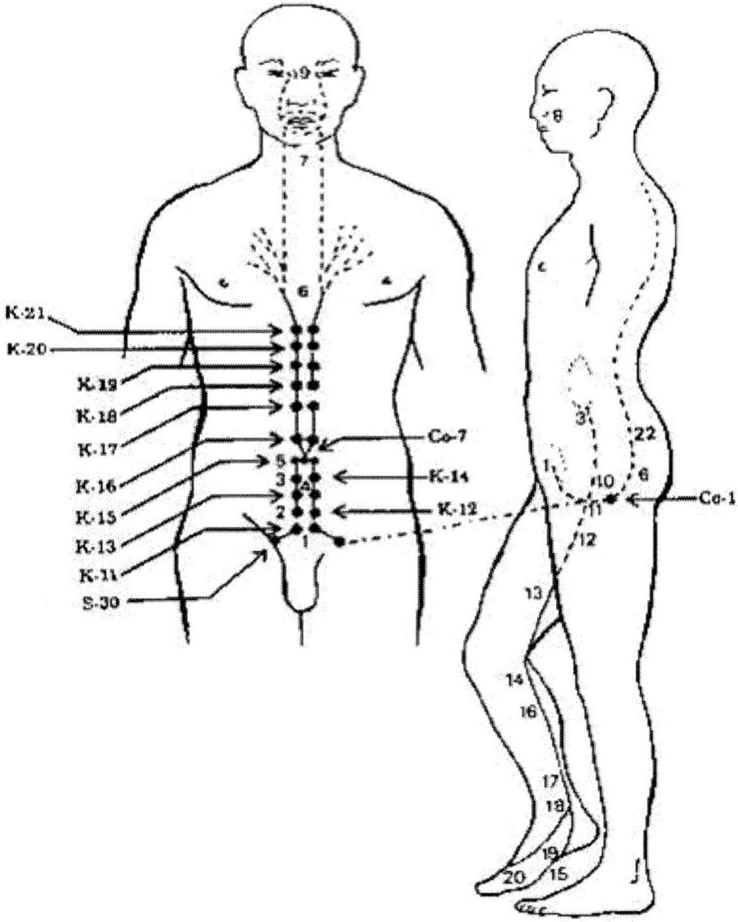

*Course#1:*

(1). Lower abdomen - (2). Emerges along the Path of Qi - (3). Tracks the course of the kidney channel - (4). Ascends through the abdomen - (5). Skirts the navel - (6). Disperses in the chest.

*Course#2:*

(6). Chest -(7). Ascends across the throat -(8). Face -(9). Nasal cavity.

*Course #3:*

(1). Lower abdomen - (10). Below the kidney - (11). Emerges along the Path of Qi - (12). Descends along the medial aspect of the thigh - (13). Popliteal fossa - (14). Medial margin of the tibia and the posterior aspect of the medial malleolus - (15). Bottom of the foot.

*Course#4:*

(16). Tibia - (17). Toward the lateral margin of the bone - (18). enters the heel - (19). Crosses the tarsal bones of the foot - (20). Big toe.

*Course#5:*

(21). Pelvic cavity - (22). Enter the spine and circulates through the back.

***This vessel intersects Huiyin (LI-1), Yinjiao (LI-7), Qichong (S-30), Henggu (K-11), Dahe (K-12), Qixue (K-13), Siman (K-14), Zhongzhu (K-15), Huangshu (K-16), Shangqu (K-17), Shiguan (K-18), Yindu (K-19), Tonggu (K-20), and Youmen (K-21).

## The Dai (Girdle) Meridian

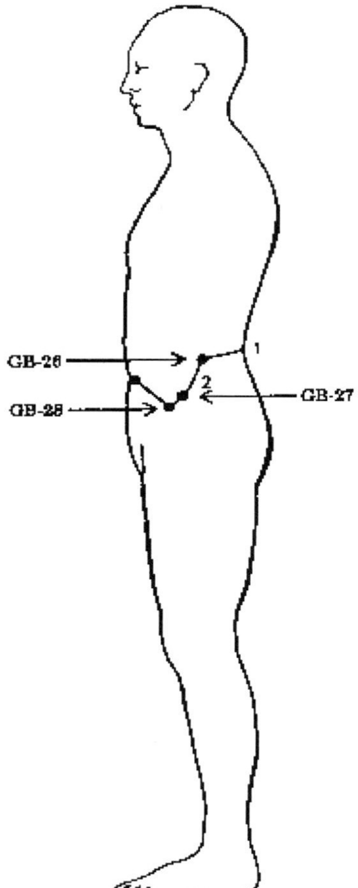

*Course:*

(1). Below the hypochondrium at the level of the 2nd lumbar vertebra -(2). Turns downward and encircles the body at the waist like a girdle.

***This vessel intersects Daimai (GB-26), Wushu (GB-27), and Weidao (GB-28).

## The Du(Governing) vessel Meridian

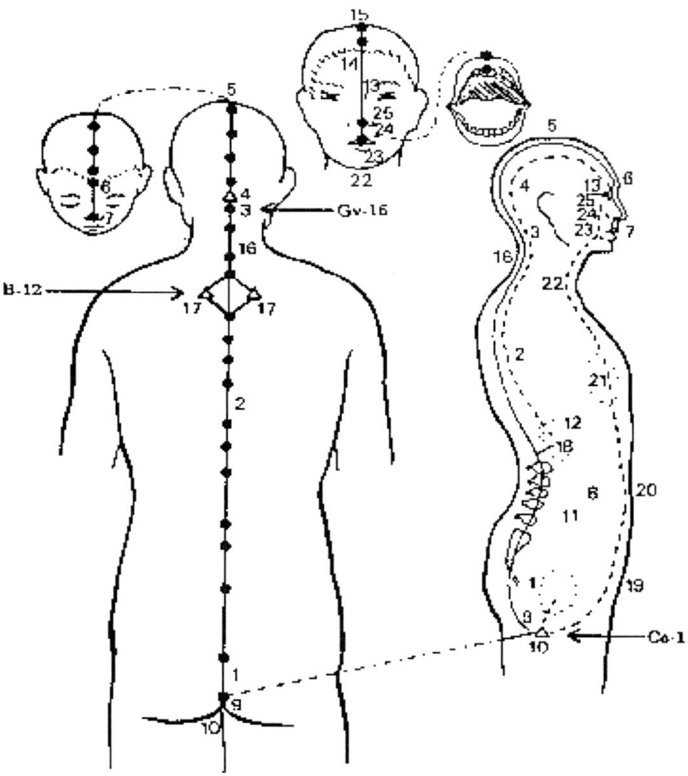

*Course #1:*

(1). Perineum - (2). Along the middle of the spine - (3). Fengfu (Gv-lG) - (4). Enters the brain - (5). To the top of the head - (6). Midline of the forehead across the bridge of the nose - (7). Upper lip.

*Course #2:*

(8). Pelvic region -(9). Descends to the genitals and perineum (10). Tip of the coccyx - (11). Gluteal region (intersects the kidney and urinary bladder channels) -(12). Returns to the spinal column and then joins with the kidneys.

*Course #3:*

(13). Inner canthus of the eye - (14). Two (bilateral) branches, ascend across the forehead - (15). Converge at the vertex (enters the brain) - (16). Emerges at the lower end of the nape of the neck - (17). Divides into two branches which descend along opposite sides of the spine to the waist - (18). Kidneys.

*Course #4:*

(19). Lower abdomen - (20). Across the navel -(21). Passes through the heart -(22). Enters the trachea -(23). Crosses the cheek and encircles the mouth - (24). Terminates at a point below the middle of the eye.

****This vessel intersects Fengmen (B-12) and Huiyin (LI-l).

*Cavities:*

Changqiang (Gv-l), Yaoshu (Gv-2), Yaoyangguan (Gv-3), Mingmen (Gv-4), Xuanshu (Gv-S), Jizhong (Gv-G), Zhongshu (Gv-7), Jinsuo (Gv-8), Zhiyang (Gv-9), Lingtai (Gv-l0), Shendao (Gv-ll), Shenzhu (Gv-12), Taodao (Gv-13), Dazhui (Gv-14), Yamen (Gv-lS), Fengfu (Gv-lG), Naohu (Gv-17), Qiangjian (Gv-18), Houding (Gv-19), Baihui (Gv-20), Qianding (Gv-21), Xinhui (Gv-22), Shangxing (Gv-23), Shenting (Gv-24), Suliao (Gv-25), Renzhong (Gv-26), Duiduan (Gv-27), and Yinjiao (Gv-28).

## The Heart Meridian

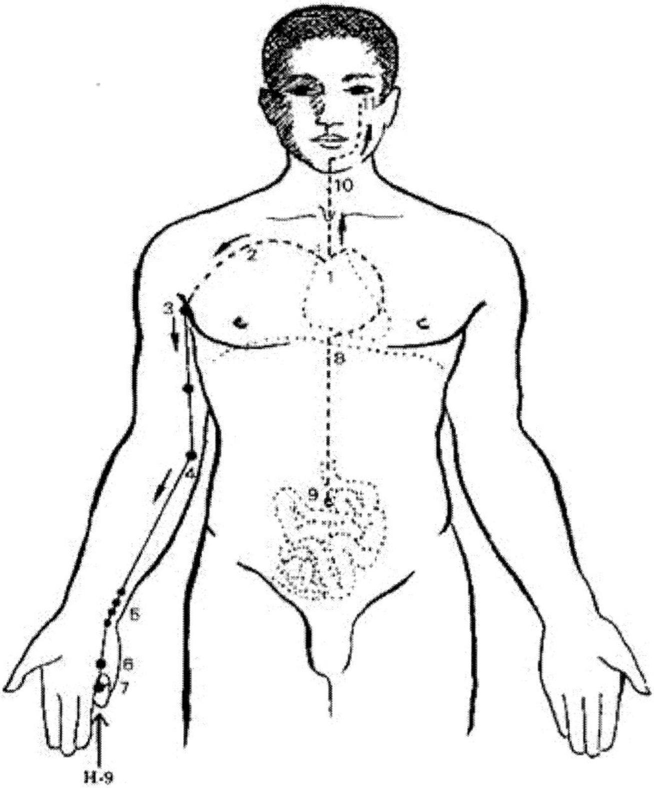

*Course #1:*

(1). Heart -(2). Lung - (3). Below the axilla -(4). Upper arm (5). Antecubital fossa - (6). Between ossa metacarpal IV and V - (7). Tip of the little finger (Shaochong, H-9).

*Course #2:*

(1). Heart- (8). Diaphragm- (9). Small intestine.

*Course #3:*

(1). Heart - (10). Throat - (11). Tissues surrounding the eye (orbital system).

*Related Viscera:*

Heart (Pertaining Organ), small intestine, lung, and kidney.

*Cavities:*

Jiquan (H-1), Qingling (H-2), Shaohai (H-3), Lingdao (H-4), Tongli (H-5), Yinxi (H-6), Shenmen (H-7), Shaofu (H-8), Shaochong (H-9).

## The Kidney Meridian

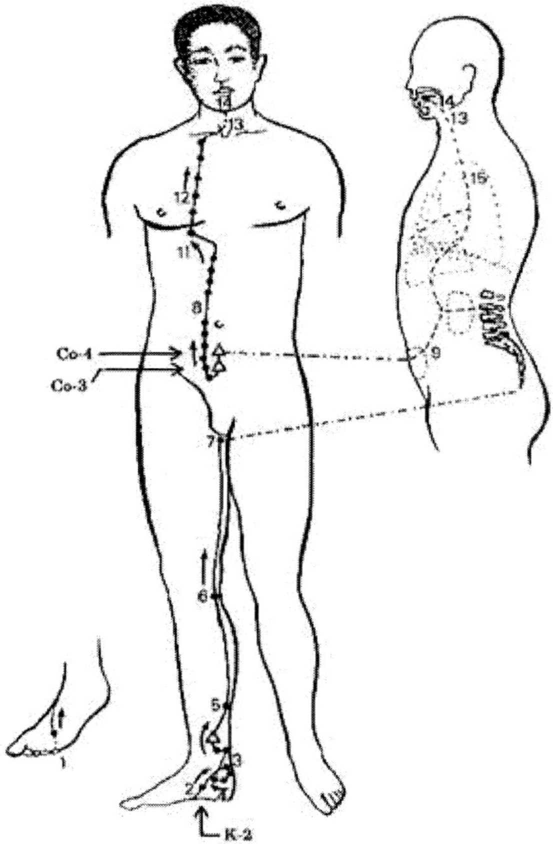

*Course #1:*

(1). Small toe - (2). Inferior aspect of the navicular tuberosity (Rangu, K-2)- (3). Behind the malleolus medialis -(4). Spreads to the heel - (5). M. gastrocnemius - (6). Medial side of the popliteal fossa - (7). Posterior aspect of the thigh - (8). Enters kidney - (9). Communicates with the urinary bladder - (10).'Guanyuan (LI-4) and Zhongji (LI-3).

*Course #2:*

(9). Kidney -(11). Liver and diaphragm -(12). Enters the lung (13). Along the throat - (14). Root of the tongue.

*Course #3:*

(12). Lung - (15). Heart and spreads to the chest.

*Related Viscera:*

Kidney (Pertaining Organ), urinary bladder, liver, lung, heart, and other organs.

*Cavities:*

Yongquan (K-1), Rangu (K-2), Taixi (K-3), Dazhong (K-4), Shuiquan (K-5), Zhaohai (K-6), Fuliu (K-7), Jiaoxin (K-8), Zhubin (K-9), Yingu (K-10), Henggu (K-11), Dahe (K-12), Qixue (K-13), Siman (K-14), Abdomen-Zhongzhu (K-15), Huangshu (K-16), Shangqu (K-17), Shiguan (K-18), Yindu (K-19), Abdomen-Tonggu (K-20), Youmen (K-21), Bulang (K-22), Shenfeng (K-23), Lingxu (K-24), Shencang (K-25), Yuzhong (K-26), and Shufu (K-27).

## The Gall Bladder Meridian

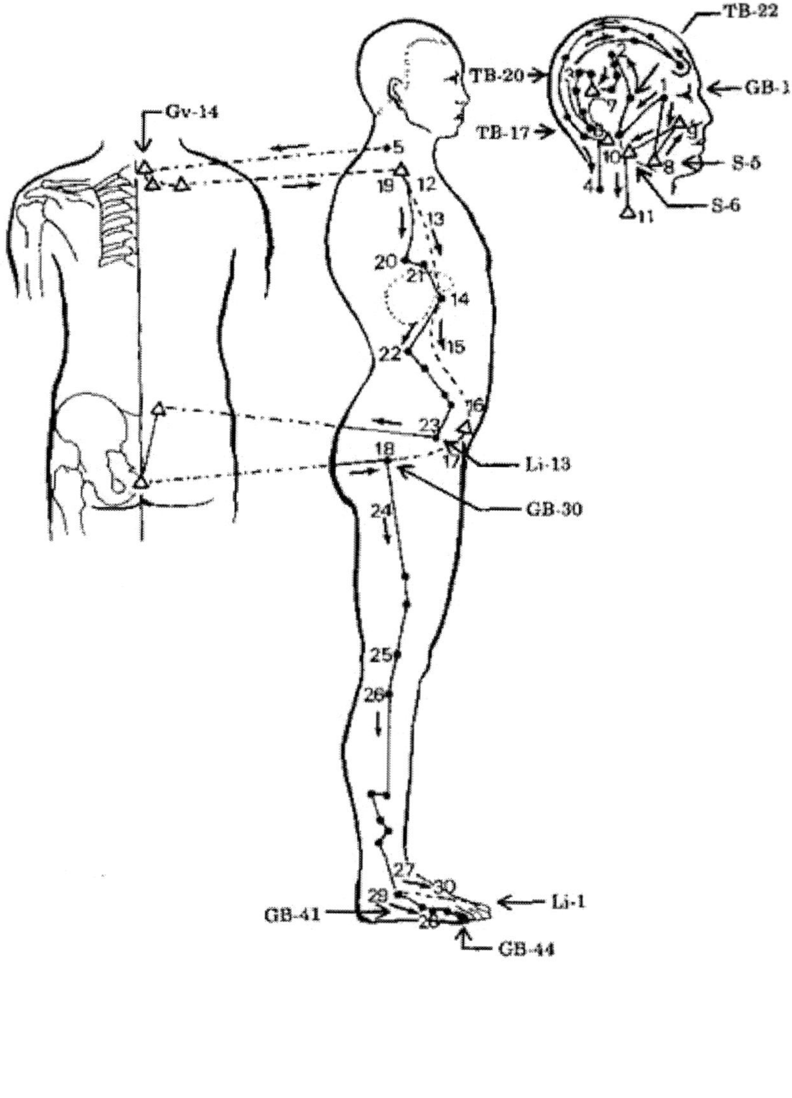

*Course #1:*

(1). Outer canthus of the eye (Tongziliao, GB-1) - (2). Nose Heliao (TB-22)- (3). Jiaosun (TB-20)- (4). Dazhui (Gv-14)- (5). Enters the supraclavicular fossa.

*Course #2:*

(6). Retro-auricular region, passes through Yifeng (TB-17) - (7). Tinggong (SI-19) and Xiaguan (S-7).

*Course #3:*

(1). Outer canthus of the eye - (8). Daying (S-5) - (9). Infraorbital region - (10). Jiache (S-6) -(11). Supraclavicular fossa -(12). Into the chest -(13). Tianchi (P-1)- (14). Communicates. with the liver -(15). Pertains to the gall bladder - (16). Inside of the hypochondrium (17). Around the genitals -(18). Hip (Huantiao, GB-30).

*Course #4:*

(19). Supraclavicular fossa - (20). Axilla - (21). Lateral aspect of the chest -(22). Through the hypochondrium - (23). Zhangmen (Li 13) - (24). Along the lateral aspect of thigh - (25). Knee - (26). Anterior aspect of the fibula - (27). Anterior aspect of the malleolus (28). Lateral side of the tip of the 4th toe or Zuqiaoyin (GB-44).

*Course #5:*

(29). Dorsum of the foot (Linqi, GB-41) - (30). Big toe (Dadun, Li-1).

*Related Viscera:*

Gall bladder (Pertaining Organ), liver, and heart.

*Cavities:*

Tongziliao (GB-1), Tinghui (GB-2), Shangguan (GB-3), Hanyan (GB-4), Xuanlu (GB-S), Xuanli (GB-G), Qubin (GB-7), Shuaigu (GB 8), Tianchong (GB-9), Fubai (GB-10), Head-Qiaoyin (GB-11), Head Wangu (GB-12), Benshen (GB-13), Yangbai (GB-14), Head-Linqi (GB-15), Muchuang (GB-16), Zhengying (GB-17), Chengling (GB-18), Naokong (GB-19), Fengchi (GB-20), Jianjing (GB-21), Yuanye (GB-22), Zhejin (GB-23), Riyue (GB-24), Jingmen (GB-25), Daimai (GB-26), Wushu (GB-27), Weidao (GB-28), Femur-Juliao (GB-29), Huantiao (GB-30), Fengshi (GB-31), Femur-Zhongdu (GB-32), Xiyangguan (GB-33), Yanglingquan (GB-34), Yangjiao (GB-35), Waiqiu (GB-36), Guangming (GB-37), Yangfu (GB-38), Xuanzhong (GB-39), Qiuxu (GB-40), Foot-Linqi (GB-41), Diwuhui (GB-42), Xiaxi (GB-43), Foot-Qiaoyin (GB-44).

## Large Intestine(Colon) Meridian

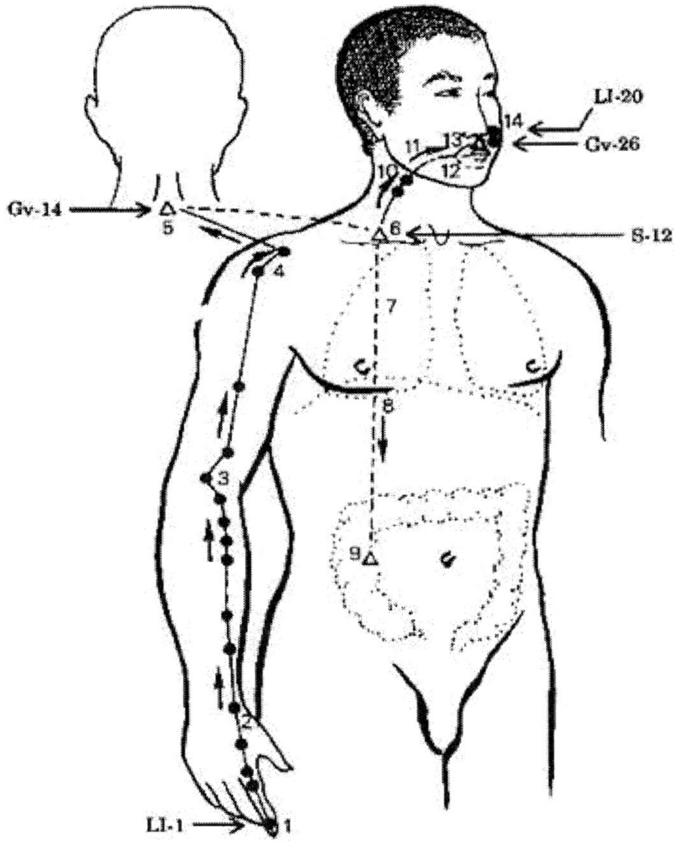

*Course #1:*

(1). Index finger (Shangyang, LI-1) -(2). Wrist -(3). Elbow - (4). Shoulder Joint - (5,. Governing vessel at Dazhui (Gv-14) - (6). Supraclavicular Fossa (Quepen, S-12) - (7). Lung - (8). Diaphragm (9). Large intestine.

*Course #2:*

(6). Supraclavicular fossa - (10). Neck - (11). Cheek - (12). Lower Gum - (13). Renzhong (Gv-26) - (14). Side of the nose (Yingxiang, LI-20).

*Related Viscera:*

Large intestine (Pertaining Organ), lung, and stomach.

*Cavities:*

Shangyang (LI-1), Erjian (LI-2), Sanjian (LI-3), Hegu (LI-4), Yangx; (LI-S), Pianli (LI-G), Wenliu (LI-7), Xianlian (LI-8), Shanglian (LI-9), Shousanli (LI-10), Quchi (LI-11), Zhouliao (LI-12), Hand-Wuli (LI-13), Binao (LI-14), Jianyu (LI-15), Jugu (LI-16), Tianding (LI-17), Futu (LI-18), Heliao (LI-19), and Yingxiang (LI-20).

## The Liver Meridian

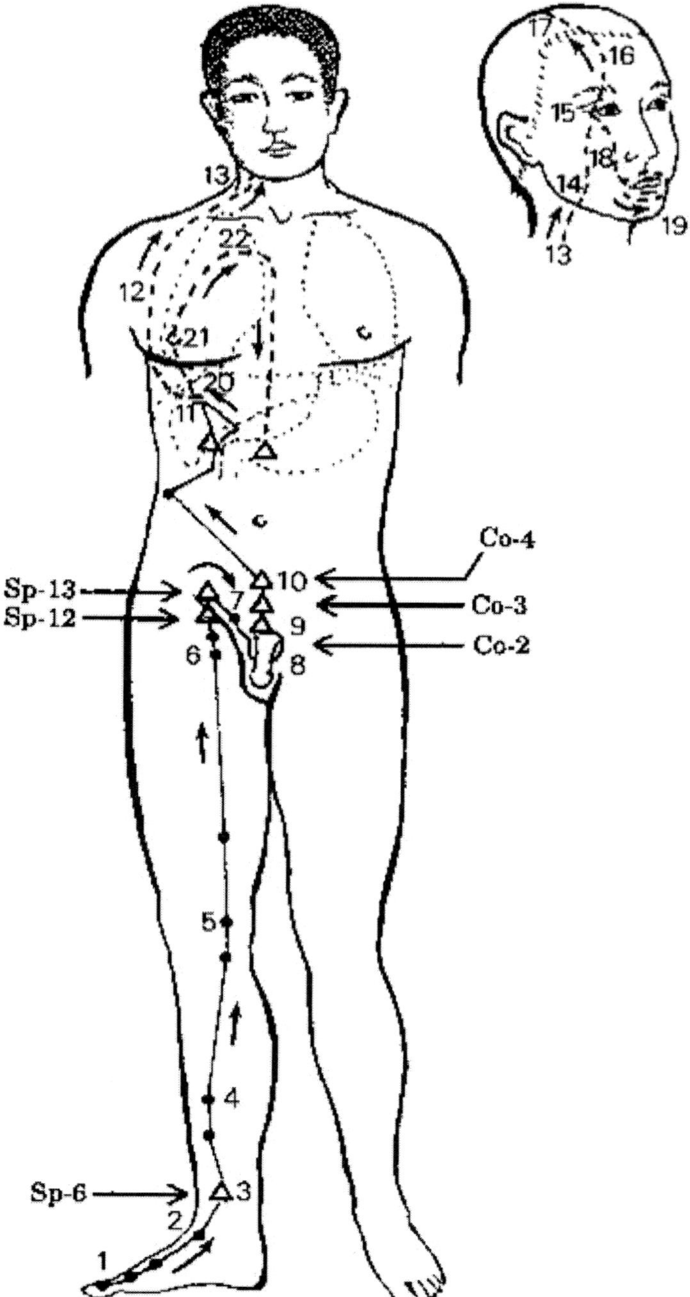

*Course #1:*

(1). Behind the nail of the big toe - (2). Malleolus medialis - (3). Sanyinjiao (Sp-6) - (4). Side of shin - (5). Side of knee - (6). Medial aspect of the thigh - (7). Chongmen (Sp-12) and Fushe (Sp-13) - (8). Pubic region - (9). Lower abdomen - (10). Qugu (CV-2), Zhongli (CV-3), and Guanyuan (CV-4) - (11). Liver - (12). Lower chest - (13). Neck posterior - (14). Upper palate - (15). Tissues of the eye - (16). Forehead -(17). Vertex.

*Course #2:*

(15). Eye - (18). Cheek - (19). Curves around the inner surface of the lips.

*Course #3:*

(20). Liver -(21). Through diaphragm -(22). Lung.

*Related Viscera:*

Liver (Pertaining Organ), gall bladder, lung, stomach, and brain.

*Cavities:*

Dadun (L-1), Xingjian (L-2), Taichong (L-3), Zhongfeng (L-4), Ligou (L-5), Tibia-Zhongdu (L-6), Xiguan (L-7), Ququan (L-8), Yinbao (L-9), Femur-Wuli (L-10), Yinlian (L-11), Jimai (L-12), Zhangmen (L-13), and Qimen (L-14).

## The Lung Meridian

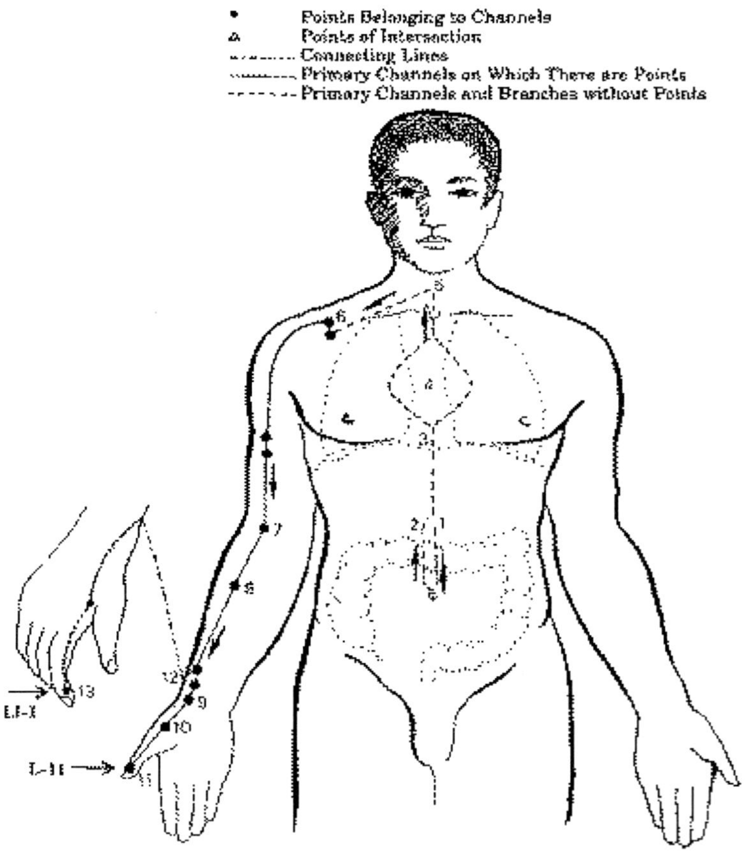

*Course #1:*

(1). Stomach (Zhong Jiao, middle triple burner) - (2). Large intestine - (3). Diaphragm - (4). Lung - (5). Throat - (6). Upper Arm (7). Mid-Elbow -(8). Forearm -(9). Wrist -(10). Thenar- (11). Pollex (Shaoshang, L-11).

*Course #2:*

(12). Above the styloid process at the wrist - (13). Index Finger (Shangyang, LI-1).

*Related Viscera:*

Lung (Pertaining Organ), large intestine, stomach, and kidney.

*Cavities:*

Zhongfu (L-1), Yunmen (L-2), Tianfu (L-3), Xiabai (L-4), Qize (L 5), Kongzui (L-6), Lieque (L-7), Jingqu (L-8), Taiyuan (L-9), Yuji (L-10), and Shaoshang (L-11).

## The Pericardium(Sex Circulation) Meridian

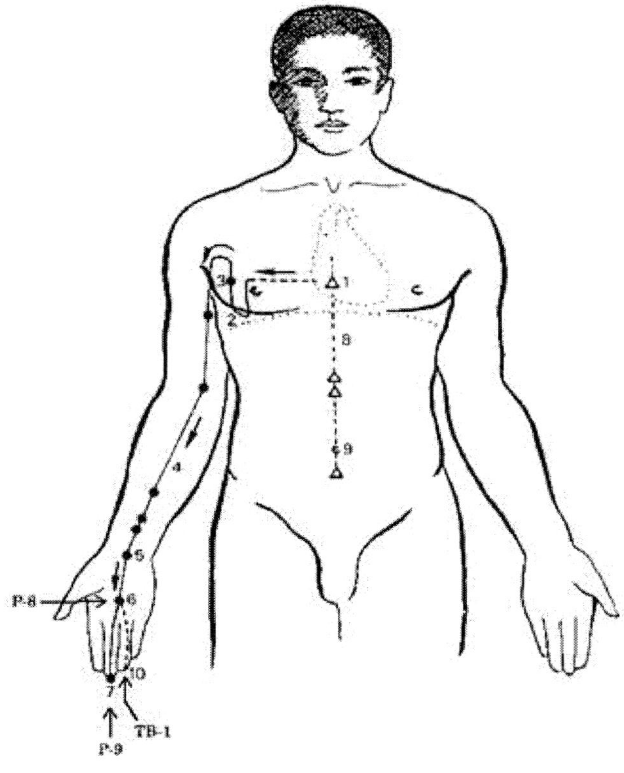

*Course #1:*

(1). Pericardium - (2). Below the armpit - (3). Axilla -(4). Forearm - (5). Wrist - (6). Palm - (7). Tip of middle finger (Zhongchong, P-9).

*Course #2:*

(1). Pericardium -(8). Diaphragm -(9). Connects triple burner (Sanjiao)

*Course #3:*

(6). Palm (Laogong, P-8) - (10). Tip of ring finger (Guanchong, TB-1).

*Related Viscera:*

Pericardium (Pertaining Organ) and triple burner (Sanjiao).

*Cavities:*

Tianchi (P-1), Tianquan (P-2), Quze (P-3), Ximen (P-4), Jianshi (P-5), Neiguan (P-6), Daling (P-7), Laogong (P-8), and Zhongchong (P-9).

## The Ren Meridian

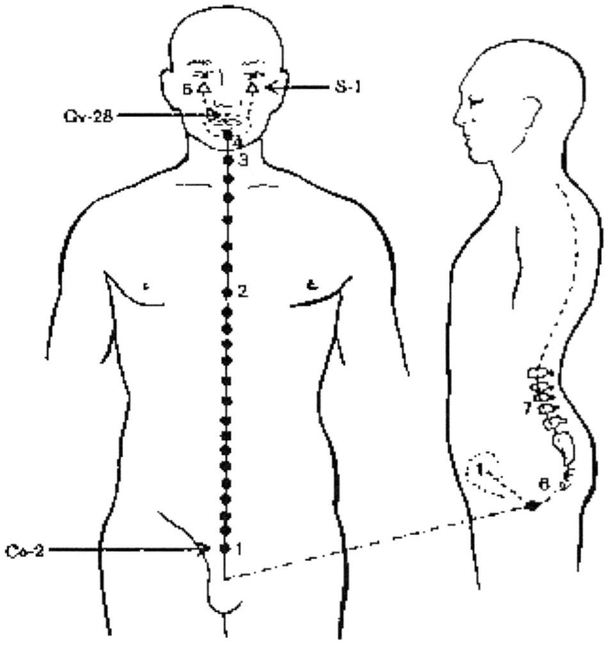

*Course #1:*

(1). Lower abdomen below Qugu (LI-2) -(2). Ascends along the midline of the abdomen and chest - (3). Crosses the throat and jaw (4). winds around the mouth - (5). Terminates in the region of the eye.

*Course #2:*

(6). Pelvic cavity - (7). Enters the spine and ascends along the back.

***This vessel intersects Chengqi (S-1) and Yinjiao (Gv-28).

*Cavities:*

Huiyin (LI-1), Qugu (LI-2), Zhongli (LI-3), Guanyuan (LI-4), Shimen (LI-5), Qihai (LI-6), Abdomen-Yinjiao (LI-7), Shenjue (Co 8), Shuifen (LI-9), Xiawan (LI-10), Jianli (LI-ll), Zhongwan (LI-12), Shangwan (LI-13), Juque (LI-14), Jiuwei (LI-15), Zhongting (LI-16), Shanzhong (LI-17), Yutang (LI-18), Chest-Zigong (LI-19), Huagai (LI-20), Xuanji (LI-21), Tiantu (LI-22), Lianquan (LI-23), and Chengjiang (LI-24).

## The San Jiao Meridian

Note: It is often referred as triple warmer, energizer, heater, burner

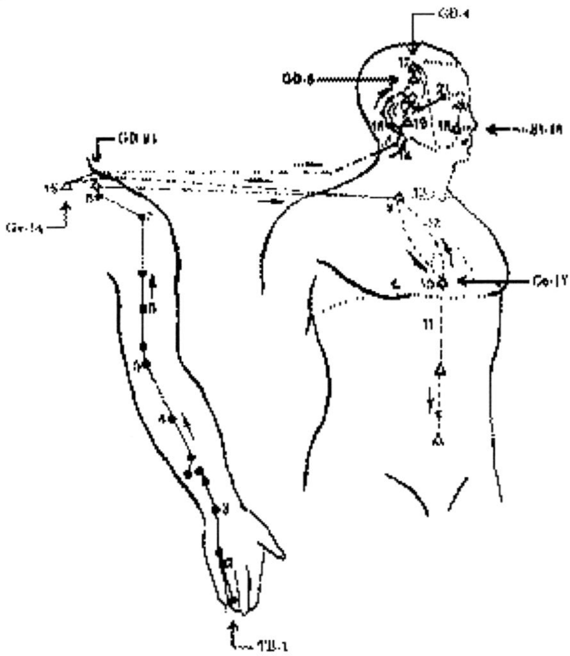

## The Small Intestine Meridian

*Course #1:*

(1). Tip of the digitus minimus (Shaoze, SI-1) - (2). Wrist - (3). Top of elbow - (4). Dorsal surface of the upper arm - (5). Shoulder (6). Circle around the superior and inferior fossa of the scapula - (7). Meets Dazhui (Gv-14)- (8). Enters the supraclavicular fossa - (9). Heart - (10). Passes along the esophagus -(11)Ä Diaphragm - (12). Stomach- (13). Small intestine.

*Course #2:*

(8). Supraclavicular fossa - (14). Neck -(15). Cheek -(16). Tongziliao (GB-1)- (17). Into the ear.

*Course #3:*

(18). Cheek -(19). Jingming (B-1)- (20). Distributes over zygoma obliquely.

*Related Viscera:*

Small intestine (Pertaining Organ), heart, and stomach.

*Cavities:*

Shaoze (SI-1), Qiangu (SI-2), Houxi (SI-3), Hand-Wangu (SI-4), Yanggu (SI-S), Yanglao (SI-G), Zhizheng (SI-7), Xiaohai (SI-8), Jianzhen (SI-9), Naoshu (SI-10), Tianzong (SI-11), Bingfeng (SI-12), Quyuan (SI-13), Jianwaishu (SI-14), Jianzhongshu (SI-15), Tianchuang (SI-16), Tianrong (SI-17), Quanliao (SI-18), Tinggong (SI-19).

## The Spleen Meridian

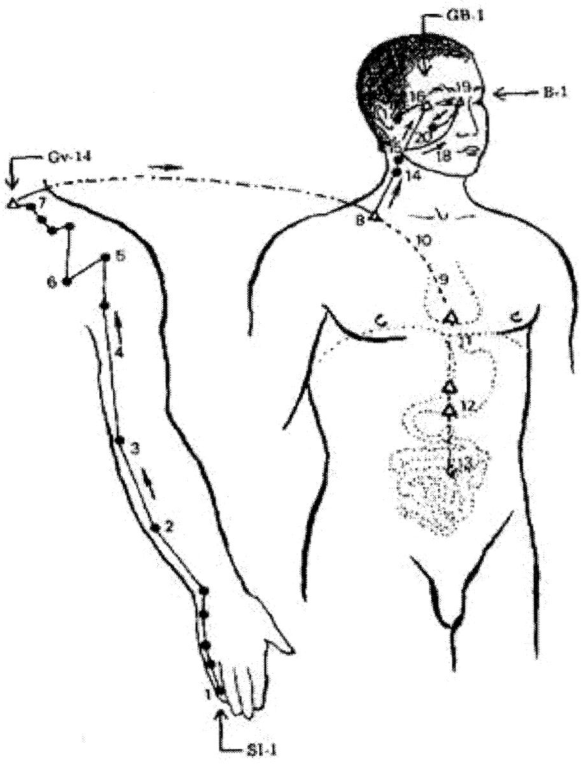

*Course #1:*

(1). Medial tip of the big toe (Yinbai, Sp-l) - (2). Anterior border of the medial malleolus - (3). Along the posterior border of the tibia (4). Medial aspect of the leg - (5). Medial aspect of the art. genus (6). Anterior medial aspect of the thigh - (7). Enter the abdomen - (8). Zhongji (LI-3) and Guanyuan (LI-4)- (9). Pertains to the spleen and communicates with the stomach - (10). Riyue (GB-24) and Qimen (Li-14) - (11). Penetrates the diaphragm through Zhongfu (L-1) - (12). Throat - (13). Root of the tongue.

*Course #2:*

(9). Stomach -(14). Through the diaphragm and disperses into the heart.

*Related Viscera:*

Spleen (Pertaining Organ), stomach, heart, lung, and intestines.

*Cavities:*

Yinbai (Sp-l), Dadu (Sp-2), Taibai (Sp-3), Gongsun (Sp-4), Shangqiu (Sp-S), Sanyinjiao (Sp-G), Lougu (Sp-7), Diji (Sp-8), Yinlingquan (Sp-9), Xuehai (Sp-10), Jimen (Sp-ll), Chongmen (Sp-12), Fushe (Sp-13), Fujie (Sp-14), Daheng (Sp-lS), Fuai (Sp-16), Shidou (Sp-17), Tianxi (Sp-18), Xiongxiang (Sp-19), Zhourong (Sp-20), Dabao (Sp-21).

## The Stomach Meridian

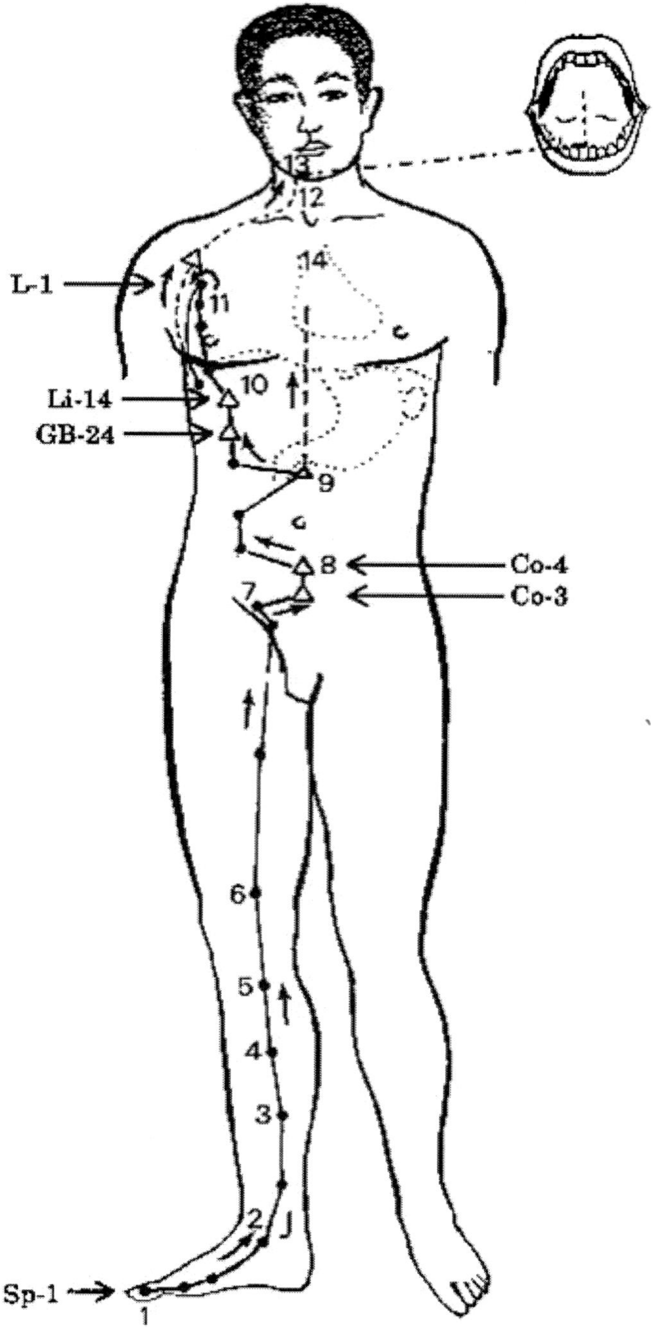

*Course #1:*

(1). Sides of the nose (Yingxiang, LI-20) - (2). Root of the nose (3). Lateral side of the nose - (4). Upper gum - (5). Renzhong (Gv-26) - (6). Chengjiang (LI-24)- (7)- Daying (S-5)- (8). Jiache (S-6)- (9) Ear- (10). Hair line -(11). Shenting (Gv-24).

*Course #2:*

(7). Daying (S-5)- (12)- Renying (S-9)- (13). Throat -(14). Into the chest - (15)- Through the diaphragm to Zhongwan(LI-12).

*Course #3:*

(16). Infraclavicular fossa - (17). Along the sides of the umbilicus - (18). Qichong (S-30). - (19)- Biguan (S-31) - (20)- Futu (S-32)- (21) Dubi (S-35) - (22). Lateral side of tibia - (23). Dorsal aspect of the foot - (24). Lateral side of the tip of the second toe (Lidui, S-45).

*Course #4:*

(25). Below the knee - (26). Lateral side of the middle toe.

*Course #5:*

(27). Dorsum of the foot (Chongyang, S-42) - (28). Along the medial margin of the hallus and emerges out at its tip (Yinbai, Sp-1).

*Related Viscera:*

Stomach (Pertaining Organ), spleen, heart, small large intestine.

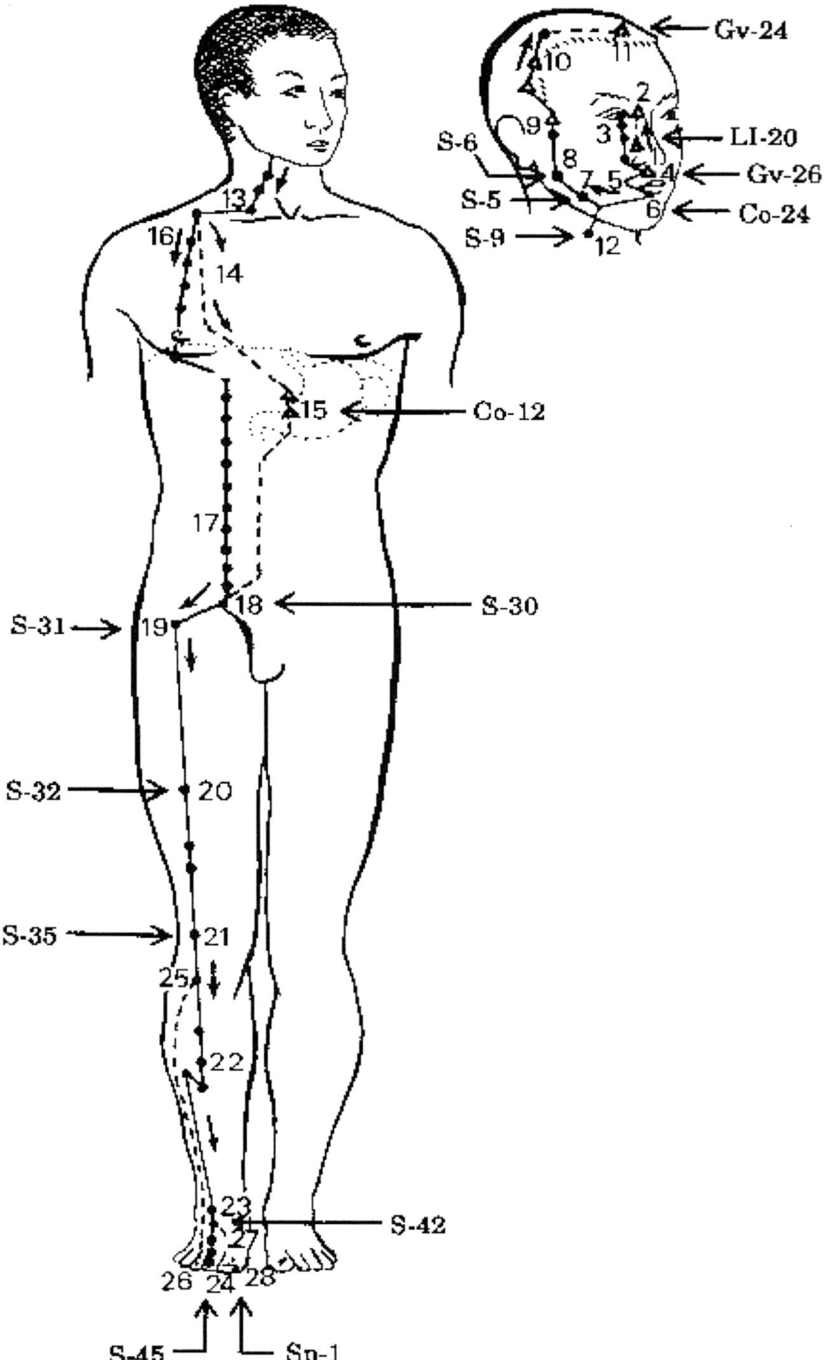

Gv-24
10
11
2
9
3
LI-20
S-6
8
7
5
4
Gv-26
S-5
6
Co-24
S-9
12
13
16
14
15
Co-12
17
18
S-30
S-31
19
S-32
20
S-35
21
25
22
23
S-42
27
26
24
28
S-45
Sp-1

*Cavities:*

Chengqi (S-1), Sibai iS-2), Juliao (S-3), Dicang (S-4), Daying (S-5), Jiache (S-Ci), Xiaguan (S-7), Touwei (S-8), Renying (S-9), Shuitu (S-10), Qishe (S-11), Quepen (S-12), Qihu (S-13), Kufang (S-14), Wuyi (S-15), Yingchuang (S-16), Ruzhong (S-17), Rugen (S-18), Burong (S-19), Chengman (S-21), Liangmen (S-21), Guanmen (S-22), Taiyi (S-23), Huaroumen (S-24), Tianshu (S-25), Wailing (S-26); Daju (S-27), Shuidao (S-28), Guilai (S-29), Qichong (S-30), Biguan (S-31), Futu (S-32), Yinshi (S-33,, Liangqiu (S-34), Dubi (S-35), Zusanli (S-36), Shangjuxu (S-37), Tiaokou (S-38), Xiajuxu (S-39), Fenglong (S-40), Jiexi (S-41), Chongyang (S-42), Xiangu (S-43), Neiting (S-44), Lidui (S-45).

## The Urinary Bladder Meridian

*Course #1:*

(1). Canthus medial -(2). Shenting (Gv-24)- (3). Baihui (Gv-20).

*Course #2:*

(3). Baihui (Gv-20)- (4). Fubai (GB-10), Head-Qiaoyin (GB-11), and Wangu (Head-Wangu, GB-12), etc.

*Course #3:*

(3). Baihui (Gv-20)- (5). Naohu (Gv-17)- (6). Neck -(7). Dazhui (Gv-14) and Taodao (Gv-13) - (8). Lumber region - (9). Kidney - (10). Urinary bladder.

*Course #4:*

(8). Lumbar region - (11). Crosses the buttock -(12). Popliteal fossa.

*Course #5:*

(6). Neck - (13). Medial side ofthe scapula - (14). Lumber region - (15). Lateral side of the thigh - (16). Popliteal fossa - (17). M. gastrocnemius - (18). Pushen (B-61)- (19). The lateral side of the tip of the small toe (Zhiyin, B-67).

*Related Viscera:*

Urinary bladder (Pertaining Organ), kidney, brain, and heart.

*Cavities:*

Jingming (B-1), Zanzhu (B-2), Meichong (B-3), Quchai (B-4), Wuchu (B-5), Chengguang (B-6), Tongtian (B-7), Luogue (B-8),

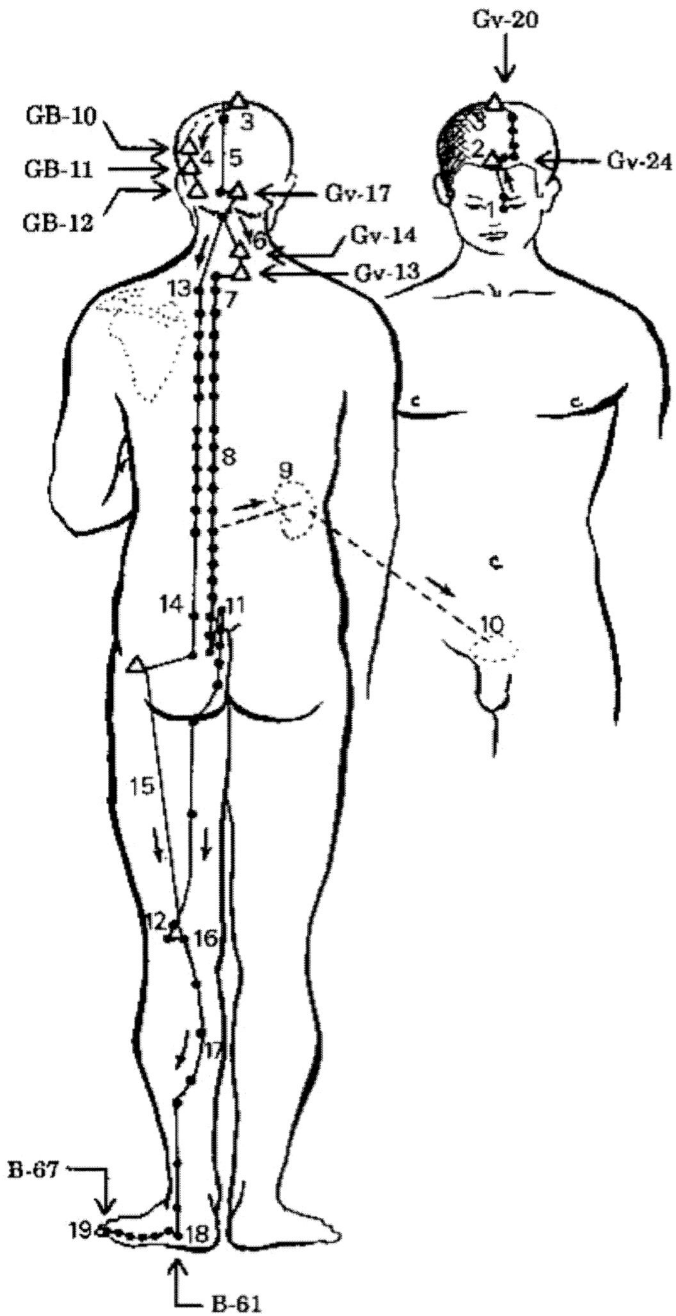
Gv-20
GB-10
GB-11
GB-12
Gv-24
Gv-17
Gv-14
Gv-13
1
2
3
4
5
6
7
8
9
10
11
12
13
14
15
16
17
18
19
B-67
B-61

Yuzhen (B-9), Tianzhu (B-10), Dashu (B-11), Fengmen (B-12), Feishu (B-13), Jueyinshu (B-14), Xinshu (B-15), Dushu (B-16), Geshu (B-17), Ganshu (B-18), Danshu (B-19), Pishu (B-20), Weishu (B-21), Sanjiaoshu (B-22), Shenshu (B-23), Qihaishu (B-24), Dachangshu (B 25), Guanyuanshu (B-26), Xiaochangshu (B-27), Pangguanshu (B 28), Zhonglushu (B-29), Baihuanshu (B-30), Shangliao (B-31), Ciliao (B-32), Zhongliao (B-33), Xialiao (B-34), Huiyang (B-35), Fufen (B 36), Pohu (B-37), Gaohuangshu (B-38), Shentang (B-39), Yixi (B-40), Geguan (B-41), Hunmen (B-42), Yanggang (B-43), Yishe (B-44), Weicang (B-45), Huangmen (B-46), Zhishi (B-47), Baohuang (B-48), Zhibian (B-49), Chengfu (B-50), Yinmen (B-51), Fuxi (B-52), Weiyang (B-53), Weizhong (B-54), Heyang (B-55), Chengjin (B-56), Chengshan (B-57), Feiyang (B-58), Fuyang (B-59), Kunlun (B-60), Pushen (B 61), Shenmai (B-62), Jinmen (B-63), Jinggu (B-64), Shugu (B-65), Foot-Tonggu (B-66), and Zhiyin (B-67).

## The Yang Qiao and Yin Qiao(Heel Vessels) Meridian

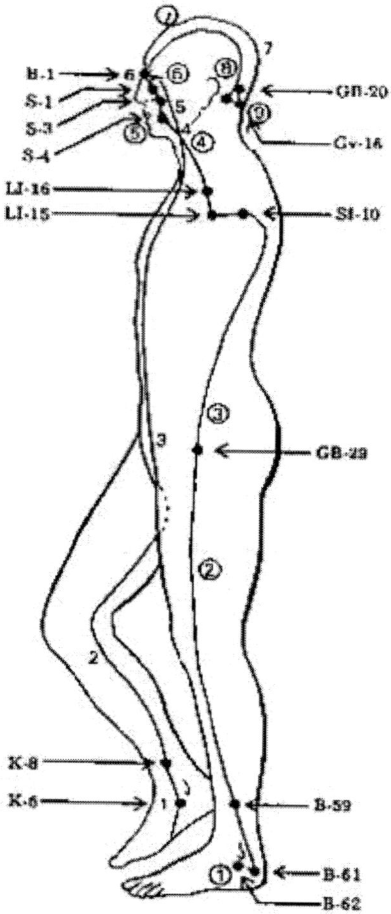

## Yang Qiao

*Course:*

(1). Below the lateral malleolus at Shenmai (B-62) - (2). Ascends along the lateral aspect of the leg - (3). Posterior aspecl; of the hypochondrium - (3). Lateral side of the shoulder - (4). Traverses the neck - (5). Passes beside the mouth -(6). Inner canthus (joins the Yin Heel vessel and the urinary bladder channel) - (7). Ascends across the forehead - (8). Winds behind the ear to Fengchi (GB-20) - (9). Enters the brain at Fengfu (Gv-lG).

***This vessel intersects Shenmai (B-62), Pushen (B-61), Fuyang (B-59), Jingming (B-1), Juliao (GB-29), Fengchi (GB-20), Naoshu (SI-10), Jugu (LI-16), Jianyu (LI-15), Dicang (S-4), Juliao (S 3), Chengqi (S-1), and Fengfu (Gv-16).

## Yin Qiao

*Course:*

(1). Zhaohai (K-6) below the medial malleolus - (2). Extends upward along the medial aspect of the leg - (3). Crossing the per ineum and chest entering the supraclavicular fossa - (4). Ascends through the throat and emerges in front of Renying (S-9)- (5). Traverses the medial aspect of the cheek - (6). Inner canthus (joins the urinary bladder channel and Yang Heel vessels) - (7). Ascends over the head and into the brain.

***This vessel intersects Zhaohai (K-6), Jiaoxin (K-8), and Jingming (B-1)

## The Yang Wei and Yin Wei Meridians

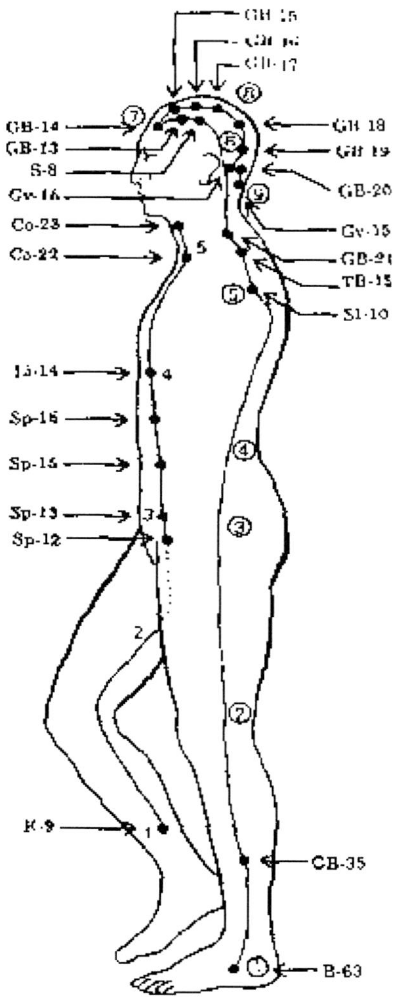

## Yang Wei

*Course:*

(1). Jinmen (B-63) on the heel -(2). Ascends along the lateral aspect of the leg - (3). Lower abdomen - (4). Slants upward across the posterior aspect of the hypochondrium - (5). Across the posterior axillary fold to the shoulder - (6). Ascends the neck and crosses behind the ear - (7). Proceeds to the forehead - (8). Doubles back over the head- (9). Fengfu (Gv-lG).

**"This vessel intersects Jinmen (B-63), Yangjiao (GB-35), Jianjing (GB-21), Fengchi (GB-20), Naokong (GB-19), Chengling (GB-18), Zhengying (GB-17), Muchuang (GB-16), Head-Linqi (GB-15), Yangbai (GB-14), Benshen (GB-13), Tianliao (TB-15), Naoshu (SI-10), Yamen (Gv-lS), Fengfu (Gv-lG), and Touwei (S-8).

## Yin Wei

*Course:*

(1). Lower leg at Zhubin (K-9) - (2). Ascending along the medial aspect of the leg - (3). Enters the lower abdomen - (4). Upward across the chest - (5). Throat (meets Tiantu (LI-22) and Liansuan (LI-23).

"'This vessel intersects Zhubin (K-9), Chongmen (Sp-12), Fushe (Sp- 13), Daheng (Sp- 15), Fuai (Sp-16), Qimen (Li 14), Tiantu (LI-22), and Lianquan (LI-23).

# EAR ACUPUNCUTRE

1. TEETH UPPER JAW
2. MOUTH
3. JAW AND TONSIL
4. TEETH LOWER JAW
5. EYE
6. INNER EAR
7. TEETH LOWER JAW
8. TONSIL
9. INNER EAR
10. FOOT
11. ANKLE
12. KNEE
13. SHENMEN - RELAX
14. WRIST
15. HIP
16. ELBOW
17. PROSTATE
18. GALL BLADDER
19. ZERO - RELAX
20. STOMACH
21. LIVER
22. SHOULDER
23. LUNG AND BRONCHI
24. HEART
25. INTERNAL NOXE
26. TOOTHACHE
27. NECK
28. ADRENAL
29. PINGCHUAN - ASTHMA
30. ENDOCRINE
31. HUNGER
32. LUMBAR VERTEBRAE
33. DIAPHRAGM
34. SUBCORTEX
35. TRIPLE WARMER
36. LARGE INTESTINE
37. SYMPATHETIC
38. EXTERNAL GENITALIA
39. UTERUS
40. KIDNEY

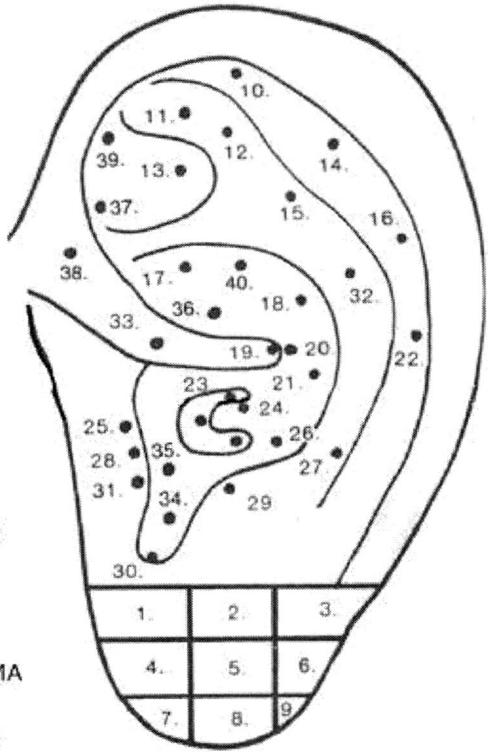


Use the same Tonify (+) Disperse (-) setting as indicated for the body points for the particular condition.

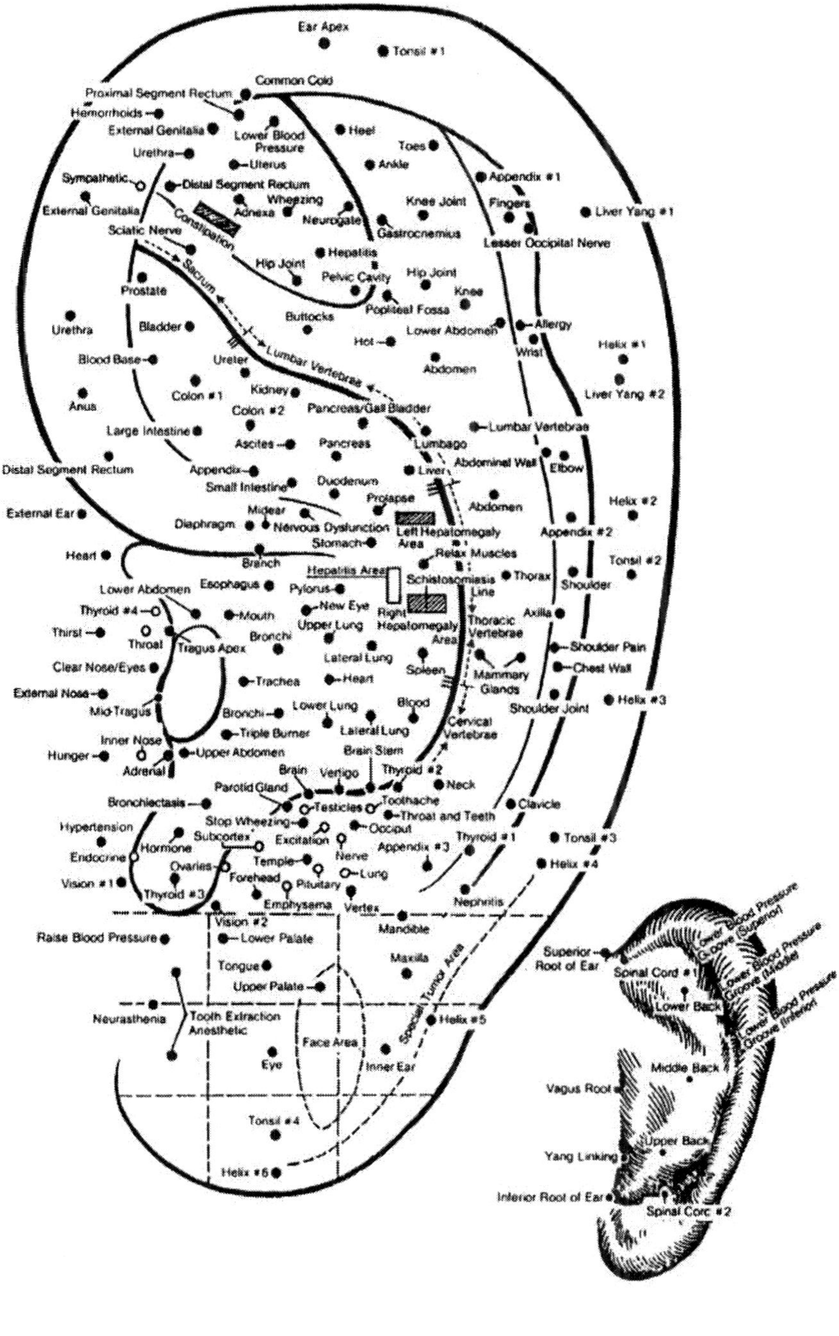
Ear Apex
Tonsil #1
Common Cold
Proximal Segment Rectum
Hemorrhoids
External Genitalia
Lower Blood Pressure
Heel
Toes
Urethra
Uterus
Ankle
Sympathetic
Distal Segment Rectum
Appendix #1
External Genitalia
Wheezing
Adnexa
Neurogate
Knee Joint
Fingers
Liver Yang #1
Sciatic Nerve
Constipation
Gastrocnemius
Lesser Occipital Nerve
Hepatitis
Hip Joint
Pelvic Cavity
Hip Joint
Sacrum
Prostate
Knee
Popliteal Fossa
Buttocks
Urethra
Bladder
Allergy
Lower Abdomen
Hot
Wrist
Helix #1
Blood Base
Ureter
Lumbar Vertebrae
Abdomen
Colon #1
Kidney
Liver Yang #2
Anus
Colon #2
Pancreas/Gall Bladder
Large Intestine
Lumbar Vertebrae
Ascites
Pancreas
Lumbago
Distal Segment Rectum
Appendix
Liver
Abdominal Wall
Elbow
Small Intestine
Duodenum
Prolapse
Abdomen
Helix #2
External Ear
Midear
Diaphragm
Nervous Dysfunction
Left Hepatomegaly Area
Appendix #2
Stomach
Heart
Branch
Relax Muscles
Tonsil #2
Hepatitis Area
Schistosomiasis Line
Thorax
Shoulder
Lower Abdomen
Esophagus
Pylorus
Thyroid #4
Mouth
New Eye
Right Hepatomegaly Area
Thoracic Vertebrae
Axilla
Thirst
Throat
Tragus Apex
Bronchi
Upper Lung
Lateral Lung
Shoulder Pain
Clear Nose/Eyes
Spleen
Mammary Glands
Chest Wall
Trachea
Heart
External Nose
Lower Lung
Blood
Shoulder Joint
Helix #3
Mid-Tragus
Bronchi
Lateral Lung
Cervical Vertebrae
Inner Nose
Triple Burner
Hunger
Adrenal
Upper Abdomen
Brain Stem
Brain
Vertigo
Thyroid #2
Neck
Parotid Gland
Toothache
Bronchiectasis
Testicles
Throat and Teeth
Clavicle
Stop Wheezing
Occiput
Hypertension
Subcortex
Excitation
Thyroid #1
Tonsil #3
Hormone
Nerve
Appendix #3
Endocrine
Temple
Ovaries
Lung
Helix #4
Vision #1
Forehead
Pituitary
Thyroid #3
Emphysema
Vertex
Nephritis
Vision #2
Mandible
Raise Blood Pressure
Lower Palate
Tongue
Maxilla
Special Tumor Area
Upper Palate
Neurasthenia
Tooth Extraction Anesthetic
Helix #5
Face Area
Eye
Inner Ear
Tonsil #4
Helix #6
Superior Root of Ear
Spinal Cord #1
Lower Blood Pressure Groove (Superior)
Lower Blood Pressure Groove (Middle)
Lower Blood Pressure Groove (Inferior)
Lower Back
Middle Back
Vagus Root
Upper Back
Yang Linking
Inferior Root of Ear
Spinal Cord #2

*Chapter Fourteen*

# Therapeutics of Common Ailments

To give emphasis on treatment listed below tne names of acupuncture points to be penetrated against each malady.

**Acute Sinusitis**

DU 20, G.B.14, Ex 3, S.I.18, L.I.4

Infection: DU 14, L.I.11, SP 6

Allergy: SP10

**Rhinitis**

DU 20, DU 24.5(Ex 1), L.I. 4, L..I.20, LU 7

Allergy: SP10

Blocked Nose: L.I.19, St 3, DU 23

Nose Bleeding: L.I.19, DU 23, DU 25, DU 26, U.B. 17, LU 9, LU 6

**Common Cold**

DU 14, DU 20, G.B.20, L.I. 4

Headache: St 8, Ex 2

Blocked Nose: L.I.19

Nasal Discharge: Ex 1, L.I. 20

Allergy: SP 20

Sore Throat: LU 11

Fever: DU 14, L.I.11

Cough: LU 7

**Acute Bronchitis**

LU 5, L..I.4

Fever: L.I.4, DU14, L.I.11, SP 6

Sore Throat: S.I.17

Chest Pain: LU 6

Excessive Sputum: St 40

Seasonal Attack/Allergy: SP 10, DU 14, Ren 6, St 36, SP 6

**Bronchial Asthma**

Ren 17, Ren 22, LU 6, S.I. 6, K 7, DU 20

Pain in Chest with Cough: LU 1

Excessive Sputum: St 40

Allergy: SP 10

Blocked Nose: L.I.19

**Acute Conjunctivitis**

DU 20, Ex 2, U.B.1,S.J.23, St 1, G.B.1, G.B.20, L.i.4, Liv 3

Immune Enhancing Points: DU14, L.I.11, SP 6

**Myopia**

DU 20, St 1, Ex 4, Ex 7, U.B.1,G.B.1, G.B.20, G.B.37,l.I.4, L.I.5, S.I.6

## *Chapter Fifteen*

# Therapeutics of Common Ailments

Suggested Points against disease conditions are given below:

**Retinitis**

DU 20, St 1, Ex 2, Ex 4, U.B. 2, U.B. 18, G.B. 14, G.B.37, L.I.4, L.I.5, S.I.6, SP 6, Liv 3

**Cataract**

DU 20, St 1, Ex 2, Ex 4, G.B. 14, U.B. 2, L.I. 4, L.I. 11, Liv 3

**Toothache, Post- Extraction Pain**

DU 20, L.I. 4, L.I. 20, S.I. 18, St 5, St 6, St 7, St 44, Ren 24, Ah-Shi Points

**Gingivitis**

DU 14, DU 20, DU 28, Ex 10, L.I. 4, L.I. 11

Allergy: SP 10

**Pharyngitis**

DU 14, DU 20, S.I. 17, Ren 23, K 3, L.I.4, L.I. 11, SP 6

**Spasms of the Esophagus and Cartia**

St 34, St 36, P 6, Ren 12, U.B. 21

**Hiccough**

DU 20, DU 26, Ren 17, Ren 22, P6, St 36

**Gastroptosis**

DU 20, L.I.4, U.B.21, P 6, SP 4, SP 6, SP 15, St 34

**Gastritis**

DU 20, U.B.21, St 25, St 34, St 36, Ren 12, P 6, SP 6

Fever: DU 14

Diarrhoea: St 37, St 39, SP 4

Flatulence: Liv 13, G.B.25, G.B. 26

**Frogen Shoulder/Tennis Elbow**

DU 20, L.I. 4, L.I. 10, L.I.11,L.I. 15, L.U. 5,Ex 10, P 3, H 3, S.I. 9, Sj 14, St 38,

Ah-Shi points

**Gastric Hyperacidity**

DU 20, St 36, St 44, P 6, U.B.21, SP 6

**Duodenal Ulcer**

DU 20, St 21, St 25, St 36, U.B.20, U.B.21, Ren 12, P 6, SP 6

**Colitis**

U.B.25, Ren 6, St 25, St 36

**Bacilliary Dysentery**

DU 14, DU 20, St 25, St 36, St 37, SP4, SP 6, L.I. 4,L.I. 11

**Constipation**

DU 20, St 25, St 36, Sj 6, Ren 12

**Diarrhoea**

DU 14, DU 20, St 25, St 36, St 37, Ren 3, Ren 6, L.I. 11, SP 4, SP 6

**Paralytic Ileus**

DU 14, U.B. 25, U.B. 27, L.I. 11, SP 6, P 6, Ren 4, Ren 12, St 25, St 32, St 36

**Headache and Migraine**

DU 20, DU 23, G.B. 14, G. B. 34, Ex 1, Ex 2, Ex 6, St 8, St 44, H 9, Ah-Shi Points

**Trigeminal Neuralgia**

DU 20, Du 26, St 2, St 3, St 4, St 6, St 7, St 44, L.I. 4, L.I. 20, Ex 2, Ex 5, G.B. 14,

U.B. 2, S.I. 18, Sj 5, Ah-Shi Points

**Facial Palsy**

DU 20, St 3, St 4, St 5, St 6, St 7, G.B. 1, G.B. 14, G.B. 34, Ex 2, Ex 3, Ex 5, Ex 6,

S.I. 18, L.I. 4

## Obesity

1. Concentrate on 'Appetite Control' ear point. This appetite control point can help one avoid overeating. Begin the session stimulating this point for 3 minutes everyday.

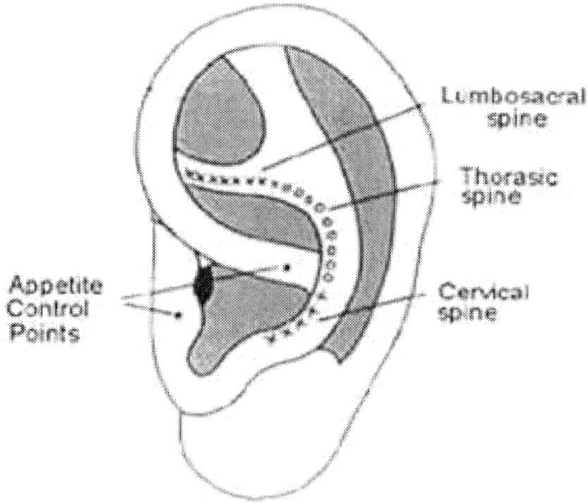


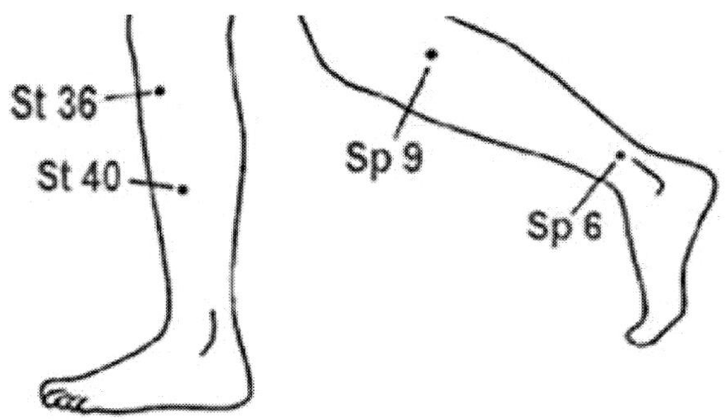


2. Spleen 6 (Sp 6) has a strengthening effect on the digestive system. Stimulate this point for about a minute.

*Caution:* Do not press this point if you are pregnant.

3. Stomach 36 (St 36) is the best point to nourish the chi and blood. It has a beneficial effect on the digestive system. Using moderate stimulation, hold for about one minute.

4. Spleen 9 (Sp 9) this point is involved with the regulation of water metabolism in the body.
5. Stomach 40 (St 40) An important point for clearing excess damp and phlegm. It is also useful for eliminating excess weight.
6. Large Intestine 11 (Li 11) is useful for clearing excess heat and damp from the body and to regulate intestinal activity.

   Li 11 stimulate for about a minute, then switch arms.
7. Liver 3 (Lv 3) prevents chii stagnation in the body and is the most important point for combating stress.

Lv 3 Start with light pressure, as this point can be sensitive, and increase as much as you can until you are using moderate to firm pressure. Press for about 1 minute.

*Pareses following a Stroke*

DU 20, Ex 5, Ex 6, St 4, St 5, St 6, St 7, St 36, L.I. 4, L.I. 10, G.B. 34

Aphasia: Ren 23, S.I. 17, H 5, L.I. 4

Upper Limb: L.I. 11, L.I. 25, Sj 3, Sj 4, Sj 14, Ex 28

Lower Limb :St 31, St 32, St 37, St 39, St 41, St 44, G. B. 30, G. B. 37, G. B. 40, SP 6,

SP 9, K 6, Ren 5, Ren 9, U. B. 20

*Peripneral Neuropathies*

Du 20, Ex 6, St 36, G. B. 34, U. B. 37

*Sequelae of Poliomyelities*

Upper Limb :L.I. 6, L. I. 11, L. I .15, S.I. 6, S.I. 10, Sj 5, L.I. 4, P 6, H 3, H 7

Lower Limb : U.B 40, U.B. 54, U.B. 57, U.B. 60, G.B. 31, G B 34, G. B. 39, St 32, St 36, St 37, St 41, K 3, SP 6

Abdominal Area : U.B. 20, U.B. 21, St 21, St 25, L.I. 11, G.B. 34

*Meniere's Disease*

DU 20, Sj 3, Sj 5, Sj 21, S.I. 6, S.I. 19, G.B. 2, G.B. 41, Liv 3, L.I. 4

Travel sickness related nausea and vomiting: St 36, P 6

*Neuralgic Bladder Dysfunction*

DU 3, DU 20, U.B. 23, U.B. 28, U.B. 32, U.B. 40, U.B. 54, U.B. 60, SP 6, SP 9, Ren 2,

Ren 3, Ren 4, St 29, St 36, H 7, K 3

*Nocturnal Enuresis*

DU 20, U.B. 23, U.B. 28, U.B. 32, U.B. 40, U.B. 62, Ren 3, Ren 4, Ren 6, St 36, SP 6,

H 7, K 3

*Intercostal Neuralgia*

DU 20, G.B. 34, Liv 3, Sj 5, Ex 6

*Cervicobrachial Syndrome*

DU 20, G.B. 20, G.B. 29,G.B. 34, L.I. 4, L.I. 11, Ex 11

*Sciatica*

U.B. 25, U.B. 40, U.B. 57, G.B. 34, G.B. 39, Ex 11

*Low Back Pain*

DU 3, DU 4, U.B. 23, U.B. 25, U.B. 40, S.I. 6, Ex 11

*Osteoarthritis*

Shoulder joint: L.I.11, L.I. 15, L.I. 16, Sj 5, Sj 14, G.B.34, S.I. 10, St 38, U.B. 57

Elbow joint:L.I. 11, L.I. 13, LU 5, G.B. 34, Sj 5, H 3

Wrist joint:L.I. 4, L.I. 11, S.I. 6, P 6, P 7

Finger joints:L.I. 4, L.I. 11, P 6, Ex 12, Ah-Shi Points

Hip joint: G.B. 29, G.B. 30, G.B.34, U.B. 40

Knee joint: St 34, St 35, G. B. 33, G.B. 34, SP 6, Sp 10, U.B. 40

Ankle joint: G.B. 34, G.B. 39, St 41, SP 6, U.B. 60

Toe joints: G.B. 34, St 36, St 41, U.B. 60, Ex 17, Ah-Shi Points

## *Chapter Sixteen*

# Infertility, Impotence and Acupuncture

There are many couples facing infertility problems, infertility actually strikes 1 in every 6 couples, some due to ovulation problems, infections or abnormalities in the female genitalia besides there are some psychological issues as well.

Most cases of undiagnosed infertility that do not respond to modern medicine may benefit from Traditional Chinese Medicine and Acupuncture.

Traditional Chinese Medicine looks at human reproductive system differently than modern medicine and by using diagnostic tools, traditional Chinese medicine can figure out what is the cause of imbalance and correct the problem. When dealing with infertility , acupuncture, herbs and dietary changes, a couple can increase overall health and improve quality of life, thereby bettering the chances of conceiving a baby. For a number of women, incorporating acupuncture traditional Chinese medicine positive results have been achieved.

One of the main causes of infertility is stress and psychological issues which contributes to unexplained infertility. Stress and psychological issues result in hormonal imbalances and prevent the flow of qi or energy within the body. By using acupuncture it is believed a woman can release qi and improve her chances of being able to conceive.

There are different reasons for female infertility, sometimes the reason is hormonal dysfunction or certain infections of reproductive organs, and many cases the exact reason is unknown. In some cases of female infertility acupressure can help.

Acupressure is actually a blend of acupuncture and pressure – a complementary medicine technique derived from acupuncture. In this technique a physical pressure is applied to acupuncture points by the hand, elbow, or with various devices.

*Constitutional Deficiency* - women with congenital meridian channel deficiencies which may have arisen from being born prematurely or having had an unhealthy mother.

*Excessive Sexual Activity* - particularly around puberty, but also in women who have had multiple child births a/or chronic deficiencies of Jing and blood can lead to malnourishment of the Bao Mai and Uterus.

*Cold or Damp* - may arise from Ying- Yang Deficiency or chronic exposures to cold/damp during menstruation can disrupt the Uterus.

Stagnations of Qi or Blood, possibly with Phlegm or damp can block the Uterus.

*Differentiation:*

Excess Pathologies

Cold in the Uterus

Blood Stagnation with Phlegm (blocked fallopian tubes fall under this differentiation)

Deficient Pathologies

Ying- Yang Deficiency

Blood Deficiency

Cold in the Uterus - Excess Condition

**Signs & Symptoms:**

Patient will likely appear pale, delayed menstruation w/dark dilute flow, pain or coldness of the lower abdomen which improves with the application of heat, aversion to cold, cold limbs, may also have weak back or knees and or profuse clear urination. Clinical indications are:

Tongue: Pale

Pulse: Deep, slow

*Suggested points:*

CV 5 - TH Mu, warm the uterus

CV 2 - warm the Uterus

CV 4 - tonify Qi

GV 4 - tonify Yang

KD 3 - tonify KD

CV 2 - warm the Uterus

CV 4 - tonify Qi

GV 4 - tonify Yang

KD 7 - tonify KD Yang

UB 23 - KD Shu

*Blood Stagnation with Phlegm - Excess Condition*

**Signs & Symptoms:**

Patient is likely to be overweight, irregular menstruation w/ clotting, delayed most likely, chest a/or hypochondriac distention, irritability, palpitation, dizziness, profuse sticky leucorrhea.

Tongue: White greasy coat with purple spots

Pulse: Deep, wiry

**Treatment Points:**

*Suggested points:*

CV 3 - resolve damp in lower abdomen

ST 30 - regulate menstruation

KD 13 - important point for infertility, influence chong mai

ST 40 - resolve phlegm

SP 6 - tonify SP, move lower abdomen

If discharge - SP 9

If profuse leucorrhea - UB 32

If hesitant flow - SP 8

Chest/hypochondriac distention - LV 3 w/PC 6

*Suggested points:*

CV 3 - resolve damp in lower abdomen

Zigong Xue - infertility

ST 28 - excess damp in the lower warmer

SP 9 - resolve damp

SP 6 - tonify SP

CV 9 - move stagnant water

LU 7 w/KD 6 - yin qiao ren mai

ST 30 - regulate menstruation

KD 14 - influence chong mai

UB 32 - move excesses in the lower warmer

TH 5 w/GB 41 - yang wei dai mai

**Treatment for Blocked Fallopian Tubes**

Use electrical stimulation from positive CV 4 to negative UB 32

**KD Yang Deficiency**

**Signs & Symptoms:**

Irregular menstruation with scanty pinkish Blood, weak back and or knees, fatigue, dizziness.

Tongue: Thin white coat

Pulse: Deep, thin, particularly weak in the ying yang position

*Suggested points:*

UB 23 - KD Shu

KD 13 - important point for infertility, influence the chong mai

KD 2 - fire point, usually used to disperse empty fire rising causing sore throat, may be used with moxa to strengthen and warm the Uterus

KD 3 - tonify KD

CV 4 - tonify Qi, Blood and Yin

**If dizziness a/or tinnitus** - TH 17

**If weak back a/or knees** - KD 10

*Suggested points:*

KD 13 - important point for infertility, influence the chong mai

KD 3 - tonify KD

UB 23 - KD Shu

UB 52 - tonify psycho-emotional aspects of the KD

KD 6 with LU 7 - yin qiao ren mai

CV 8 - strongly tonify Yang

CV 4 - tonify Yang

GV 4 - tonify Yang

**KD Yin Deficiency**

*Signs & Symptoms:*

Irregular menstruation, sore back, constipation, mallor flush, night sweats, heat in the 5 palms, insomnia, dry throat, dizziness, vertigo

Tongue: Red with or without coat

Pulse: Floating, empty, rapid

**Suggested points:**

CV 4 - tonify Yin

CV 7 - influence chong mai

KD 3 - tonify KD

KD 13 - important point for infertility - influence chcng mai

LU 7 with KD 6 - yin qiao ren mai

SP 6 - tonify Yin

UB 52 - strengthen will power or life force

**Blood Deficiency**

*Signs & Symptoms:*

Delayed menstruation w/scanty, pinkish flow, emaciation, sallow complexion, fatigue, dizziness, may also have palpitations a/or insomnia if HT Blood is deficient

Tongue: Pale, possibly swollen

Pulse: Deep, thin, weak

**Suggested points:**

CV 4 - tonify Yin & Blood

KD 13 - important point for infertility, influence the chong mai

Zigong Xue - infertility

SP 6 - tonify SP

ST 36 - tonify ST/SP

UB 18 - LV Shu

UB 20 - SP Shu

If signs of hot Blood - SP 10

If insomnia/palpitations - HT 7

If dizziness - GV 20

**Suggested points:**

Points as above plus the following

UB 23 - KD Shu

UB 17 - hui meeting of the Blood, instead of UB 18 above

There are specific points on the body (shown on the pictures) that can help balance hormonal dysfunction naturally, which can in some cases lead to normalization of hormonal status and woman can completely avoid taking any medications for hormonal stabilization.

Acupuncture can be used in fertility problems and can also be used to relieve menstrual pain, support the sexual reproductive system, and to detoxify the body. Applying acupuncture on specific points increases blood circulation to the reproductive organs and increases oxygenation to the tissues. Often the blockage is caused by the presence of toxins that accumulate as a result of poor diet, medications, stress, and poor sleep. In such conditions, the hormonal balance within the body is compromised leading to poor ovulation cycles.

Acupuncture can improve your chances of conceiving because it stimulates blood flow to the reproductive organs and releases toxins, congestion and inflammation, hormonal regulation and balance, while stimulating ovulation and helping oxygenate the uterus in preparation for pregnancy.

Symptoms of stagnation of the liver are often associated with infertility in Traditional Chinese Medicine. If you suffer from PMS, irregular cycles, headaches before your period, cold hands and feet, mood swings, low energy, one may benefit from using acupressure.

For female infertility, acupuncture promotes a smooth menstruation and facilitates the conception process.

Started generally on the 14 th day of a woman's menstrual cycle, on selected points of guan-yuan & xie -hai, apply fine needles with a reinforcing technique; needle retention is for 3 to 5 minutes, once every four days. This is applied for all types of infertility.

On selected points of he-gu, san-yin-jiao, zhong-ji, zi-gong & nei-ting, apply fine needles and use a rotation method in insertion. Reinforcing technique is applied in he-gu and san-yin-jiao especially. Needles are manipulated until the arrival of qi (deqi) , as opposed to using needle retention of a certain time and repeat this process once every four days. This is applied for infertility associated with menstrual problems.

On selected points are ge-yu, di-ji, xie-hai, san-yin-jiao, guan-yuan, zhong-ji & zi-gong, apply fine needles using an even technique for 15 minutes of needle retention time on the abdominal points , this should be done once every four days for functional infertility.

On selected points of guan-yuan, zi-gong, zhong-ji, qi-hai & shi-men, apply fine needles by even technique until arrival of qi (deqi). Needle retention lasts for one hour on each of the points once every four days, this is applied for infertility due to an inverted uterus.

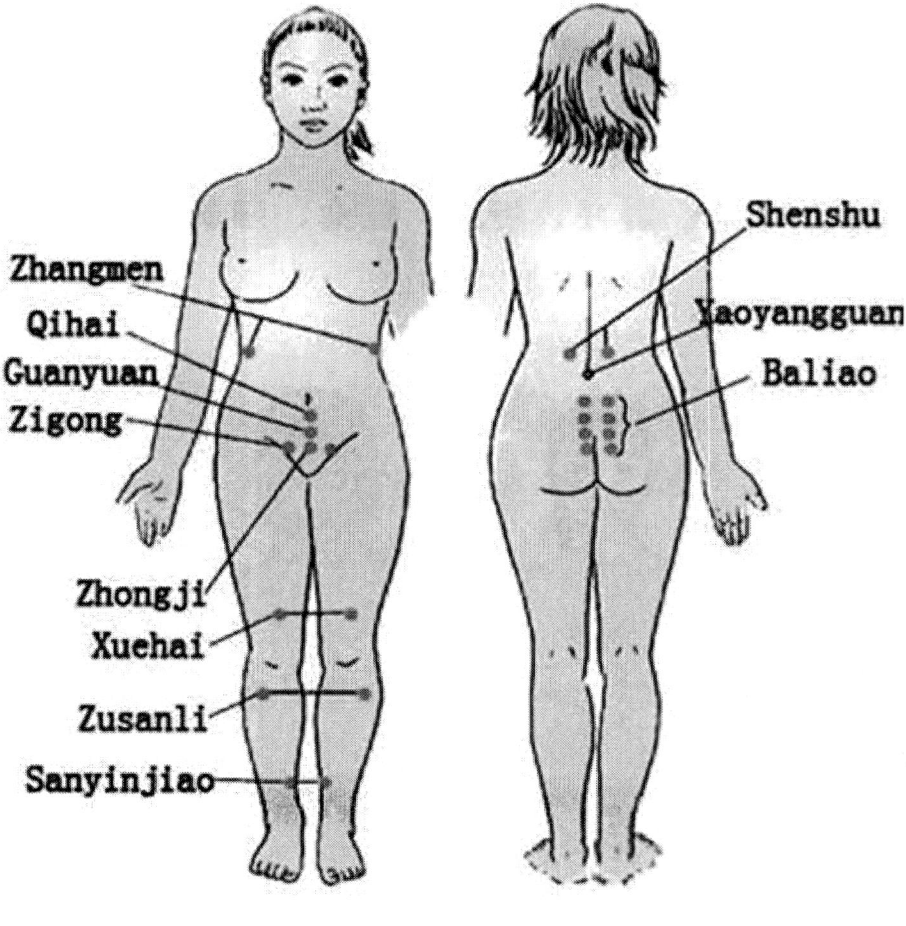
Zhangmen
Qihai
Guanyuan
Zigong
Zhongji
Xuehai
Zusanli
Sanyinjiao
Shenshu
Yaoyangguan
Baliao

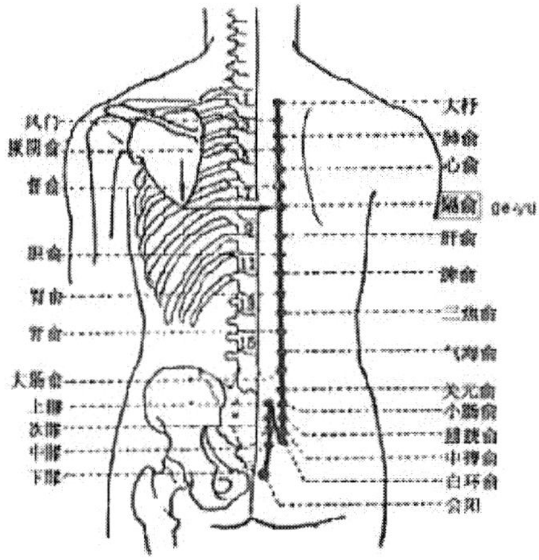
风门
厥阴俞
督俞
胆俞
胃俞
肾俞
大肠俞
上髎
次髎
中髎
下髎
大杼
肺俞
心俞
膈俞 ge-yu
肝俞
脾俞
三焦俞
气海俞
关元俞
小肠俞
膀胱俞
中膂俞
白环俞
会阳

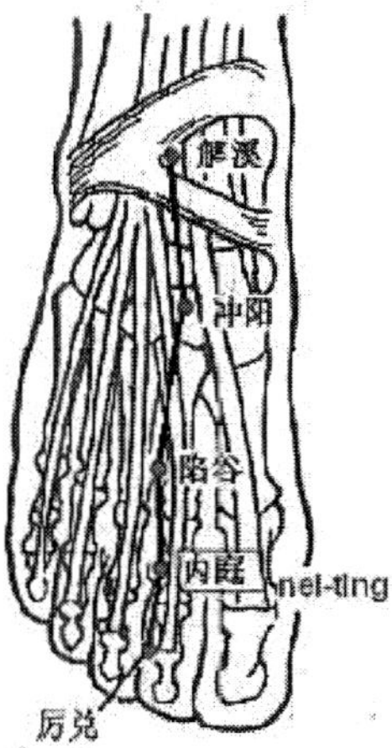
解溪
冲阳
陷谷
内庭 nei-ting
厉兑

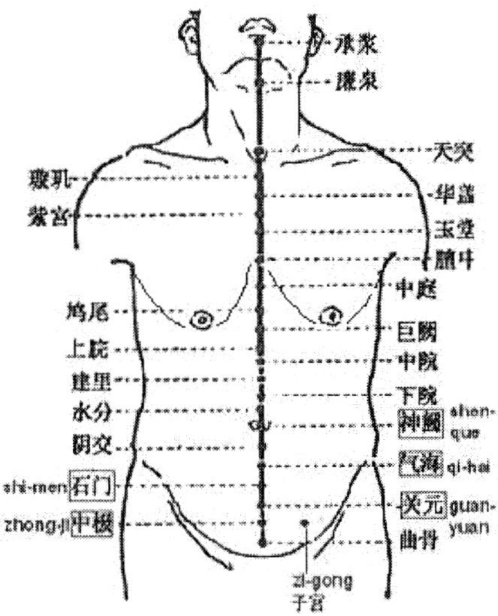
承浆
廉泉
天突
璇玑
紫宫
华盖
玉堂
膻中
中庭
鸠尾
巨阙
上脘
中脘
建里
下脘
水分
神阙 shen-que
阴交
气海 qi-hai
shi-men 石门
关元 guan-yuan
zhong-ji 中极
曲骨
zi-gong
子宫

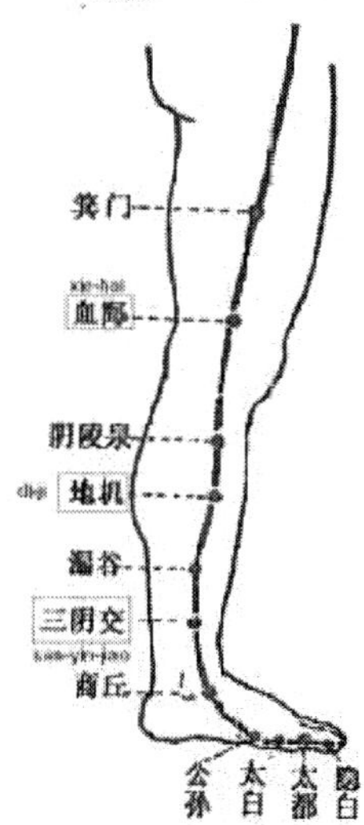
箕门
xie-hai
血海
阴陵泉
diji 地机
漏谷
三阴交
san-yin-jiao
商丘
公孙
太白
太都
隐白

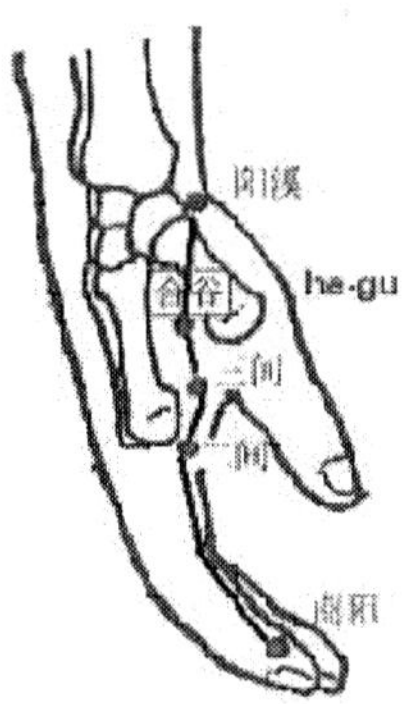
阳溪
合谷 he-gu
三间
二间
商阳

**Kidney Channel**

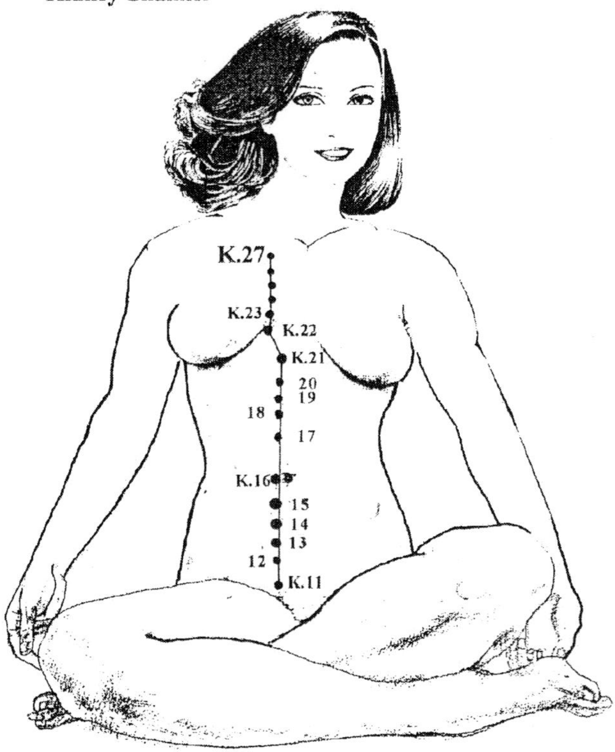

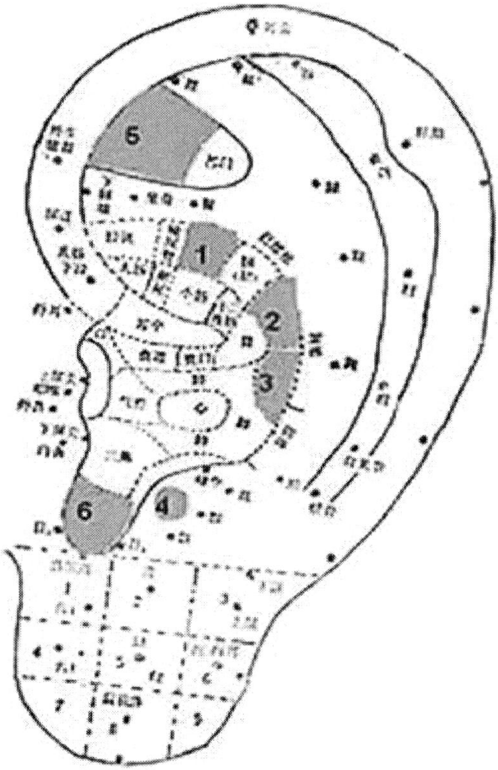


## 2. Auricular Acupuncture Therapy

This involves needling points in the ear that correspond to different organ systems in the body. The ear points can be needled with conventional needles, sometimes, small seeds or specialized "press" needles are used.

The usual selected auricular points for fertility treatment are the kidneys, liver, spleen, ovary, uterus and endocrine system. Each time three to five points are selected and strong stimulation is applied on them.

*Common aural points for infertility*

1. Kidney
2. Uterus
3. Liver

4. Spleen
5. Ovary
6. Endocrine

*Unexplained infertility*

Unexplained infertility is, by definition, when a couple has not conceived after 12 months of intercourse without opting for any contraception methods.

There are many causes of infertility, including the following:

*For the male:*

1. Impaired production and function of sperm, low sperm concentration. Normal sperm concentration is greater than or equal to 20 million sperm per milliliter of semen. A count of 10 million or fewer sperm per milliliter of semen indicates low sperm concentration, and the chances of conception lessen. A count of 40 million sperm or higher per milliliter of semen indicates increased fertility; also, if a sperm changes its shape and mobility or is slow, the sperm may not be able to reach or penetrate the egg.
2. The malfunction of the Hypothalamic-Pituitary-Gonadal Axis: if the axis is not working properly, the male hormone level will be disturbed and the sperm will be both low in count and slow in activity.
3. The testes system, including transportation and maturation.

*For the female:*

1. Fallopian tube damage or blockage.
2. Endometriosis.
3. Ovulation disorders.
4. Early menopause.
5. Polycystic ovary syndrome.
6. Fibroid in the uterine.

Even though there are many women who cannot conceive because of the above reasons, there are also 15 % of couples who cannot conceive due to unexplained reasons.

## Acupuncture Points:

Zhong Ji (Ren 3), Guan Yuan (Ren 4), Gui Lai (Stomach 29), Chong Men (Spleen 12), and Fushe (Spleen 13). This group of acupuncture points adjusts the hormonal level of the entire body. Zhong Ji and Guan Yuan (Ren 3 and Ren 4) directly stimulate the uterus, which makes the uterus muscle very relaxed, and will increase the chance of conception and easy implantation. Stimulation of the point Fushe (Spleen 12), and Chongmen (Spleen 13)both points bilateral and adjacent to the ovary and uterus will directly adjust the ovary's hormonal secretion cycle, in turn increasing the activity of the pituitary, adrenal and ovary axis and increasing the chance of conception. Gui Lai (Stomach 29) is also adjacent to the ovary and uterus, which assists the first four points in adjusting the entire female hormone system.

The second group is on the back eight-liao points.

Eight-liao points (eight points on both sides of the sacral area) directly stimulate the pudendal nerve and the pelvic splanchnic nerve. These nerves will stimulate the uterus and ovaries and help increase the chance of conception, as well as adjust the entire hormonal system of the female reproductive system.

The two groups above of key acupuncture points will be alternatively treated during each day's visit, in addition to the Hegu Large Intestine 4, Quchi Large Intestine 11, San Yin Jiao Spleen 6, Xue Hai Spleen 10 and Tai Chong Liver 3 all of which will help adjust the hormone environment in the entire body and thus aid conception.

## Acupuncture for Male Infertility

Infertility statistics claim that women are unfairly blamed for being responsible for rise in infertility. Several studies show that approximately 40% of infertility problems are caused by male infertility factor such as low sperm count, problems with sperm motility and issues that concern sperm size and shape. Additionally, lifestyle of men and women is another factor that can contribute to increased level of fertility related problems. Approximately 15-20 % of all cohabiting couples are infertile. In 50 % of cases, it is the male factor that is responsible for the infertility (Kumar and Clark 1994).

There are many causes of male infertility, such as:

Infection such as mumps and prostatitis

Physical injury

Exposure to toxic substances or drugs

Varicoceles

Impotence or Libido problem

Impotence means that the penis in adult cannot erect or erect insufficiently for sexual intercourse. According to TCM. impotence is caused by intemperance of sexual Fife and decline of fire in mingmen (gate of life) ; or by over-anxiety that impairs the heart and spleen and leads to as-thenia of the thoroughfare vessel; or by downward migra-tion of damp-heat in the liver and kidney that leads to flac-cidity of the genitalia. Clinically impotence is usually of asthenia syndrome.

*1. Impairment of the heart and spleen*

Frigidity in sexual life, or insufficiency of erection, palpitation and susceptibility to fright, insomnia and am-nesia, lusterless complexion, spiritual lassitude and fa-tigue, shortness of breath and spontaneous sweating, light-colored tongue with white fur, thin and weak pulse.

*2. Decline of fire in mingmen (gate of life)*

Impotence, or premature ejaculation, thin and cold semen, blackish eyelids and complexion, dizziness, cold sensation in the body and spiritual lassitude, aching loins and tinnitus, light-colored tongue, deep and thin pulse.

*3. Downward migration of damp-heat*

Burning sensation in the urinary tract, yellow and scanty urine, profuse whitish secreta from the external orifice of urethra, bitter taste and dryness of mouth, thirst and desire to drink water, retention of dry feces, red tongue, yellow and greasy tongue fur, slippery and rapid pulse.

But in many men there is no apparent cause of the infertility.

In order to achieve the qi, were needles manipulated for approximately 10 minutes, and then they were left in place for another 25 minutes.

*Suggested Acupuncture points:*

Bl23, Bl28, Du4, then St29, St36, Sp6, Ren3 and Ren2

Lu7, Li4, Li11, St30, St36, Sp6, Sp9, Sp10, Ht7, Bl20, Bl23, Bl33, Ki6, Ki7, P6, Lv5, Lv8, Ren1, Ren2, Ren4, Ren6 and Du4.

Specific combinations of the above points may be selected according to the principles of TCM , also the points may be divided up into two broad categories:

1. Deficiency of the kidneys, Ki3, Bl23, Ki11 and Bl52.
2. Damp-heat in the genital system, Sp9, Lv5, Li11, St28, Gb41.

Points for both syndromes are: Sp6, Ren4, Lu7, Ki6, St30.

Some other points that may be used for less common categories of TCM in regard to male infertility are :

Li4, St36, Sp10, Ht7, Bl20, P6, Ren1, Ren2, Ren6, Du4, Du20, Gb20, Lv3, Ki7, Gb27.

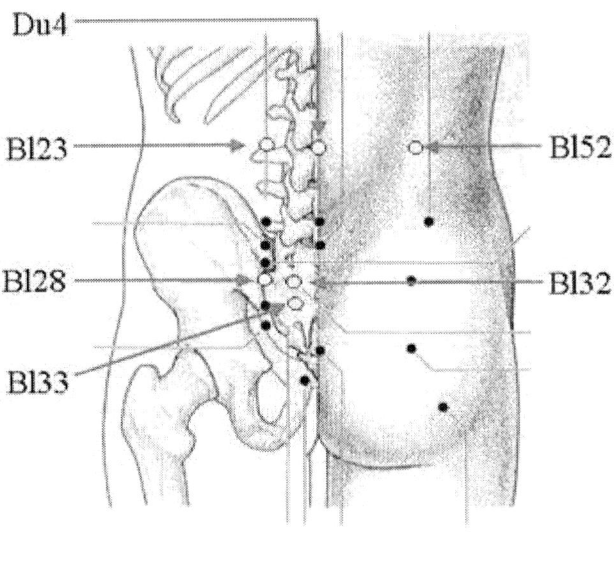


Back Acupuncture points

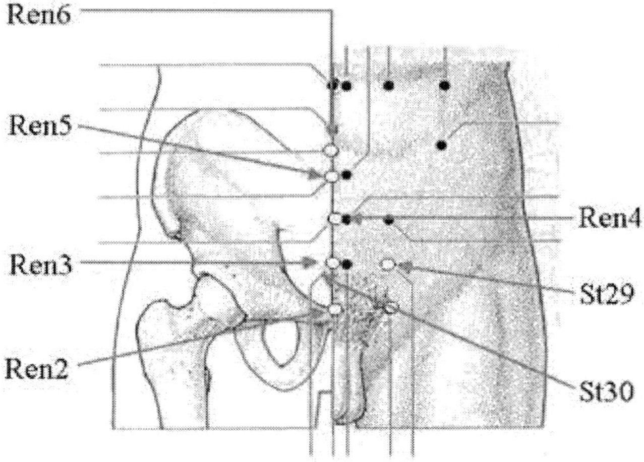


Abdomen Acupuncture points

The following acupuncture points were used as main points: *Guan yuan* (Ren 4), *shen shu* (UB 23, bilateral), *ci liao* (UB 32, bilateral), *tai cong* (Liv 3, bilateral), and *tai xi* (KI 3, bilateral). Secondary points included *zhu san li* (ST 36, bilateral), *xue hai* (SP 10, bilateral), *san yin jiao* (SP 6, bilateral), *gui lai* (ST 29, bilateral), and *bai hui* (Du 20). Needles are to be inserted to a depth of between 15 and 25 millimeters, depending on the region of the body being treated. Needles were manipulated for 10 minutes to achieve *de qi*, then left in place for another 25 minutes before being removed.

Studies indicate that while acupuncture appeared able to improve the overall quality and structural integrity of sperm, it was ineffective against some common sperm pathologies. It has been observed that despite the inability of acupuncture to significantly reduce some sperm abnormalities, the treatment could be used to improve overall sperm quality, leading to the possibility of increased fertility.

## *Chapter Seventeen*

# Acupuncture in Hairfall

For who are facing falling and thinning of hair, is such a very serious problem that not only affects the beauty but has indepth psychological impacts.

Hair loss is caused by various factors such as poor food balance and bad shampoo method. The main causes are heredity and psychological stress. Is there any effective acupressure point for stopping such fallen hair?

In China, it is believed that blood raises hair. The deep black hair is a proof whose blood is abundant because blood carries nutritive substance to hair. So, it is important for the measure against hair loss to improve the flow of the blood of the head first.

The acupuncture point that has an effect in improving the blood circulation of a head is the "Paihui" located in the top of the head. It is believed that stimulating paihui point will help reduce hair loss.

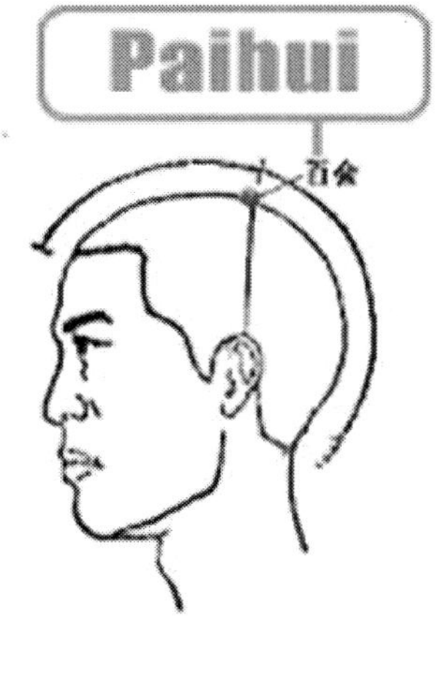

**Paihui**

The "Paihui" is located in the top of the head, at which the extension from a nose crosses the extension top of an ear on either side.

*Stimulation method*

Use slight stimulation on the "Paihui." also stimulate the portion from which hair tends to fall. And finally please give a stimulus uniformly to the whole head. Generally, perform the above method for 2 to 3 minutes, once a day. Extra care is necessary as deep penetration may damage the scalp.

In addition, it is still more effective if "a head massage" is practiced.

*Head massage*

With five fingers of one hand, push the "Paihui" and its surroundings lightly in the vertical direction. It is because many acupuncture points that have an effect to hair loss exist in the surroundings of the "Paihui."

In a study by Y.H.Chang, M.T.Hiseh and C.R.Wu of Department of Acupuncture, China Medical College Hospital, Taichung, Taiwan (1999) it has been observed that acupuncture at Pai-Hui affects the memory storage process and has preventive and immediate therapeutic effects. So it's worth to give it a try after all it has rewarding effects on memory storage.

## *Chapter Eighteen*

# Does Acupuncture Hurts

Acupuncture is an art and science of healing that was developed in China over the last several thousand years and has now become quite popular in the West. It is based on the use of needles inserted into the body as a means of unblocking or harmonizing the flow of chi, or energy, in the body, which forms the basis for both good health and ill health.

"Chi" is energy in the body, or life force, and there are different kinds of chi in the body. The idea is that the needles are put in specific points to affect different systems in the body. Chinese doctors look at the body a little bit differently than Western doctors. Where a Western doctor may look at the physiology of the organs, the Chinese look at the different organs in terms of their jobs, or functions. And there are jobs that the organs do in relation to each other, and the needles will help give the body signals to help the organs do their jobs better and in more harmony to bring a person back to balance.

Chinese doctors and acupuncture practitioners get trained in how to feel the chi in the different channels in the body.

Western science has already noticed that certain acupuncture points have different electrical resistances than areas just around those points, so they know there is something special there. Western science has mapped out currents in the body that are separate from the nervous system current, for example. So they've gotten pieces of it and can explain parts of how it works, but they haven't gotten the whole picture yet from a Western, technological point of view.

As children we get lots of injections, and those needles are much thicker and they're hollow, so they actually tear the skin, and it's much more painful. Acupuncture needles are very thin, some are even hair thin, and often painless.

How deep the needles may go in depends on the area of the body. They can go anywhere from 0.1 cm to two or three inches. For example, you would go deeper into the buttocks than into the chest region.

Look at which functions are not working properly, and which organs or which systems are being affected, choose the needle points based on that information,oneI might use six to ten points, so anywhere from 12 needles or ten needles, depending on the condition of the patient. Then the patient lies in a relaxed position and I put the needles in the points, and the patient stays there for 15 or 20 minutes. During that time, Acupuncturist may leave the room, or may stay in the room and do other things like acupressure and gentle touch therapy just to move the energy, and maybe put on some nice music and dim the lights.

People most often need more than one treatment. A common misconception about acupuncture is that is cures magically. There are a lot of people, especially those with acute problems, who will get a lot of benefit after the first time, but people should really expect to go two, three, four times, typically.

Acupuncture is an invasive technique, and therefore not without risk. Hematoma may result from accidental puncture of any circulatory structure. Nerve injury can result from the accidental puncture of any nerve. Brain damage or stroke is possible with very deep needling at the base of skull. Also rare but possible is pneumothorax from deep needling into the lung, and kidney damage from deep needling in the low back. Needling over an occult sternal foramen (an undetectable hole in the breastbone which can occur in up to 10% of people) may result in a potentially fatal haemopericardium. There are clear warnings in responsible texts on acupuncture regarding both the depth to which needles may be inserted, and with regard to the angle at which needles may be inserted. Both these instructions are clearly intended to prevent acupuncture needles from penetrating the lungs, the abdominal cavity, etc.

Needles that are not properly sterilized can transfer diseases such as HIV and hepatitis. In the United Kingdom, British Acupuncture Council (BAcC) members observe the Code of Safe Practice which lays down stringent standards of hygiene and sterilisation for other equipment - members use single-use pre-sterilised disposable needles, which are permanently withdrawn from service after being used in treatment. Similar standards apply in most jurisdictions in the United States. Needles are sometimes stored in alcohol, but alcohol does not kill the virus causing hepatitis C. Also, acupuncture needles are very thin and can break, making surgical removal necessary. Sometimes, when treating pain or using acupuncture as an anesthetic, a mild electrical current is applied to the needles. This stimulates the nerve cells in the area of the needles so that they become depleted of the chemicals needed to transmit signals (please note this is not an acupuncture effect!). Prolonged stimulation of nerve cells in this way can cause irreversable damage.

Severe injury from acupuncture is extremely rare, but not unheard of. Well-trained, licensed and experienced acupuncturists are less likely to injure a patient. However, in many countries anyone can call himself an acupuncturist, there are no legal requirements with regard to training and education, nor are licensing boards regulated in any way, making it very hard to assess the actual value of licenses and training of acupuncturists. The NIH consensus panel made the following statement about the risks associated with acupuncture: "Adverse side effects of acupuncture are extremely low and often lower than conventional treatments."

Acupuncture involves the insertion of very fine needles through the skin and tissues at specific points on the body. There is no injection of any substance and the treatment itself causes minimal discomfort. "Classical" acupuncture was developed in China as a system of diagnosing and treating pain and disease. It defines acupuncture as one component of Traditional Chinese Medicine which aims to balance energy and blood in the body in order to keep it functional and healthy. Although proven successful for hundreds of years without the benefit of modern medical knowledge, it is only in recent years that the scientific and medical communities of Europe and North America have begun to study acupuncture to understand and explain its effectiveness. "Anatomical" acupuncture refers to a more modern approach taken today by the Acupuncture Foundation of Canada Institute (AFCI) and other western trained acupuncture therapists. When combined with a knowledge of anatomy, physiology, modern therapists can use acupuncture effectively.

Modern technology has allowed variations in acupuncture treatment. Electro-acupuncture involves stimulation of inserted needles with gentle electrical impulses. Rubber electrodes or moistened cotton-tipped applicators can also be used to deliver electrical stimulation to acupuncture points (transcutaneous electrical nerve stimulation or T.E.N.S.). Low power laser may also be used instead of needles to stimulate appropriate points.

Acupuncture stimulates the body to produce its own pain relieving chemicals called "endorphins." These chemicals mimic morphine by attaching to opiate receptor sites found throughout the nervous system. Endorphins help to block pathways that relay pain messages from the body to the brain, resulting in relief of pain, general relaxation and biochemical restoration of the body's own well-being.

Acupuncture is very effective in treating a variety of painful disorders, both acute and chronic.

The World Health Organization has identified the benefits of acupuncture in the treatment of a wide range of medical problems including:

Digestive disorders: gastritis, hyperacidity, spastic bowel, constipation, diarrhea

Respiratory disorders: sinusitis, bronchitis, asthma

Neurological and muscular disorders: headaches, neck and back pain, neuralgia, frozen shoulder, tennis elbow, tendonitis, sciatica, arthritis

Urinary, menstrual and reproductive disorders

Addiction, insomnia

In treating any illness or affliction, a correct diagnosis is important before any decisions are made regarding therapy. Once the diagnosis is established, a qualified practitioner can advise whether acupuncture is appropriate

One of the most striking aspects of acupuncture is the almost complete absence of adverse effects and complications from its use. Most patients find that the treatments are relaxing and cause minimal discomfort.

People with pacemakers should avoid electrical stimulation unless approved by their cardiologist. Women in early pregnancy and haemophiliacs should be treated with caution.

The AFCI recommends that only sterile disposable needles be used, preventing any risk of transmission of the AIDS or hepatitis viruses when sterile disposable needles are used.

People experience differing sensations with acupuncture. Most patients feel only minimal discomfort as the needles are inserted: some feel no pain at all. Once the needles are in place, there should be no significant discomfort.

Acupuncture needles are extremely fine and are made from stainless steel. Two or three needles would fit inside the barrel of a regular hollow needle used for injections.

The number of treatments will vary with each individual and the condition being treated. For acute problems, only a few treatments may be required. In some cases, one treatment will be sufficient.

For complex or longstanding conditions, one or two treatments a week for several weeks may be recommended with less frequent treatment as improvement occurs. Treatment sessions usually last between 15 and 30 minutes. Relief may be immediate or occur within a few hours, or after a few days.In some conditions, several sessions may be required before improvement is noticed Eighty to ninety percent of patients respond well to acupuncture with noticeable improvement. Acupuncture can be used as the only form of therapy or it may be combined successfully with other forms of medical or physical therapy.

Acupuncture is used successfully on cats, dogs, horses and other animals. These animal patients do not understand or believe in the process that helps them get better. A positive attitude towards wellness may reinforce the effects of any type of treatment. A neutral or negative attitude ("I don't know if I really believe in this") will not block the effects of acupuncture.

Is there any special advice to follow before an acupuncture treatment?

Acupuncture treatment can be done at any time. Patients are advised not to eat unusually large meals before or after treatments. It is best to avoid alcohol or sedatives for four hours prior to treatment. Pain medications may be taken as required.

If possible, a short rest after treatment is desirable, but not essential. Some patients feel unusually relaxed and prefer to plan activities accordingly. Strong exercise is not recommended immediately after treatment.

For painful conditions, avoid strenuous activity for 48 hours after treatment. Alcohol, and ideally caffeine and cigarettes, should be avoided for at least two hours. Medication, as directed by your physician, may be taken as required.

Improperly performed acupuncture can cause fainting, local hematoma (due to bleeding from a punctured blood vessel), pneumothorax (punctured lung), convulsions, local infections, hepatitis B (from unsterile needles), bacterial endocarditis, contact dermatitis, and nerve damage. The herbs used by acupuncture practitioners are not regulated for safety, potency, or effectiveness. There is also risk that an acupuncturist whose approach to diagnosis is not based on scientific concepts will fail to diagnose a dangerous condition.

The adverse effects of acupuncture are probably related to the nature of the practitioner's training. A survey of 1,135 Norwegian physicians revealed 66 cases of infection, 25 cases of punctured lung, 31 cases of increased pain, and 80 other cases with complications. A parallel survey of 197 acupuncturists, who are more apt to see immediate complications, yielded 132 cases of fainting, 26 cases of increased pain, 8 cases of pneumothorax, and

45 other adverse results . However, a 5-year study involving 76 acupuncturists at a Japanese medical facility tabulated only 64 adverse event reports (including 16 forgotten needles and 13 cases of transient low blood pressure) associated with 55,591 acupuncture treatments. No serious complications were reported. The researchers concluded that serious adverse reactions are uncommon among acupuncturists who are medically trained.

More recently, members of the British Acupuncture Council who participated in two prospective studies have reported low complication rates and no serious complications among patients who underwent a total of more than 66,000 treatments . An accompany editorial suggests that in competent hands, the likelihood of complcations is small. Since outcome data are not available, the studies cannot compare the balance of risks vs benefit. Nor do the studies take into account the likelihood of misdiagnosis (and failure to seek appropriate medical care) by practitioners who use traditional Chinese methods.

Acupuncture anesthesia is not used for surgery in the Orient to the extent that its proponents suggest. In China physicians screen out patients who appear to be unsuitable. Acupuncture is not used for emergency surgery and often is accompanied by local anesthesia or narcotic medication.

"Chinese medicine," often called "Traditional Chinese Medicine (TCM)," encompasses a vast array of folk medical practices based on mysticism. It holds that the body's vital energy (chi or qi) circulates through channels, called meridians, that have branches connected to bodily organs and functions. Illness is attributed to imbalance or interruption of chi.. Ancient practices such as acupuncture, Qigong, and the use of various herbs are claimed to restore balance.

Traditional acupuncture, as now practiced, involves the insertion of stainless steel needles into various body areas. A low-frequency current may be applied to the needles to produce greater stimulation. Other procedures used separately or together with acupuncture include: moxibustion (burning of floss or herbs applied to the skin); injection of sterile water, procaine, morphine, vitamins, or homeopathic solutions through the inserted needles;

applications of laser beams (laserpuncture); placement of needles in the external ear (auriculotherapy); and acupressure (use of manual pressure). Treatment is applied to "acupuncture points," which are said to be located throughout the body. Originally there were 365 such points, corresponding to the days of the year, but the number identified by proponents during the past 2,000 years has increased gradually to about 2,000 . Some practitioners place needles at or near the site of disease, whereas others select points on the basis of symptoms. In traditional acupuncture, a combination of points is usually used.

Qigong is also claimed to influence the flow of "vital energy." Internal Qigong involves deep breathing, concentration, and relaxation techniques used by individuals for themselves. External Qigong is performed by "Qigong masters" who claim to cure a wide variety of diseases with energy released from their fingertips. However, scientific investigators of Qigong masters in China have found no evidence of paranormal powers and some evidence of deception. They found, for example, that a patient lying on a table about eight feet from a Qigong master moved rhythmically or thrashed about as the master moved his hands. But when she was placed so that she could no longer see him, her movements were unrelated to his. Falun gong, which China recently banned, is a Qigong varient claimed to be "a powerful mechanism for healing, stress relief and health improvements."

# *Chapter Nineteen*

# Related Therapies

**Moxibustion:**

The Chinese ideogram, symbol or character for "acupuncture" is a combination of the characters for "needle" and "moxibustion." While many people have a concept of the needles involved in acupuncture, moxibustion is not as commonly known. Moxibustion is the burning of small cones of mugwort herb (moxa) on or near the skin, usually at acupoints.

Most moxa therapy has been administered by acupuncturists and moxibustionists. But, the long history of moxibustion practiced in Japan includes folk medicine, where the local Zen monk applied moxibustion or family members treated each other. Although Moxibustion is a clinical specialty in Japan today, it is still common to have patients apply some form of moxibustion to themselves or a family member as a form of home therapy.

Moxibustion is often used for chronic conditions. Chinese classic literature states, "Moxibustion tonifies (nourishes) the deficiency of the Source Chi." In stubborn conditions, it can be the only thing that works.

Moxibustion is hot, but the heat can feel very good. After a moxa treatment you feel comfortably warm and refreshed like you just took a bath. You can feel the warmth penetrating into the core of your body.

Acupuncturists frequently use moxibustion at the end of an acupuncture treatment to increase the effectiveness of the treatment. Most treatment protocols in Japanese Acupuncture still include the use of moxa. Occasionally, the practitioner will limit the treatment to moxibustion, no needles.

Moxa stimulates the immune system through the skin in a variety of ways. Moxa cones are placed on the skin and the heat slowly penetrates into the body. The heat first brings an inflammation response to the area. Second, a beneficial chemical contained in the moxa herb has a potent effect on increasing immune cell migration. Third, moxibustion increases regulatory mechanisms to stimulate distant lymph tissues and organs to increase the body's overall immune response. (If you want the details, email me and I'll send you more info).

Moxa stimulation activates a local cascade of effects including an increased circulation of white blood cells. From local stimuli, the effects of moxibustion spread outward throughout the whole body. This results in a definite immunological enhancement.

With its calming heat, acupoint stimulation, and immune system activation, moxibustion has been successfully employed for thousands of years, and has been scientifically shown to be beneficial.

## Cupping

In this process hollow cups made of horn, glass, wood or bamboo are prepared partially air free through burning spirit moistened cotton inside it and then it is attached or applied to the specific points of the body with care, when cooled it automatically holds itself with the body parts through suction.

## Electro Acupuncture

Instead of mechanical stimulation to obtain deqi, electronic stimulators are attached with acupuncture needles to send electronic impulses to obtain improved, painless sensation.

## Acupressure

Instead of insertion of needles pressure is applied by fingers or any blunt sticks on acupuncture points. It has been found useful in stress mamagement, asthma, headache, insomnia,aches and pain, digestive and circulatory disorders.

## Chromotherapy

Application of choosen colours on the acupuncture points also gives fruitful results.

### Hammering

It is a process in which some needles are fitted one end of a stick and mild strokes are applied on the skin especially on ah-shi points or large joints.

### Hydrotherapy

Hydrotherapy is probably of Chinese origin, since cold baths were used for fevers as early as 180 BC. The inoculation of smallpox matter, in order to produce a mild but immunizing attack of the disease, was practiced in China from ancient times and came to Europe about 1720.

### Holistic Medicine

A doctrine of preventive and therapeutic medicine that emphasizes the necessity of looking at the whole person—his body, mind, emotions, and environment—rather than at an isolated function or organ and which promotes the use of a wide range of health practices and therapies. It has especially come to stress responsibility for "self-healing," or "self-care," by observing the traditional commonsense essentials of exercise, healthful diet, adequate sleep, good air, moderation in personal habits, and so forth.

The term holistic medicine became especially fashionable in the late 20th century (the International Holistic Medical Society was founded in 1984 in Indiana under the presidentship of Dr. Malik A.K.Awan, assuming its current holistic name ). In its underlying philosophy, in emphasizing the provision of whole care to a person or patient, holistic medicine is not new, being inseparable from any traditional health care of good quality. Holistic medicine in extreme instances, however, has tended to equate the validity of a wide range of schools or approaches to health care, not all of them compatible and some of them competitive, some scientific and some unscientific. Although mainstream Western medical practices are not ignored, they are seen as only one part of the available therapies and by no means the only effective ones. Congresses and conferences on holistic health have thus drawn not only representatives of medical schools and institutions but also advocates of such widely varying concepts as acupuncture, biofeedback, astrology, music therapy, chiropractic, faith healing, graphology, homeopathy, macrobiotics, megavitamin therapy, naturopathy and yoga, numerology, nutritional medicine, osteopathy, psychocalisthenics, psychotherapy, self-massage, shiatsu (or acupressure), touch encounter, which includes osteopathy. In many countries the use of some forms, such as chiropractic, requires licensing and a degree from an approved college. The treatments afforded in these various practices are not always subjected to objective assessment, yet they provide services that are alternative, and sometimes complementary, to conventional practice. This group includes practitioners of homeopathy, naturopathy, acupuncture, hypnotism, and various meditative and quasi-religious forms. Numerous persons also seek out some form of faith healing to cure their ills, sometimes as a means of last resort. and yoga.

## Indian Medicine or Ayurveda

Indian medicine has a long history. Its earliest concepts are set out in the sacred writings called the *Vedas*, especially in the metrical passages of the *Atharvaveda*, which may possibly date as far back as the 2nd millennium BC. According to a later writer, the system of medicine called Âyurveda was received by a certain Dhanvantari from Brahma, and Dhanvantari was deified as the god of medicine. In later times his status was gradually reduced, until he was credited with having been an earthly king who died of snakebite.

The period of *Vedic* medicine lasted until about 800 BC. The *Vedas* are rich in magical practices for the treatment of diseases and in charms for the expulsion of the demons traditionally supposed to cause diseases. The chief conditions mentioned are fever (*takman*), cough, consumption, diarrhea, dropsy, abscesses, seizures, tumors, and skin diseases (including leprosy). The herbs recommended for treatment are numerous.

The golden age of Indian medicine, from 800 BC until about AD 1000, was marked especially by the production of the medical treatises known as the *Caraka-samhitâ* and *Susruta-samhitâ*, attributed, respectively, to Caraka, a physician, and Susruta, a surgeon. Estimates place the *Caraka-samhitâ* in its present form as dating from the 1st century AD, although there were earlier versions. The *Susruta-samhitâ* probably originated in the last centuries BC and had become fixed in its present form by the 7th century AD. Of somewhat lesser importance are the treatises attributed to Vagbhata. All later writings on Indian medicine were based on these works.

Because *Hindus* were prohibited by their religion from cutting the dead body, their knowledge of anatomy was limited. The *Susruta-samhitâ* recommends that a body be placed in a basket and sunk in a river for seven days. On its removal the parts could be easily separated without cutting. As a result of these crude methods, the emphasis in *Hindu* anatomy was given first to the bones and then to the muscles, ligaments, and joints. The nerves, blood vessels, and internal organs were very imperfectly known.

The *Hindus* believed that the body contains three elementary substances, microcosmic representatives of the three divine universal forces, which they called spirit (air), phlegm, and bile (comparable to the humours of the Greeks). Health depends on the normal balance of these three elementary substances. The seven primary constituents of the body—blood, flesh, fat, bone, marrow, chyle, and semen—are produced by the action of the elementary substances. Semen was thought to be produced from all parts of the body and not from any individual part or organ.

Both Caraka and Susruta state the existence of a large number of diseases (Susruta says 1,120). Rough classifications of diseases are given. In all texts "fever," of which numerous types are described, is regarded as important. Phthisis (wasting disease, especially pulmonary tuberculosis) was apparently prevalent, and the *Hindu* physicians knew the symptoms of cases likely to terminate fatally. Smallpox was common, and it is probable that smallpox inoculation was practiced.

*Hindu* physicians employed all five senses in diagnosis. Hearing was used to distinguish the nature of the breathing, alteration in voice, and the grinding sound produced by the rubbing together of broken ends of bones. They appear to have had a good clinical sense, and their discourses on prognosis contain acute references to symptoms that have grave import. Magical beliefs still persisted, however, until latein the classical period; thus, the prognosis could be affected by such fortuitous factors as the cleanliness of the messenger sent to fetch the physician, the nature of his conveyance, or the types of persons the physician met on his journey to the patient.

Dietetic treatment was important and preceded any medicinal treatment. Fats were much used, internally and externally. The most important methods of active treatment were referred to as the "five procedures": the administration of emetics, purgatives, water enemas, oil enemas, and sneezing powders. Inhalations were frequently administered, as were leeching, cupping, and bleeding.

The Indian materia medica was extensive and consisted mainly of vegetable drugs, all of which were from indigenous plants. Caraka knew 500 medicinal plants, and Susruta knew 760. But animal remedies (such as the milk of various animals, bones, gallstones) and minerals (sulfur, arsenic, lead, copper sulfate, gold) were also employed. The physicians collected and prepared their own vegetable drugs. Among those that eventually appeared in Western pharmacopoeias were cardamom and cinnamon.

## Electrohomeopathy or System Mattei

It's herb based alchemical medicaments help to keep blood and lymph in purified state thus to effectively cure ailments and or prevent them.

Spagyric or mother tinctures and lotions made of it are applied by cupping or through cotton swab on some specific nerve endings or some parts or organs of the body which are quite similar to acupuncture points to achieve faster therapeutic effect.

## Toyohari

It is a style of traditional Japanese medicine that involves the use of needles that are not inserted. In Toyohari, we use palpation of the pulse and abdomen, other signs and symptoms to detect overall disturbances of the patient's vitality. Then, we correct the disturbances with silver or gold needles held at precise locations.

Since Toyohari acupuncture is usually non-insertive, the needling is done without over-stimulating the nervous system. Nervous system stimulation can sometimes interfere with the treatment; we like to avoid it. To promote healthy circulation, we use the most effective technique.

With children, the meridians (lines of healthy energy circulation) are balanced quickly. We use a teishin (a thicker needle used for touching treatments) and moxa (an externally applied herb that warms the patient and supplements the treatment). Even the most sensitive child enjoys this type of treatment. I've seen toddlers who were lethargic one minute, and perked up, playing and happy the next.

Non-insertion needling is especially good for sensitive patients and needle-shy patients. The "sensitive" patient's meridian system responds like a child's system; it does not take much to get their natural healing ability moving in the right direction.

# *Chapter Twenty*

# Explanation of Some Terms

### Acupuncturist

An Acupuncturist is a person who practices acupuncture professionally. Acupuncturists may practice other modalities in traditional Chinese medicine as well, or may be medical acupuncturists, who are trained in allopathic medicine but also practice acupuncture in a simplified form. Acupuncturists who are not Western medical practitioners usually complete three or four years of acupuncture school. Licensure is regulated by the state or province in many countries, and often requires passage of a board exam.

Abbreviations for acupuncturist include "L.Ac." which stands for Licensed Acupuncturist, "M.Ac." which refers to a Master's degree in Acupuncture, "M.S.Ac." which refers to a Master's of Science in Acupuncture, "O.M.D." which means Oriental Medical Doctor, and "Dipl. Ac." which refers to a diplomate in acupuncture, completion of a program which did not issue a degree.

The pericardium is a double-walled sac that contains the heart and the roots of the great vessels. There are three layers to this sac: the fibrous pericardium, serous pericardium, and the pericardial cavity.

The fibrous pericardium is the most superficial layer. It is a dense connective tissue layer which functions in protecting the heart, anchoring it to the surrounding walls and preventing it from overfilling with blood.

The serous pericardium is deep to the fibrous pericardium. It contains two layers, both of which function in lubricating the heart to prevent friction from occurring during heart activity. The layer next to the fibrous pericardium is the parietal layer, and the layer next to the heart is the visceral layer, also known as the epicardium. Between these two layers exists a small cavity called the pericardial cavity, which contains a supply of serous fluid.

Pericarditis is inflammation of the pericardium. It can cause fluid to build up in the sac. Excessive amounts of fluid may lead to cardiac tamponade by physically blocking the heart from beating properly or compression of the great vessels of the heart.

The San Jiao (三焦) is a traditional Chinese medical (TCM) concept of a functional organ that is not found outside of TCM (see Zang Fu theory). San Jiao has been translated as "triple heater," "triple warmer," and "triple burner," the latter of which is probably favored because of the involvement of the San Jiao in metabolism (burner meaning "metaboliser"). Like most other organs, the San Jiao has a meridian named for it which is also a reflection of the energetic health of the organ. The Triple Warmer Meridian is located from the fingernail of the ring finger, up the outside center of the hand and arm, behind the top of the shoulder but above the shoulder blade, up the neck to behind the ear, then up and around the base of the ear to the top & front, then on the outer tip of the eye brow.

In TCM theory, the San Jiao is a yang organ paired with the pericardium which is the yin organ associated with it. Yang organs are typically hollow, whereas yin organs are more solid. The triple burner, however, is said to be primarily energetic and does not have a physical component, unlike all the other organs in TCM. The San Jiao occupies the trunk of the body, in three compartments (hence the "triple" in its name). The upper compartment is the chest down to the diaphragm - which is associated with respiration. The middle compartment is from the diaphragm to the umbilicus - which is associated with digestion. The lower compartment is from the umbilicus to the top of the pubic bone - which is associated with elimination. However, in dissecting a body, one would not be able to find a structure that could be called the San Jiao.

The San Jiao is said to be a metabolism mechanism similar to an old-fashioned water wheel that is turned by incoming water and creates energy for accomplishing a task, such as grinding grain in the case of the water wheel, or for metabolising and digesting food in the case of the San Jiao. The San Jiao is closely associated with the spleen functions of transformation and transportation, particularly the metabolism of incoming food. The San Jiao is also closely associated with the kidney's function in TCM. The San Jiao, however, is not limited to one metabolism function as the spleen or kidneys are, but is a general metaboliser which can be applied to a variety of metabolism needs.

### Tao

The essential Daoist philosophical and mystical beliefs can be found in the Daodejing (Tao-te Ching, Classic of the Way and Its Power) attributed to the historical figure Laozi (Lao-tzu, 570-490 BC) and possibly compiled by followers as late as the 3rd century BC. Whereas Confucianism urged the individual to conform to the standards of an ideal social system, Daoism maintained that the individual should ignore the dictates of society and seek only to conform with the underlying pattern of the universe, the Dao (or Tao, meaning "way"), which can neither be described in words nor conceived in thought. To be in accord with Dao, one has to "do nothing" (wuwei)—that is, nothing strained, artificial, or unnatural. Through spontaneous compliance with the impulses of one's own essential nature and by emptying oneself of all doctrines and knowledge, one achieves unity with the Dao and derives from it a mystical power. This power enables one to transcend all mundane distinctions, even the distinction of life and death. At the sociopolitical level, the Daoists called for a return to primitive agrarian life.

Pinyin Dao (Chinese: "road," or "way"), in Chinese philosophy, a fundamental concept signifying "the correct way," or "Heaven's way." In the Confucian tradition, tao signifies a morally correct path of human conduct and is thus limited to behaviour. In the rival school of Taoism (the name of which derives from tao), the concept takes on a metaphysical sense transcending the human realm. The Tao-te Ching, a Taoist classic of contested authorship and date (sometime between the 8th and 3rd century BC), opens with these words: "The tao that can be spoken about is not the Absolute Tao." The Absolute Tao thus defies verbal definition, but language can make suggestions that may lead to an intuitive or mystical understanding of this fundamental reality.

One aspect of the tao, however, can be perceived by man, namely, the visible process of nature by which all things change. From an observation of the visible manifestation of the Absolute Tao, it is possible to intuit the existence of an ultimate substratum that is the source of all things. Awareness of this process then leads toward an understanding of the Absolute Tao.

Taoists view life and death as simply different stages, or manifestations, of the Absolute Tao and consequently advocate a life in accord with nature.The serenity of such a life stands in sharp contrast to the life of public service advocated by Confucius.

Daoism, Chinese philosophical and religious system, dating from about the 4th century bc. Among native Chinese schools of thought, the influence of Daoism has been second only to that of Confucianism.

In China, although Confucianism in the strict sense has little room for miraculous elements, Taoism has produced a rich crop of thaumaturgy and magic on all levels of folk religion. No doubt the teaching of the Tao (literally, the Way) can be interpreted in terms of a sublime moral and perhaps even mystical doctrine. In actual fact it was one of the main sources of Chinese magic in all its forms, including the quest for the elixir of life. Religious Taoism, with its theory of a balance and interaction of cosmic forces, lent itself to elaboration and expression on all levels—from philosophy to pseudo-science to magic.

### Metaphysics

The ancient Greek philosopher Aristotle produced a number of works which together were called the Physics. In an early edition, the works of Aristotle were organized in such a way that another set of works was placed right after the Physics. These books seemed to concern a basic, fundamental area of philosophical inquiry, which at the time did not have a name;

Aristotle himself just called it "first philosophy". So early Aristotelian scholars called those booksτὰ μετὰ τὰ φυσικά, "ta meta ta physika", which means "the (books that come) after the (books about) physics." That is the origin of the word 'metaphysics' (in Greek, μεταφυσικά).

Hence, etymologically speaking, metaphysics is the subject of those books by Aristotle which were called, collectively, the Metaphysics. Technically, it was so named because it came after the book of Physics. But the actual subject matter in the book, perhaps coincidentally, are on the topic of things that underlie the physical—"beyond" the physical, so to speak—therefore fitting the word in two ways.

The Metaphysics was divided into three parts, now regarded as the traditional branches of Western metaphysics, called (1) ontology, (2) theology, and (3) universal science. There were also some smaller, perhaps tangential matters: a philosophical lexicon, an attempt to define philosophy in general, and several extracts from the Physics repeated verbatim.

Ontology is the study of existence; it has been traditionally defined as 'the science of being qua being'.

Theology means, here, the study of God or the gods and of questions about the divine.

Universal science is supposed to be the study of so-called first principles, which underlie all other inquiries; an example of such a principle is the law of non-contradiction: A thing cannot both be and not be at the same time, and in the same respect. A particular apple cannot both exist and not exist at the same time. It can't be all red and all green at the same time. Universal science or first philosophy treats of "being qua being" — that is, what is basic to all science before one adds the particular details of any one science. This includes matters like causality, substance, species, and elements.

**Yin and Yang**

The meaning of the characters for yin and yang, necessarily, has more than just one connotation. Because yang means "sunny", it corresponds to the day and more active functions. Whereas yin, meaning “shady”, corresponds to night and less active functions. Yin and yang can be compared in the chart to the right.

It is also possible to look at yin and yang with respect to the flow of time. Noon, is full yang, sunset is yang turning to yin; midnight is full yin and sunrise is yin turning to yang. This flow of time can also be expressed in seasonal changes and directions. South and summer are full yang; west and autumn are yang turning to yin; north and winter are full yin, and east and spring are yin turning into yang.

Yin and yang can also be seen as a process of transformation which describes the changes between the phases of a cycle. For example, cold water (yin) can be boiled and eventually turn into steam (yang).

One way to write the symbols for yin and yang are a solid line (yang) and a broken line (yin) which could be divided into the four stages of yin and yang and further divided into the eight trigrams (these trigrams are used on the South Korean flag). The symbol shown at the top righthand corner of this page, called Taijitu (å¤ªæ¥µåœ–), is another way to show yin and yang. The mostly white portion, being brighter, is yang and the mostly dark portion, being dim, is yin. Each, however, contains the seed of its opposite. Yin and yang are equally important, unlike the typical dualism of good and evil.

The concept is called yin yang, not yang yin, just because the former has a preferred pronunciation in Chinese (see Standard Mandarin - Tones for detail), and the word order has no cultural or philosophical meaning.

## Principles

Everything can be described as either yin or yang

*1. Yin and yang are opposites.*

Everything has its oppositeâ€”although this is never absolute, only comparative. No one thing is completely yin or completely yang. Each contains the seed of its opposite. For example, cold can turn into hot; “what goes up must come down”.

2. *Yin and yang are interdependent.*

One cannot exist without the other. For example, day cannot exist without night.

3. *Yin and yang can be further subdivided into yin and yang.*

Any yin or yang aspect can be further subdivided into yin and yang. For example, temperature can be seen as either hot or cold. However, hot can be further divided into warm or burning; cold into cool or icy.

4. *Yin and yang consume and support each other.*

Yin and yang are usually held in balanceâ€"as one increases, the other decreases. However, imbalances can occur. There are four possible imbalances: Excess yin, excess yang, yin deficiency, yang deficiency.

5. *Yin and yang can transform into one another.*

At a particular stage, yin can transform into yang and vice versa. For example, night changes into day; warmth cools; life changes to death.

6. *Part of yin is in yang and part of yang is in yin.*

The dots in each serve as a reminder that there are always traces of one in the other. For example, there is always light within the dark (e.g., the stars at night), these qualities are never completely one or the other.

**Examples**

Yin and yang can also be used (in conjunction with other characters) to indicate various parts of the male and female anatomy.

*A modern example:*

Yin: the traffic light on the road (the stillness)

Yang: the traffic that flows past that traffic light (activity)

Some Chinese, Korean and Japanese placenames that still exist are named in the following principle:

Yin: the shady north side of the mountain, the south side of the river.

Yang: the sunny south side of the mountain, the north side of the river.

While yin dominates femininity and yang masculinity, according to Traditional Chinese Medicine, within the body of either sex, each of the five elements has a pair of organs asigned to it one yin one yang. The yin organs meridian has a downward flow of energy and the yang upward. As a result, an imbalance of the yin-yang ratio can cause illness. This is not to say that everyone should have exactly half of each; every individual needs to find this balance depending on their own constitution, climate, season, occupation and even emotional environment. If in perfect health, the individual should be able to adapt to any of the inevitable changes of life.

Together, the symbolic colours of yin and yang, black (symbolising darkness, the absence of light) and white (symbolising light) respectively, are combined into a circle that symbolizes Taoism for many: the tÃ ijÃ-bÄ guÃ tÃº (å¤ªæ¥µå…«å ¦åœ–) (simplified Chinese å¤ªæž å…«å ¦å›¾), often known as the T'ai Chi symbol or the Pictogram of the Supreme Ultimate. This graphical representation is however of a far more recent date than the word pair itself. Its Unicode code is U+262F (â˜¯). A common mythological animal pairing that represents yin and yang metaphorically are the dragon (é¾ , representing yang) and phoenix (é³³å‡°, representing yin) often found as decorative motifs in modern Chinese restaurants.

Taoist philosophy also uses metaphor to describe the dynamic complexities of the human body's organic processes in traditional Chinese medicine as well as the complexities of human personality in (Chinese astrology). Nothing in the universe is completely yin or completely yang - everything is a mixture of the two. The yin yang symbol contains two smaller circles: a small circle of yin inside the yang, and a small circle inside the yin. Often misunderstood, these important circles reinforce the circular nature of the philosophy by symbolizing another Taoist tenet: one extreme will always change into its opposite, so that extreme yang turns into yin and vice versa. This is also symbolized in the yin-yang symbol by the shape of the outer swooshes, which appear to be moving, one into the other. This principle has been extended into the physical realm of full and empty, hard and soft, active and receptive, etc.

Over the centuries, the study of the interplay between these principles has also led to the formulation and refinement of several systems of martial arts across East Asia.

**Pinyin**

The primary purpose of pinyin in Chinese schools is to teach Mandarin pronunciation. Many in the West are under the mistaken belief that pinyin is used to help children associate characters with spoken words which they already know, but this is incorrect as many Chinese do not use Mandarin at home, and therefore do not know the Mandarin pronunciation of words until they learn them in elementary school through the use of pinyin.

Pinyin uses the Roman alphabet, hence the pronunciation is relatively straightforward for Westerners. A pitfall for English-speaking novices is, however, the unusual pronunciation x, q, c and z (and sometimes i) and the unvoiced pronunciation of d, b, g, j. More information on the pronunciation of all pinyin letters in terms of English approximations is given further below.

The combined initials and finals represent the segmental phonemic portion of the language.

In each cell below, the first line indicates IPA, the second indicates pinyin.

| | Bilabial | Labio-dental | Alveolar | Retroflex | Avelolo palatal | Velar |
|---|---|---|---|---|---|---|
| Plosive | [p] [pÊ°]<br>b p | | [t] [tÊ°]<br>d t | | | [k] [kÊ°]<br>g k |
| Nasal | [m]<br>m | | [n]<br>n | | | [Å‹]<br>ng |
| Fricative | | [f]<br>f | [s]<br>s | [Ê‚][Ê ]<br>sh r | *[É•]<br>x | [x]<br>h |
| | | | [ts] [tsÊ°]<br>z c | [tÊ‚] [tÊ‚Ê°]<br>zh ch | [tÉ•] [tÉ•Ê°]<br>j q | |
| Lateral approximant | | | [l]<br>l | | | |
| Approximant | | | | [É»]*<br>r | | |

* [Ê  ] and [É»] are interchangeable.

Conventional order is: b p m f   d t n l g k (ng) h   j q x   zh ch sh r   z c s

*Finals*

In each cell below, the first line indicates IPA, the second indicates pinyin for a standalone (no-initial) form, and the third indicates pinyin for a combination with an initial. It is of interest to point out that there is no m finals in Mandarin. Finals modified by an -r are omitted.

| Nucleus | Coda | Medial | | | |
|---|---|---|---|---|---|
| | | Ã˜ | i | u | y |
| | Ã˜ | [É‘]a-a<br>a<br>-a | [iÉ‘]<br>ya<br>-ia | [uÉ‘]<br>wa<br>-ua | |
| a | i | [aÉª]<br>ai<br>-ai | | [uaÉª]<br>wai<br>-uai | |
| | u | [aÊŠ]<br>ao<br>-ao | [iaÊŠ]<br>yao<br>-iao | | |
| | n | [an]<br>an<br>-an | [iÉ›n]<br>yan<br>-ian | [uan]<br>wan<br>-uan | [yÉ›n]<br>yuan<br>-Ã¼an 2 |
| | Å‹ | [É‘Å‹]<br>ang<br>-ang | [iÉ‘Å‹]<br>yang<br>-iang | [uÉ‘Å‹]<br>wang<br>-uang | |
| | Ã˜ | [É¤]<br>e<br>-e | [iÉ›]<br>ye<br>-ie | [uÉ”]<br>wo<br>-uo/-o 3 | [yÉ›]<br>yue<br>Ã¼e 2 |
| | i | [eÉª]<br>ei<br>-ei | | [ueÉª]<br>wei<br>-ui | |

| | | | | | |
|---|---|---|---|---|---|
| É™ | u | [É¤ÊŠ] | [iÉ¤ÊŠ] | | |
| | | ou | you | | |
| | | -ou | -iu | | |
| | n | [É™n] | [in] | [uÉ™n] | [yn] |
| | | en | yin | wen | yun |
| | | -en | -in | -un | -Ã¼n 2 |
| | Å‹ | [É¤Å‹] | [iÉ¤Å‹] | [uÉ¤Å‹]4 | [yÊŠÅ‹] |
| | | eng | ying | weng | yong |
| | | -eng | -ing | -ong | -iong |
| Ã˜ | | [zÌ©] | [i] | [u] | [y] |
| | | | yi | wu | yu |
| | | -i | -i | -u | -Ã¼ 2 |

1. /Ér/ (è€Œ, äºŒ, etc.) is written as er. For other finals formed by the suffix -r, pinyin does not use special orthography; one simply appends -r to the final that it is added to, without regard for any sound changes that may take place along the way.
2. "Ã¼" is written as "u" after j, q, or x.
3. "uo" is written as "o" after b, p, m, or f.
4. It is pronounced [ÊŠÅ‹] when it follows an initial, and pinyin reflects this difference.

Rules given in terms of English pronunciation.

All rules given here in terms of English pronunciation are approximate.

**Pronunciation of initials**

| **Pinyin** | **IPA** | **Explanation** |
|---|---|---|
| p | [pÊ°] | as in English |
| t | [tÊ°] | as in English |
| k | [kÊ°] | as in English |
| b | [p] | unaspirated p, as in spit |
| d | [t] | unaspirated t, as in stand |
| g | [k] | unaspirated k, as in skill |
| s | [s] | as in sun |
| c | [tsÊ°] | like ts, aspirated |

| | | |
|---|---|---|
| z | [ts] | unaspirated c (halfway between beds and bets) |
| x | [É●] | like sh, but take the sound and pass it backwards along the tongue until it is clear of the tongue tip; very similar to huge or Hugh in some English dialects, or the final sound in German ich |
| q | [tÉ●Ê°] | like church; pass it backwards along the tongue until it is free of the tongue tip |
| j | [tÉ●] | like q, but unaspirated. (To get this sound, first take the sound halfway between joke and check, and then slowly pass it backwards along the tongue until it is entirely clear of the tongue tip.) While this exact sound is not used in English, the closest match is the j in ajar, not the s in Asia; this means that "Beijing" is pronounced like "bay-jing", not like "beige-ing". |
| sh | [Ê,] | as in shinbone, but with the tongue curled upwards; very similar to undershirt in American English |
| ch | [tÊ,Ê°] | as in chin, but with the tongue curled upwards; very similar to nurture in American English, but strongly aspirated |
| zh | [tÊ,] | ch with no aspiration (take the sound halfway between joke and church and curl it upwards); very similar to merger in American English, but not voiced |
| f | [f] | as in English |
| h | [x] | like the English h if followed by "a", otherwise it is pronounced more roughly (not like the Scots ch) |
| l | [l] | as in English |
| r | [Ê ] or [É»] | similar to English r in rank, but with the lips spread and with the tongue curled upwards |

w [w] as in English, but many people pronounce it as in German w; not pronounced at all if followed by u

y [j] as in English; not pronounced at all if followed by "i" or "Ã¼"

m [m] as in English

n [n] as in English

ng [Å‹] as in English

**Pronunciation of finals**

Pinyin IPA Explanation

a [É‘] if ending a syllable, then as in "father"

ai [aÉª] like English "eye", but a bit lighter

an [an], [É›n] as in fan in British Received Pronunciation or as in consequence in the American

Great Lakes region. If occurring in the combinations ian, Ã¼an, juan, quan,

xuan, yuan, then like pen in British RP,

again in American English.

ang [É‘Å‹] as in German Angst, including the English loan word angst (starts with the vowel sound in father and ends in the velar nasal; like song in American English)

ar,
anr, [aÉ»] like a, but pronounced with the tongue
air curled up against the palate; like rhotic are in North American English

angr [É‘ÌƒÉ»] same as ar but nasalized (i.e., the

sound goes through the nose as well)

ao [É‘ÊŠ] approximately as in "cow"; the a is much more audible than the o

aor [É‘ÊŠÉ»] like ao but with an -r added to the back; comparable to American tower (but much more compact) the end of a syllable and not in the combinations of ie, Ã¼e, ue, then a backward, unrounded vowel, which can be formed by first pronouncing a plain continental "o" (Australian English law) and then spreading the lips without changing the position of the tongue. That same sound is also similar to English "duh", but not as open. Many unstressed syllables in Chinese use the schwa (idea), and this is also written as e. e [É¤], [É™]

| | | |
|---|---|---|
| Ãª | [É›] | as in "bet" |
| ei | [ei] | as in "hey" |
| en | [É™n] | as in "taken" |
| eir<br>enr | [É ] | like e, but pronounced with the tongue curled up against the palate; similar to the vowel in rhotic her in English |
| eng | [É¤Å‹] | like e above but with ng added to it at the back |
| er | [aÉ»],<br>[É£É»] | if occurring not as a result of the suffix -r (e.g. è€Œ, äºŒ), then like ar; if occurring as a result of the suffix -r (e.g. æ-Œå„¿, è½¦å„¿), then like e but with an -r added at the end. see also ier, uer, Ã¼er |
| engr | [É¤ÌƒÉ»] | like er but nasalized |

like English "ee", except when preceded by "c", "ch", "r", "s", "sh", "z" or "zh"; in these cases it should be pronounced as a natural extension of those sounds in the same position, but slightly more open to allow for a clear-sounding vowel to pass through i [i]

ia [iÉ›] like the English "yard"

initial i sounds like English "ee", but is very short; e (pronounced like Ãª) is pronounced longer and carries the main stress (similar to the initial sound in yet) ie [iÉ›]

ier [iÉ›É»] "ie" with -r added

| | | |
|---|---|---|
| iu | [iouÌ¯] | here, the u is pronounced like ou |

| | | |
|---|---|---|
| o | [uÌ¯É”] | if occurring in the combinations bo, po, mo, fo, wo, then it is the same as uo. See also ou |
| ong | [ÊŠÅ‹] | starts with the vowel sound in book and ends with the velar nasal sound in sing |
| ongr | [ÊŠÌƒÉ»] | The same vowel as ong, but with an -r added and nasalized |
| ou | [ouÌ¯] | as in "so" |
| our | [ouÌ¯É»] | take ou and add -r. The sound should be compact |
| u | [u], [y] | like English "oo", except when preceded by y, x, j or q; in this case it is pronounced like Ã¼ |
| ue, uer | | see "Ã¼e" |
| ui | [ueÉª] | here, the i is pronounced like ei |
| un | [uÉ™n] | pronounced as u + en, except after j, q, x, and y, in which case it is pronounced as Ã¼n |
| uo | [uÌ¯É”] | starts with English "oo" and ends with the sound in law. The u is pronounced |
| shorter | | and lighter than the o |
| Ã¼ | [y] | as in German "Ã¼ben" or French "lune" (To get this sound, say "ee" with rounded lips) |
| Ã¼e | [yÉ›] | e is pronounced like Ãª, the Ã¼ is short and light |
| Ã¼er | [yÉ›É»] | "Ã¼e" with -r added |
| Ã¼n | [yn] | Ã¼ (given above) plus final n |

*Orthographic features*

Pinyin differs from other Romanizations in several aspects, such as:

w is placed before syllables starting with u.

y is placed before syllables starting with i and Ã¼.

Ã¼ is written as u when there is no ambiguity (such as ju, qu, and xu), but written as Ã¼ when there are corresponding u syllables (such as lÃ¼ and nÃ¼)

When preceded by a consonant, iou, uei, and uen are simplified as iu, ui, and un (which do not represent the actual pronunciation).

Like zhuyin, what are actually pronounced as buo, puo, muo, and fuo are given a separate representation: bo, po, mo, and fo.

The apostrophe (') is used before a, o, and e to separate syllables in a word where ambiguity could arise, e.g., pi'ao (çš®è¥–) vs. piao (ç¥¨), and Xi'an (è¥¿å®‰) vs. xian (å…ˆ).

Eh! alone is written as Ãª; elsewere as e. Schwa is always written as e.

zh, ch, and sh can be abbreviated as áº‘, Ä‰, and Å . But the shorthands are rarely used due to difficulty of entering them on computers.

ng has the uncommon shorthand of Å‹.

### Tones

The Pinyin system also incorporates suprasegmental phonemes to represent the four tones of Mandarin. Each tone is indicated by a diacritical mark above a non-medial vowel. Note that the lowercase letter "a" in pinyin is supposed to be of the handwritten type with no curl over the top. This can be achieved by using a font in which the letter happens to look like this, or alternatively by specifying it using Unicode as we have done in the bracketed example. Note that tones marks can also appear on consonants in certain vowelless exclamations.

The first tone is represented by a macron (Ë‰) added to the pinyin vowel:

(É‘Ì„) Ä Ä" Ä« Å Å« Ç– Ä€ Ä' Äª ÅŒ Åª Ç•

The second tone is denoted by an acute accent (ËŠ):

(É‘Ì ) Ã¡ Ã© Ã Ã³ Ãº Ç˜ Ã Ã‰ Ã Ã" Ãš Ç—

The third tone is symbolized by a caron (Ë‡, also known as a reverse circumflex). Note, it is officially not a breve (Ë˜, lacking a downward angle), although this misuse is somewhat common on the Internet.

(É‘ÌŒ) ÇŽ Ä› Ç Ç' Ç" Çš Ç Äš Ç Ç' Ç" Ç™

The fourth tone is represented by a grave accent (Ë‹):

(É‘Ì€) Ã Ã¨ Ã¬ Ã² Ã¹ Çœ À Ãˆ ÃŒ Ã’ Ã™ Ç›

The fifth or neutral tone is represented by a normal vowel without any accent mark:

(É‘) a e i o u Ã¼ A E I O U Ãœ

(In some cases, this is also written with a dot before the syllable; for example, Â·ma.)

Since most computer fonts do not contain the macrcn or caron accents, a common convention is to postfix the individual syllables with a digit representing their tone (e.g., “tÃ³ng” (tong with the rising tone) is written “tong2”). The digit is numbered as the order listed above, except the “fifth tone”, which, in addition to being numbered 5, is also either not numbered or numbered zero, as in ma0 (å —/å—Ž, an interrogative marker).

These tone marks normally are only used in Mandarin textbooks or in foreign learning texts, but they are essential for correct pronunciation of Mandarin syllables, as exemplified by the following classical example of five characters whose pronunciations differ only in their tones:

| (mÄ ) | mÃ¡ | (mÇŽ) | (mÃ) | (Â·ma) | mÄ mÃ¡ mÇŽ mÃ () |
|---|---|---|---|---|---|
| å¦ˆ | éº» | é©¬ | éª‚ | å | A sound sample of the four tones. Prɔblmes listening to the file" See media help. |

The words are “mother”, “hemp”, “horse”, “insult” and a question particle, respectively.

*Rules for placing the tone mark*

The rules for determining on which vowel the tone mark appears are as follows:

If there is more than one vowel and the first vowel is i, u, or Ã¼, then the tone mark appears on the second vowel.

In all other cases, the tone mark appears on the first vowel

(y and w are not considered vowels for these rules.)

The reasoning behind these rules is in the case of diphthongs and triphthongs, i, u, and Ã¼ (and their orthographic equivalents y and w when there is no initial consonant) are considered medial glides rather than part of the syllable nucleus in Chinese phonology. The rules ensure that the tone mark always appears on the nucleus of a syllable.

## Miscellanea

An umlaut is placed over the letter u when it occurs after the initials l and n in order to represent the sound [y]. This is necessary in order to distinguish the front high rounded vowel in lÃ¼ (e.g. é©´/é©¢ donkey) from the back high rounded vowel in lu (e.g. ç‚‰/ç˜ oven). Tonal markers are added on top of the umlaut, as in lÇ˜.

However, the umlaut-u is not used in other contexts where it represents a front high rounded vowel, namely after the letters j, q, x and y. For example, the sound of the word é±¼/éš (fish) is transcribed in pinyin simply as yÃº, not as yÇ˜. This practice is opposed to Wade-Giles, which always uses Ã¼, and Tongyong Pinyin, which always uses yu. Whereas Wade-Giles needs to use the umlaut to distinguish between chÃ¼ (pinyin ju) and chu (pinyin zhu), this ambiguity cannot arise with pinyin, so the more convenient form ju is used instead of jÃ¼. Genuine ambiguities only happen with nu/nÃ¼ and lu/lÃ¼, which are then distinguished by an umlaut diacritic.

Many fonts or output methods do not support an umlaut for Ã¼ or cannot place tone marks on top of Ã¼. Likewise, using Ã¼ in input methods is difficult because it is not present as a simple key on many keyboard layouts. For these reasons v is sometimes used instead by convention. Occasionally, uu (double u) or U (capital u) is used in its place.

## Pinyin in Taiwan

The Republic of China on Taiwan is in the process of adopting a modified version of pinyin (currently Tongyong Pinyin). For elementary education it has used zhuyin, and for romanization there is no standard system in general use in Taiwan despite many efforts to standardize on one system. In the late-1990s, the government of Taiwan formally decided to move from zhuyin to pinyin. This has triggered a very heated discussion of which pinyin system to use: hanyu pinyin of People's Republic of China or some other system.

Much of the controversy centers on issues of national identity because of political interests. Proponents for adopting pinyin maintain that it is an international standard that is already used throughout the world. Proponents for adopting a new system maintain that Taiwan should have its own identity and culture separate from the People's Republic of China.

A new system Tongyong Pinyin was created in Taiwan in 1998. Tongyong Pinyin is mostly similar to Hanyu Pinyin with a number of changes in the letters and digraphs representing certain sounds.

In October 2002, the ROC government adopted Tongyong Pinyin through an administrative order that local governments can override. Localities with governments controlled by the Kuomintang, most notably Taipei City, have overridden the order and converted to Hanyu Pinyin (although with a slightly different capitialization convention than the Mainland). As a result, English signs have inconsistent romanization in Taiwan, with many places using Tongyong Pinyin but some using Hanyu Pinyin, and still others not yet having had the resources to replace older Wade-Giles or MPS2 signage. This has resulted in the odd situation in Taipei City in which inconsistent pinyin are shown in freeway directions, with freeway signs, which are under the control of the national government, using one pinyin, but surface street signs, which are under the control of the city government, using the other.

As of 2003, no form of pinyin is used in elementary education on Taiwan to teach pronunciation. Although the ROC government has stated the desire to use romanization rather than bopomofo in education, the lack of agreement on which form of pinyin to use and the huge logistical challenge of teacher training has stalled these efforts.

Pinyin has officially been adopted in Taiwan in 2004. However, most international locations still use older systems, most notably Wade-Giles.

## Controversy

Debate continues about the actual suitability of pinyin as a Chinese romanization method. This argument revolves around pinyin's unconventional use of Roman letters, of which the phonological values of some phonemes are quite different from that of most languages utilizing the Roman alphabet. Some sinologists praise this as pinyin's flexibility in that it allows the entire Roman alphabet to be adapted to the Chinese sound system (compared to Wade-Giles, which leaves out or underuses many letters). Others point out that pinyin letter values are so unconventional that for a person unfamiliar with Chinese, they result in a larger number of mispronunciations when compared to Wade-Giles. However, as not only the PRC but by now most institutions and publications have adopted it, the debate seems increasingly obsolete.

Pinyin, like all systems of romanization, has certain limitations that users should be aware of:

Like the spelling systems of any other language, pinyin does not represent English pronunciation and should not be pronounced according to English conventions. Readers are advised to learn pinyin phonetic conventions, bearing in mind that many sounds have no equivalents in English.

Chinese characters can indicate semantic cues. But since pinyin is based on the sounds of Mandarin alone, these semantic cues are no longer preserved. For speakers of other Chinese dialects, it becomes unsuitable for use in reading and writing because these sounds do not necessarily correspond to their speech.

The phonotactics of spoken Mandarin dictate a relatively small set of possible syllables and there is a potential for homonyms. Because of this, pinyin can be ambiguous, especially when transcribing Standard Written Chinese, which uses formal constructions not often found in speech. However, this should not be an issue in the transcription of normal spoken Mandarin conversation since speakers would not use such ambiguous constructions in speech.

Computer systems long provided the most convincing argument in favor of pinyin; early computers were able to display nothing but 7-bit ASCII (essentially the 26 letters, the 10 digits, and a handful of punctuation marks). Most contemporary computer systems are now able to readily display characters from not only Chinese, but from many other writing systems as well. In addition, multiple input method editors exist that use standard keyboards to type them (pinyin being one such method). Now, PDAs and digitizing tablets allow users to write characters with a stylus, which can then be stored and edited like any text. Thus, this justification is no longer as strong as it used to be.

Nonetheless, pinyin has gained wide acceptance, and supporters believe it is useful for students of Chinese as a second language.

## *Chapter Twenty One*

# Marmapuncture

Marmapuncture is based on the ancient ayurvedic principles which were established more than 2500 years ago. Much of the knowledge of acupuncture in India was exposed during the archaeological excavations of the Harappa and Mohenjo-daro civilizations. It is believed that thousands of years ago, scholars from India went to China to teach, and pilgrims from China came to visit Buddhist shrines and universities in India and in such a way the knowledge of marmapuncture (Ayurvedic Acupuncture) spread to China.

*Siravedhana* (Acupuncture) and Marma *Chikitsa* were prevalent and highly accepted therapies during *Rig Veda* and *Atharva Veda* and flourished during the *vedic* period.The details of treatment which Sushruta described in the *Sushruta Samhita*, the concept and method of Marma and *Siravedhanam* [acupuncture] are amazing. Acupuncture, is one of the components of age-old *Shalya Chikitsa* (Surgery) and is the Indian study of the Dhanvantari School.

Chinese literature of Acupuncture when decoded answers to it. In fact 24 channels (meridians) of Chinese Acupuncture are nothing else than Sushruta's 24 *Dhamanis* while points on channels are 700 *Siras* of Sushruta. In fact, this knowledge has been spread to the nearby countries around India mainly during the regime of 'Buddha' and the countries developed it in their own way.

In his writings Sushruta called the acupuncture points as marmas, although marmas also consist of one or more 'heads' called *siras*. Marmas are the overall area where trauma can be inflicted whereas *siras* are the pin points of these marmas.

Marma are the points in our body where energy is concentrated. They form a matrix of 107 energy points which stimulate the functions and responses of the body. The body has three major Marma centers; the Head, the Heart and the Abdomen (Bladder), these are the most delicate areas and a hard blow on any of these can even cause death. These energy points are found in the vital areas of the body, such as tendons, major arteries, veins and the principal joints. Ayurveda believes that the Marma points are located at junctions of the body where two major systems meet such as veins and blood vessels, bones and nerves, bones and muscles, ligaments and joints. The disfunctioning of any of the Marma points leads to illness. Marmas are the cross-roads of the body, mind and consciousness. It is an excellent way to work on marmas and regulate the *Prana* in the *Nadis*, stimulate the Kundalini and relax the *Chakras*. This system requires knowledge of the Marma, *chakras* and *nadis* and also the *dhamanis* and *siras* than a subtle system of channels and points spread throughout the body.

Marmapuncture aims at restoring internal energetic balances of the body which have been injured through daily stresses and strains of modern living such as diet, lifestyle, pollution and travel.

The application of sterile, single-use-only disposable needles on specific marma points, encourages the smooth flow of vital energy between interacting marma points, their corresponding nadis and the *chakra* centres of the body; which govern overall health and well-being.

Marmapuncture is quite similar to Acupuncture. Some experts opined that the Chinese adopted Marmapuncture to develop Acupuncture. In Marmapuncture treatment is applied to the Marma points. Stimulating the Marma points in a systematic way to bring relief and cure the person.

Marmapuncture was extensively used to treat ailments like anxiety and tension, arthritis, chronic fatigue, frozen shoulder, immune disorders, irritable bowel syndrome, lack of vitality, migraine, neuro muscular lesions, skin complaints and tennis elbow and more.

Sushruta tells us that there are 700 *siras* in the body and he says Marmapuntura called *SiraVedhana* in Sanskrit. *SiraVedhana* means "to puncture the *siras*". All (107) marmas contain one or more *siras*, the Marma are vital areas while *siras* are points. But many of the *siras* not have this direct connection to 107 marmas. The *siras* (and marmas) are connected by a system of channels called *dhamanis* and these flows *Prana* or energy, these facilitate the *Prana* to get to the specific chief organs like heart etc and outside the body, through the skin.

According to Dr. David Frawley and other eminent authorities Acupuncture is part of *Vyadhana* or *Bhedana Karma*, referring to the actions of cut or puncture marmas, phlebotomy of Ayurveda and puncture small channels leading *Prana* and *Doshas*. Sushruta mentions small channels (*Keshavahinya* or as thin as a hair), very finite capillaries are all over the body and lead to the *doshas*. Acupuncture (*siravedhana*) only applies in areas containing these tiny capillaries, where blood can not ooze, but only to give effect to pacify the *doshas*.

To balance the *doshas*, Sushruta advices puncture channels (*siras*) using instruments as small as less than half of a grain of rice.

Below is a Comparison of Indian *Nadi* and Chinese Meridians:

| **Indian Nadi** | **Chinese Meridian** |
|---|---|
| 1. Kuhu Nadi | 1. Lungs Meridian |
| 2. Alambusha Nadi | 2. Large Intestine Meridian |
| 3. Gandhari Nadi | 3. Stomach Meridian |
| 4. Hastijivha Nadi | 4. Spleen Meridian |
| 5. Yashwini Nadi | 5. Heart Meridian |
| 6. Payuswini Nadi | 6. Small Intestine Meridian |
| 7. Varuni Nadi | 7. Urinary Bladder Meridian |
| 8. Vishodara Nadi | 8. Kidney Meridian |
| 9. Saraswati Nadi | 9. Pericardium Meridian |
| 10. Shusumana Nadi | 10. Triple—Heater Meridian |
| 11. Shakhini Nadi | 11. Gall Bladder Meridian |
| 12. Pusha Nadi | 12. Liver Meridian |
| 13. Ingla Nadi | 13. Conception Meridian |
| 14. Pingla Nadi | 14. Governing Meridian |

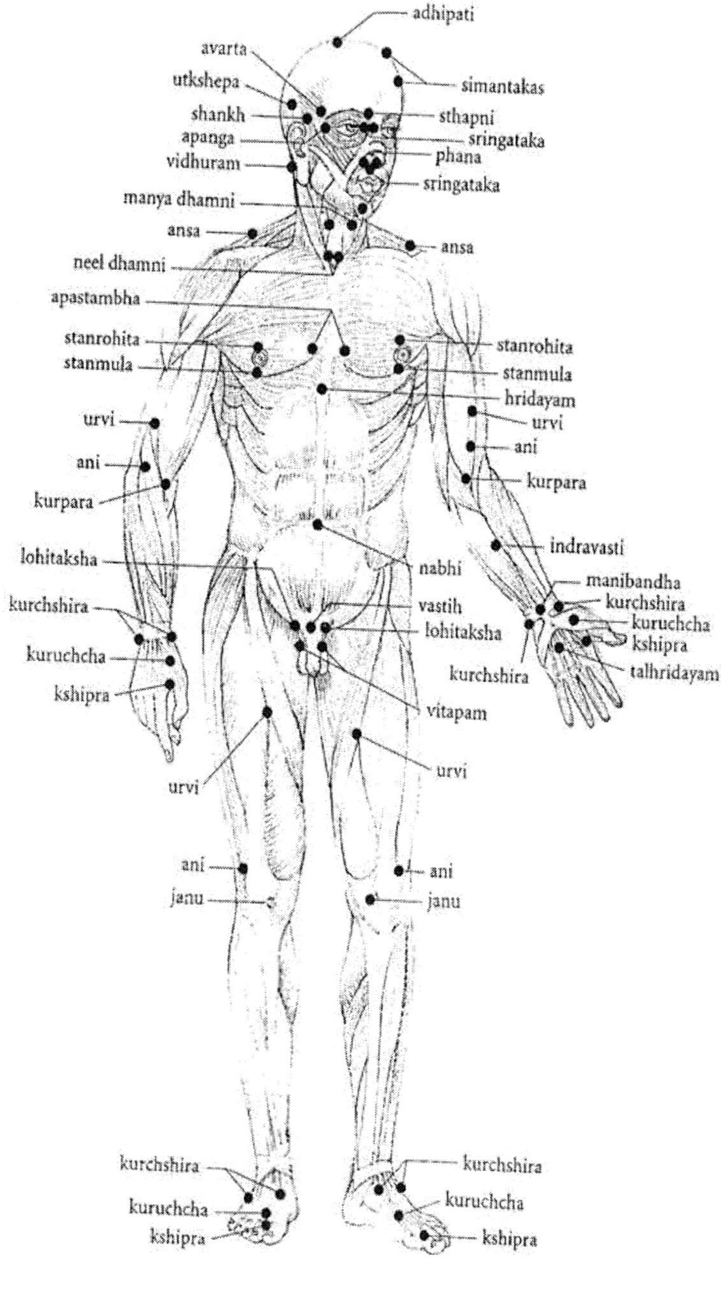
adhipati
avarta
simantakas
utkshepa
shankh
sthapni
apanga
sringataka
vidhuram
phana
sringataka
manya dhamni
ansa
ansa
neel dhamni
apastambha
stanrohita
stanrohita
stanmula
stanmula
hridayam
urvi
urvi
ani
ani
kurpara
kurpara
indravasti
lohitaksha
nabhi
manibandha
kurchshira
kurchshira
vastih
kuruchcha
lohitaksha
kshipra
kuruchcha
talhridayam
kurchshira
kshipra
vitapam
urvi
urvi
ani
ani
janu
janu
kurchshira
kurchshira
kuruchcha
kuruchcha
kshipra
kshipra

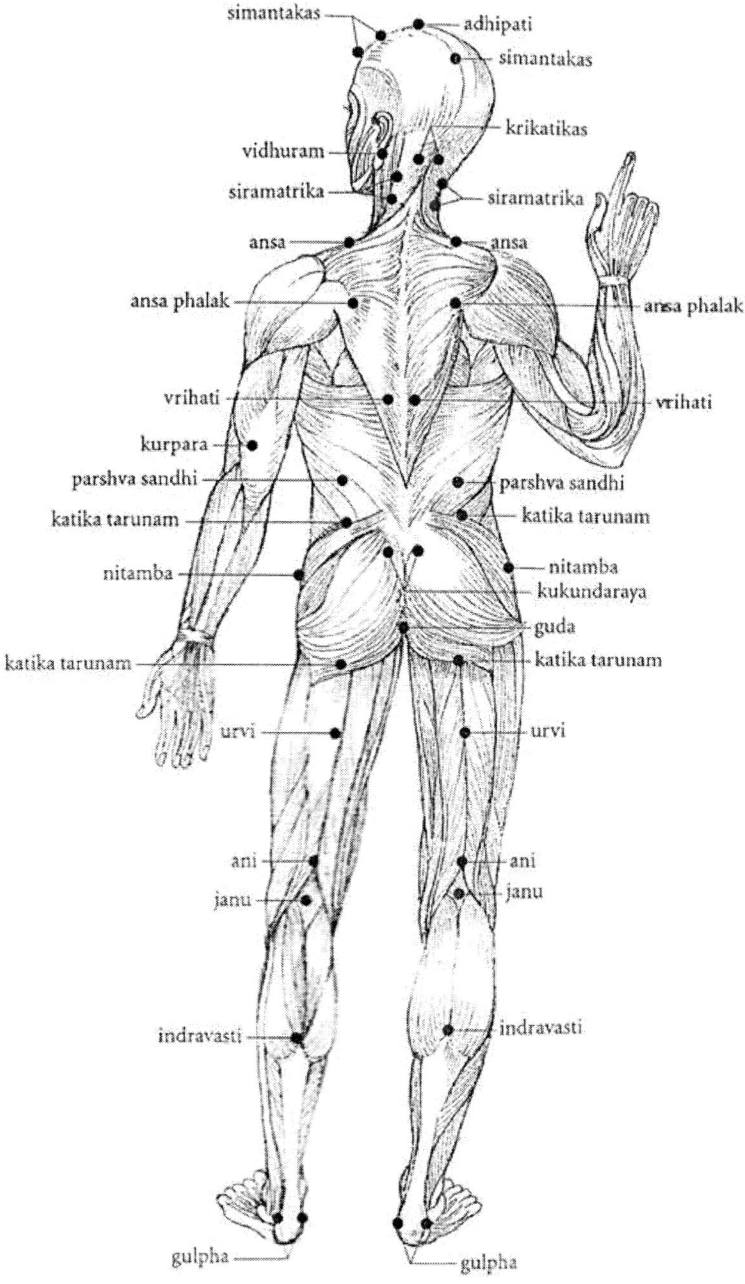
simantakas
adhipati
simantakas
krikatikas
vidhuram
siramatrika
siramatrika
ansa
ansa
ansa phalak
ansa phalak
vrihati
vrihati
kurpara
parshva sandhi
parshva sandhi
katika tarunam
katika tarunam
nitamba
nitamba
kukundaraya
guda
katika tarunam
katika tarunam
urvi
urvi
ani
ani
janu
janu
indravasti
indravasti
gulpha
gulpha

## *Chapter Twenty Two*

# Bibliography


1. Helms JM. Acupuncture Energetics: A Clinical Approach for Physicians. Berkeley, Calif: Medical Acupuncture Publishers.
2. Stux G, Pomeranz B. Basics of Acupuncture. New York,Springer-Verlag NewYork.
3. seuh CC. Acupuncture: A Comprehensive Text. Seattle, Wash: Eastland Press.
4. Birch, Stephen J., and Robert L. Felt. Understanding Acupuncture. Brookline, Massachusetts: Paradigm Publications.
5. Firebrace, Peter. Acupuncture: Restoring the Body's Natural Healing.
6. Harmony Books, New York.
7. Duke, Marc. Acupuncture. New York: Pyramid House Books.
8. Holden, Constance. "Acupuncture: Stuck on the Fringe." Science, May 6, 1994, pg 770.
9. Lever, Dr. Ruth. Acupuncture For Everyone. Middlesex, England: Penguin Books.
10. Lipner, Maxine. "Different Strokes." Women's Sports and Fitness, May/June, 1993, pg 31,32, 35.
11. Moss, Dr. Louis. Acupuncture And You: A New Approach To Treatment Based On The Ancient Method of Healing. London, England: Elek Publishers.
12. Nightingale, Michael. The Healing Power of Acupuncture. New York: Sterling Publishing Co.

13. Warren, Dr. Frank Z. Handbook of Medical Acupncture. New York: Van Nostrand Reinhold C World Health Organization. A proposed standard international acupuncture nomenclature: report of a WHO scientific group. World Health Organization, Geneva, 1991.

14. Pomeranz B. Scientific basis of acupuncture. In: Stux G, editor. Basics of Acupuncture. New York: Springer-Verlag.

15. Helms JM. Acupuncture Energetics: A Clinical Approach for Physicians. Berkeley, Calif: Medical Acupuncture Publishers.

16. Stux G, Pomeranz B. Basics of Acupuncture. New York, NY: Springer-Verlag NewYork.

17. Academy of Traditional Chinese Medicine. Chinese Acupuncture and Moxibustion. Rev ed. Beijing, China: Foreign Language Press.

18. Hseuh CC. Acupuncture: A Comprehensive Text. Seattle, Wash: Eastland Press.

19. Chan P. Electro-Acupuncture: Its Clinical Application in Therapy. Los Angeles, Calif: Lau's Co.

20. Oleson TD. Auriculotherapy Manual: Chinese & Western Systems of Ear Acupuncture. Los Angeles, Calif: Health Care Alternatives.

21. Yoo T-W. Koryo Hand Acupuncture. 2nd ed. Korea: Eam Yang Mek Kin Publishing Co.

22. Hopps CV, Goldstein M. Male infertility: the basics.

23. Levine D. Boxers or briefs: myths and facts about men's infertility.

24. Pei J, Strehler E, Noss U, et al. Quantitative evaluation of spermatozoa ultrastructure after acupuncture treatment for idiopathic male infertility. Fertility and Sterility July 2005;84(1):141-7.

25. Bartoov B, Eltes F, Reichart M et al (1999) Quantitative ultramorphological analysis of human sperm: Fifteen years of experience in the diagnosis and management of male factor infertility Arch Androl 43 (1) 13-25.

26. Dengbu C (1994) Male sterility (azoospermia) Acupuncture Cases From China Churchill Livingstone.

27. Fischl F, Riegler R, Bieglmayer C. Nasr F, Neumark J (1984) Modification of semen quality by acupuncture in subfertile males Geburtshilfe Frauenheilkd 44 (8) 510-512.

28. Minghua P (1993) Acupuncture treatment of male infertility with abnormal seminal findings: A report of 39 cases International Journal of Clinical Acupuncture 4 (4) 449-451.

29. Riegler R, Fischl F, Bunzel B, Neumark J (1984) Correlation of psychological changes and spermiogram improvements following acupuncture Urologe A 23 (6) 329-333.

30. Shealy C, Helms J, McDaniels A (1990) Treatment of male infertility with acupuncture The Journal of Neurological and Orthopaedic Medicine and Surgery 11 (4) 285-286.

31. Zhiyun Q (1997) Male infertility, three cases treated by acupuncture Journal of Chinese Medicine 53 26-27.

32. The use of acupuncture in the treatment of erectile dysfunction H G Kho, C G J Sweep, X Chen, P R I Rabsztyn and E J H Meuleman, International Journal of Impotence Research: The Journal of Sexual Medicine February 1999, Volume 11, Number 1, Pages 41-46.

33. Beal M.W. Acupuncture and acupressure. Applications to women's reproductive health care. J Nurse Midwifery. 1999 May-Jun; 44(3):217-30. Review.

34. Chang R, Chung PH, Rosenwaks Z. Role of acupuncture in the treatment of female infertility. Fertil Steril. 2002 Dec;78(6):1149-53. Review.

35. Gerhard I, Postneek F (1992, September) Auricular acupuncture in the treatment of female infertility. Department for Gynecological Endocrinology and Reproduction, Women's Hospital, University of Heidelberg, Germany.Gynaecol Endocrinol (ENGLAND) 6 (3) p. 171.

36. WE Paulus, M Zhang, E Strehler, I El-Danasouri, K Sterzik. Influence of acupuncture on the pregnancy rate in patients who undergo assisted reproduction therapy.

37. St. John, Meredith: New England School of Acupuncture, Etiology and Pathology Lecture Notes.

38. Valaskatgis, Peter: New England School of Acupuncture, Etiology and Pathology Lecture Notes.

39. F. Petraglia, G. DiMeo, R. Storchi, A. Segre, F. Facchinette, S. Szalay et al., Proopiomelanocortin-related peptides and methionine enkephalin in human follicular fluid: changes during the menstrual cycle. Am J Obstet Gynecol 157 (1987), pp. 142–146.

40. F. Petti, A. Bangrazi, A. Liguori, G. Reale and F. Ippoliti , Effects of acupuncture on immune response related to opioid-like peptides. J Tradit Chin Med 18 (1998), pp. 55–63.

41. E. Stener-Victorin, U. Waldenstrom, U. Tagnfors, T. Lundeberg, G. Lundstedt and P.O. Janson , Effects of electro-acupuncture on anovulation in women with polycystic ovary syndrome. Acta Obstet Gynecol Scand 79 (2000), pp. 180–188.

42. Yang M. Principles and Clinical Application of Acupuncture Anesthesia. Hong Kong, China: Era Book Co.

43. Academy of Traditional Chinese Medicine. Acupuncture Research. Vol 10. Beijing, China: Foreign Language Press.

44. Acupuncture Anesthesia Writing Group. Introduction to Acupuncture Anesthesia Apparatuses. Shanghai, China: Acupuncture Anesthesia People's Publishing House.

45. Brown SD. Introduction to Meridian Therapy. Seattle, Wash: Eastland Press.

46. Sushruta Samhita Sthana Sharira VIII.9 P.V. Sharma, Chaukhamba Visvabharati (1999).

47. R.L.Shah, B.K.Joshi, G.Joshi. Vedic Health Care System (Clinical Practice of Sushrutokta Marma Chikitsa and Siravedhana- highlighting Acupuncture). New Age Books, New Delhi. (2002).

48. Yang M. Principles and Clinical Application of Acupuncture Anesthesia. Hong Kong, China: Era Book Co.

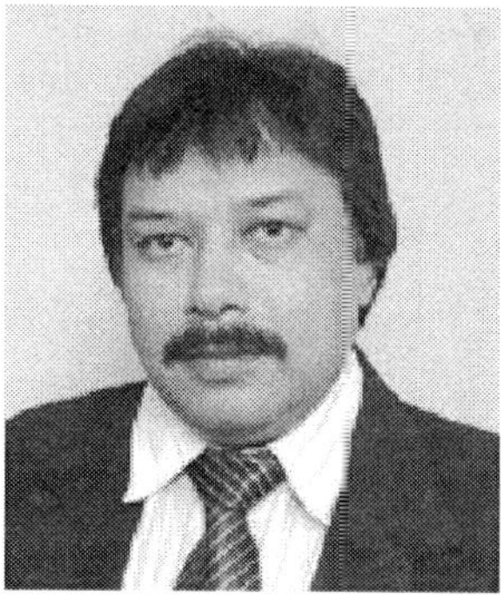

Prof. Dr.Debasish Kundu, a Ph.D in Pastoral Counselling from American University, is a renowned authority on Complementary and Alternative Medicine (CAM), he is a Visiting Professor of Khulna Homeopathic Medical College & Hospital, affiliated to Ministry of Health, Peoples Republic of Bangladesh, A Vice President of American Nutritional Medical Association, CA, U.S.A. He has authored and edited numerous books and journals on CAM, Sexology and Homeotherapeutics.

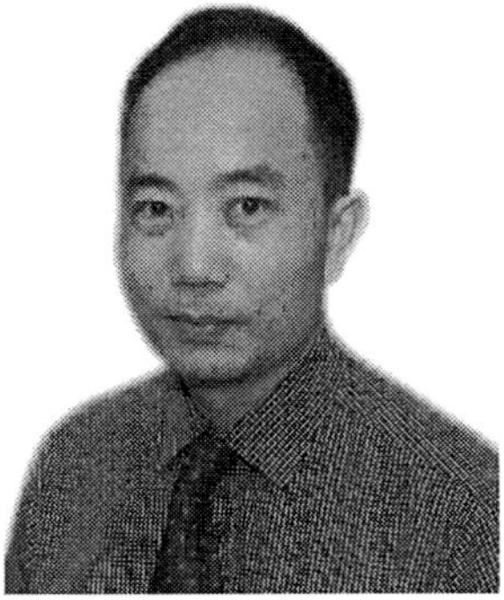

Prof. Dr Choo Led Sin, a Ph.D. in Chinese Medicine Study (China), he is the First Elected World Expert of Manipulative Medicine and Traditional Therapy (2012), Vice Chairman of the World Manipulative Medical Association, Vice Chairman of TCM Diagnosis Specialty Committee of World Federation of Chinese Medicine Societies, President of World Spinal Health Association of Singapore, Vice Chairman of International Fu Yang Health Association, Visiting Professor of World Spinal Health Science Research Institute, He is the Governing Council Member of American Nutritional Medical Association, CA, USA, Assistant Secretary of Singapore Acupuncture Association, he is also a Senior Researcher of Malaysia Chinese Medical Sciences Research Center, Life Honorary President of Professional Manipulative Therapist Association (Singapore).

Manipulative Medicine Consultant of Professional Manipulative Therapist Association (Singapore), Vice Chairman of National Spinal Manipulative Therapist Academic Committee of China, Senior Researcher of Malaysia Chinese Medical Sciences Research Centre, Academic Consultant of Malaysia Acupuncture Academy, Academic Consultant of TCM Training Centre of Penang Malaysia, Academic Consultant of Indonesia Chinese Medicine Society Jakarta TCM College, Life Honorary Consultant of Japan Holistic Manipulative Therapy Association.